Assessments in Occupational Therapy Mental Health

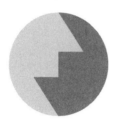

An Integrative Approach

SECOND EDITION

Assessments in Occupational Therapy Mental Health

An Integrative Approach

Second Edition

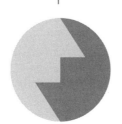

Edited by
Barbara J. Hemphill-Pearson, DMin, OTR, FAOTA

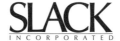

Delivering the best in health care information and education worldwide

www.slackinc.com

ISBN: 978-1-55642-773-2

Library of Congress Cataloging-in-Publication Data

Assessments in occupational therapy mental health / [edited by] Barbara J. Hemphill-Pearson. -- 2nd ed.
    p. ; cm.
 Includes bibliographical references and index.
 ISBN 978-1-55642-773-2
 1. Occupational therapy. 2. Mentally ill--Rehabilitation. 3. Psychology, Pathological--Diagnosis. I. Hemphill-Pearson, Barbara J.
 [DNLM: 1. Occupational Therapy--methods. 2. Mentally Disabled Persons--rehabilitation. 3. Needs Assessment. WM 450.5.O2 A8456 2008]

RC487.A87 2008
616.89'165--dc22

                        2007031264

Published by: SLACK Incorporated
                 6900 Grove Road
                 Thorofare, NJ 08086 USA
                 Telephone: 856-848-1000
                 Fax: 856-853-5991
                 www.slackbooks.com

Printed in the United States of America.

Last digit is print number: 10 9 8 7 6 5 4 3 2

Dedication

To a very dear friend and colleague, Elizabeth Moyer, MS, OTR/L, FAOTA, I dedicate this edition of *Assessments in Occupational Therapy Mental Health*. In 1978, at the occupational therapy national conference in San Diego, Beth was the first elected chairperson of the mental health specialty section. When I met her, she was looking for research to be presented at the meeting of the mental health specialty section. I informed her of my assessment research and that I had it with me. She gave me 15 minutes to present my research. She gave me what turned out to be my first national presentation. I am forever grateful, because after that opportunity, I realized support from my colleagues and received my first publishing contract with SLACK Incorporated. If it were not for her encouragement and support in my early days as an educator, author, and researcher, I would not have received recognition for my work and contribution to the occupational therapy profession.

Contents

Acknowledgments

I want to acknowledge all my friends, relatives, and colleagues who gave me courage and the support needed to accomplish this task. I especially want to thank those who looked at the manuscript and gave editorial suggestions. Also, I want to extend my appreciation to the authors who contributed to this project. Through medical crises, deaths, and emotional turmoil these authors kept their dedication and commitment to this project. Without them this project could not have been realized. In addition, I want to acknowledge Christine Urish, who examined the manuscript periodically. She has sharp eyes and a sense of detail. It is with great pleasure that Christine will take the major role in future editions.

About the Editor

Dr. Hemphill received her B.S. in occupational therapy from the University of Iowa. She received her M.S. degree in occupational therapy from Colorado State University. During her tenure as a therapist at Ft. Logan Mental Health Center, she was fortunate to work with Dr. Maxwell Jones, the founder of the Therapeutic Community Concept in mental health. She began her teaching career at Cleveland State University. She stayed there until she became associate professor and tenured in the department of occupational therapy at Western Michigan University. She retired emeritus after 19 years. In addition to her degrees, she has an earned Doctor of Ministry degree from the Ecumenical Theological Seminary in Detroit.

Dr. Hemphill has served on the editorial boards of the *Occupational Therapy Practice* journal and the *American Journal of Occupational Therapy* and presently serves on the editorial board of the *Occupational Therapy in Mental Health* journal. She has given numerous international, national, and state peer-reviewed papers. Her papers include two at the World Federation for Occupational Therapy; one entitled "Holism in Occupational Therapy Mental Health" and the second entitled "Occupational Therapy and Spirituality: A Global Perspective." She has given numerous papers at the national occupational therapy conferences. Among them are: "Methods in Spirituality: An Educational Experience," "Spirituality in the Treatment Setting," and "Spirituality in the Health Care Setting."

Her publication record has spanned over 25 years. Her most proud accomplishment is edited books on the topic of mental health assessment. Among them are the *Evaluative Process in Psychiatric Occupational Therapy*, which was translated into Japanese; *Mental Health Assessment in Occupational Therapy*; and *Assessments in Occupational Therapy Mental Health*. She has published in the *American Journal of Occupational Therapy*, *Occupational Therapy in Health Care*, *Occupational Therapy Practice*, and *Occupational Therapy in Mental Health*. The topics range from marketing, to depression, to deinstitutionalization. She was recognized for her contributions to education, research, and publications, and her awards include a Fellow of the American Occupational Therapy Association and Fellow of the Michigan Occupational Therapy Association.

Dr. Hemphill continues to contribute to her profession after retirement. She has taught courses in spirituality to occupational therapy students on-line and in the classroom. Her ministry is in the community. She has taught spirituality courses to senior centers and retirement homes. She also taught a series of courses about C.S. Lewis, and a PBS course entitled "A Question of God," a debate between Freud and C.S. Lewis.

About the Contributors

Susan Baptiste, MHSc, OTReg (Ont)
Professor, School of Rehabilitation Science
Faculty of Health Sciences
McMaster University
Hamilton, Ontario, Canada

Brent Braveman, PhD, OTR/L, FAOTA
Clinical Professor
Director of Professional Education,
Occupational Therapy Program
Department of Occupational Therapy
College of Applied Health Sciences
University of Illinois at Chicago
Chicago, IL

Sara J. Brayman, PhD, OTR/L, FAOTA
Professor and Chair
Occupational Therapy Department
Brenau University
Gainesville, GA

Harriett Davidson, MA, OTR
Associate Professor
School of Occupational Therapy
Institute of Health Sciences
Texas Woman's University
Houston, TX

Anne E. Dickerson, PhD, OTR/L, FAOTA
Professor and Chair
Department of Occupational Therapy
East Carolina University
Greenville, NC

Sandra Edwards, MA, OTR, FAOTA
Professor, Emeritus
Western Michigan University
College of Health and Human Services
Occupational Therapy Department
Kalamazoo, MI

Kristjana Fenger, MSc, OT
Assistant Professor
Faculty of Health Sciences
The University of Akureyri
Iceland

Kirsty Forsyth, PhD, OTR
Senior Lecturer
Queen Margaret University
Edinburgh, Scotland

Kristine Haertl, PhD, OTR/L
Associate Professor
Department of Occupational Science and
Occupational Therapy
The College of St. Catherine
St. Paul, MN

James Hinojosa, PhD, OTR/L, FAOTA
Professor and Chair
Department of Occupational Therapy
Steinhardt School of Education
New York University
New York, NY

Margo B. Holm, PhD, OTR/L, FAOTA, ABDA
Professor and Director of Post-Professional
Education
Occupational Therapy Department
School of Health and Rehabilitation
Sciences
University of Pittsburgh
Pittsburgh, PA

Gary Kielhofner, DrPH, OTR/L, FAOTA
Professor and Wade/Meyer Chair
Department of Occupational Therapy
College of Applied Health Sciences
University of Illinois at Chicago
Chicago, IL

James P. Klyczek, PhD, OTR
President
Niagara County Community College
State University of New York
Sanborn, NY

Jessica Kramer, MS, OTR/L
MOHO Clearinghouse
Department of Occupational Therapy
University of Illinois at Chicago
Chicago, IL

Sandra M. Newman, MS, OTR/L
Lead Clinician, Outpatient Rehabilitation
John Randolph Medical Center
Hopewell, VA

Marilyn S. Page, MA, OTR/L
Assistant Professor Emeritus
School of Allied Health Professions
College of Medicine and Public Health
The Ohio State University
Columbus, OH

Nancy J. Powell, PhD, OTR, FAOTA
Program Director
Occupational Therapy Program
Grand Valley State University
Cook-DeVos Center for Health Sciences
Grand Rapids, MI

Cindee Quake-Rapp, PhD, OTR
Professor and Chair
Department of Occupational Therapy
Western Michigan University
Kalamazoo, MI

Kathlyn L. Reed, PhD, OTR, MLIS, FAOTA
Associate Professor
School of Occupational Therapy
Texas Woman's University
Houston, TX

Frances Reynolds, PhD
Reader in Psychology
School of Health Sciences & Social Care
Brunel University
Uxbridge, UK

Joan C. Rogers, PhD, OTR/L, FAOTA
Professor
Occupational Therapy, Psychiatry, Nursing
School of Health and Rehabilitation
Services
Chairperson, Department of Occupational
Therapy
University of Pittsburgh
Pittsburgh, PA

Victoria P. Schindler, PhD, OTR, BCMH,
FAOTA
Program Director and Associate Professor

Richard Stockton College of New Jersey
Pomona, NJ

Emily Schulz, PhD, OTR/L, CFLE
Research Consultant
University of Alabama at Birmingham
Division of Preventative Medicine
Birmingham, AL

Roger O. Smith, PhD, OT, FAOTA
Associate Professor and Director of
Occupational Therapy
Department of Health Sciences
University of Wisconsin-Milwaukee
Milwaukee, WI

Elizabeth Stanton, PhD, OTR/L
Associate Professor
D'Youville College
Buffalo, NY

Franklin Stein, PhD, OTR, FAOTA
Editor, *Occupational Therapy International*
Professor Emeritus
Department of Occupational Therapy
Unniversity of South Dakota
Vermillion, SD

Christine K. Urish, PhD, OTR/L, BCMH
Professor
Associate of Occupational Therapy
St. Ambrose University
Davenport, IA

Janet H. Watts, PhD, OTR/L
Emeritus Associate Professor
Department of Occupational Therapy
Virginia Commonwealth University
Richmond, VA

Virginia K. White, PhD, OTR, FAOTA
Professor Emerita
School of Occupational Therapy
Texas Woman's University
Houston, TX

Foreword

When asked to write this Foreword, I was flattered by the request. I was exceptionally honored because this is a new edition of a text that has been respected for its content and influence on mental health practice. Prior editions have influenced all areas of occupational therapy practice, including information that is fundamental to occupational therapy.

This text is devoted to mental health practice. This new edition is significantly revised, with chapters written by experts from a wide range of specialty areas in occupational therapy. The revisions elucidate the authors' perspectives so that they can be incorporated into mental health practices. Most exciting, the text proposes an integrated approach to assessing multiple systems.

Occupational therapy begins with the evaluation of a client. What therapists learn about clients through evaluation guides the direction and focus of interventions. Evaluation data guides therapists in selecting the appropriate theoretical approach for intervention and is used to establish functional, realistic goals.

Addressing psychosocial issues is at the core of occupational therapy. One cannot understand a client without a basic understanding of the person's mental health status. Mental health is so fundamental that it provides the framework by which to understand the client, regardless of the person's disabilities or impairments. Occupational therapists are distinctively prepared to evaluate the whole person in the context of his or her daily life. Therapists are concerned with the person's ability to function and engage in occupations.

The selection and use of a specific assessment is critical to the intervention process. During the initial assessment, therapists interact with clients to develop a positive therapeutic relationship. Occupational therapists use assessment tools to learn about the client in his or her life. Therapists learn about the client's abilities and disabilities, as well as about his or her beliefs and performance skills. The process of evaluation does not produce a natural environment. Therefore, a therapist must learn to skillfully create a situation to learn about the client as a whole person. This is not easy when the therapist often must administer standardized assessments or ask specific, probing questions.

In this text, a holistic approach is proposed that uses concepts from the *Occupational Therapy Practice Framework: Domain and Process*. Consistent with this document, a therapist begins by conducting an occupational profile before assessing occupational performance. The approach requires that the therapist attend to the whole person as one, as opposed to an individual divided into his or her physical, mental, social, and spiritual selves. The ultimate goal is to understand the client as a real, complex person.

Today, one cannot discuss evaluation or assessment without considering accountability and related concerns. Accountability refers to a therapist interpreting assessment data in order to obtain an accurate estimation of the client's performance, skills, and deficits. The therapist then makes reasonable and skilled decisions about intervention based on sound reasoning and clinical judgment. This process takes time and clinical experience to develop. It begins by understanding the evaluation process and becoming competent in using standardized and nonstandardized methods of data collection. Finally, it requires that a therapist make judgments and be able to justify those decisions.

This book provides information that will support a therapist's development of evaluation responsibilities. The chapters in this text present a thorough process for approaching client evaluation. The reasoning process is explored in a way that will be helpful to both the novice and the experienced therapist. For all readers, the text provides information that can be used to scrutinize evaluation procedures and practices. The text provides a sound foundation for a holistic, integrated approach to client assessment.

James Hinojosa, PhD, OTR/L, FAOTA
Professor and Chair
New York University, Steinhardt School of Education
New York, NY

Preface

It has been 25 years since the first edition of the *Evaluative Process in Psychiatric Occupational Therapy* was published. This text was an effort to bring together information about assessment tools that were developed by occupational therapists. The purpose was to, through a collaborative effort, bring together assessments that were being developed and presented through workshops, seminars, conferences, unpublished manuscripts, and published journals. It was hoped that this project would encourage research that resulted in an increased number of assessments and more developed assessments. Each subsequent edition has introduced new assessments and offered updated information about assessments in mental health. I believe that the original purpose has been accomplished.

In keeping with the original purpose, in the present text there is a common thread of research, chapters written by the assessments' developers, without intention to present or endorse a particular theoretical frame of reference or theory. The authors do not impose criteria for the assessments' usefulness or research development. I believe that it is the practitioner who determines the credibility of an instrument and adds fuel for student research.

The information presented in each chapter will cover: a) the theoretical base, which will include the historical development, rationale for its development, behaviors assessed, appropriate patient use, and review of the literature; b) how the instrument is administered, which will include the procedures, problems with administering, and the materials needed; c) utilization, including the presentation of a case study and interpretation of the results; d) statistical analysis and recent studies; and e) suggestions for further research. Some of the assessments that have appeared in previous writings appear in this text. Others have been updated. As in the past, chapters summarizing assessments that occupational therapists are using are included. The assessments that are updated include Client-Centered Assessment, Role Change Assessment, Performance Assessment of Self-Care Skills, The Comprehensive Occupational Therapy Evaluation, Vocational Assessments Used in Mental Health, The Bay Area Functional Performance Evaluation, The Assessment of Occupational Functioning, The Role Checklist, OT FACT, and The Stress Management Questionnaire. Summary chapters include assessments used with the Model of Human Occupation and assessments used in pediatrics. Instead of having individual chapters on each one, it was efficient to present these assessments in a summary chapter. The purpose is to introduce them to the therapist in hopes that they will be used and research will be conducted. All assessments will appear in their current state of development. Each author was asked to use the language from the current *Occupational Therapy Practice Framework*.

Spirituality has become an area of concern and has been recognized in occupational therapy as an integral part of the triad of holism. Spiritual concerns are a part of the concern for health and should not be ignored by professionals in health care, including occupational therapy. Spirituality should therefore be included in the assessment process. An assessment entitled OT-QUEST is presented and included in this text. In addition, closely aligned to spirituality is wellness. A chapter summarizing assessments in wellness is also new to this text.

New to this project are assessments that are recognized as using media that allow patients to project their inner selves, hence called projective media. In keeping with the integrative approach to assessment, projective media is included in two chapters: the use of journal work and the use of painting and activities for the purpose of permitting patients to express inner thoughts for either diagnostic or treatment. Two chapters entitled

Journaling as an Assessment Tool in Mental Health and *Expressive Media as Assessment in Mental Health* are included in this text.

Traditionally, the last section of this text includes a chapter on research. The purpose is to present concepts that are used to further develop assessments in occupational therapy. The chapter in this book includes the use of the curve analysis. It is used to achieve further validity of an instrument. New in this section is a unit discussing evidence-based research in mental health.

Over the past 5 years, the research on developing assessments has been scarce, hence the need for summary chapters. Therapists in mental health are just not developing new assessments or conducting research on assessments that have been developed over the last 10 years. Assessments such as the Kohlman Evaluation of Living Skills and The Milwaukee Evaluation of Daily Living Skills are two examples. The authors recognize the need for updating their evaluations. The assessments were not ready at the time of this publication. Other assessments—Build-A-City, the Cognitive Adaptive Skills Evaluation, and the Adolescent Role Assessment—have not received enough interest to receive research attention. It seems that therapists are using assessments that are already developed – have the validity and necessity for use in practice; thus, there is an added need for summary chapters. The pressure to show improvement and patient turnover leaves little time for research, and it is possible that clinicians are not motivated to collect data to further develop assessments. Instead, they may be turning to already established assessments. In addition, there are currently fewer therapists practicing in mental health settings; therefore, there is a lack of manpower to do assessment research. It was hoped by this author that graduate education would add impetus to the research in assessment development in mental health. This has not been realized. Perhaps the lack of time, funding, commitment, and manpower is preventing therapists from developing and conducting further research on existing assessments in occupational therapy.

There seems to be a controversy in the occupational therapy profession over the use of the terms *patient* and *client*. Patient is used in this textbook. The use of patient is a more understood and universal term than client. It is not meant to be associated with the medical model or any model that is used in the medical profession. This text maintains a neutral position on any practice model, theory, or frame of reference. In Chapter 3, the title and content refers to client-centered evaluation. *Client-centered* is a specific term used in occupational therapy to refer to a specific evaluation and treatment reference. It seems inappropriate to use patient in this case, as the evaluation is recognized as client-centered.

The editor wishes to thank Lisa Thorne for her expertise in computer technology and editing ability, and is also grateful for her organizational skills and editorial knowledge. I also want to acknowledge my authors. They were very patient and did their best to meet my deadlines despite illnesses and adverse conditions. I want to commend the new authors who were willing to contribute and write about a topic dear to their heart. The contribution of each is immeasurable.

Barbara J. Hemphill-Pearson, DMin, OTR, FAOTA
Editor

PART I
INTRODUCTION

THE PATIENT'S PROFILE: AN INTEGRATIVE APPROACH

Barbara J. Hemphill-Pearson, DMin, OTR, FAOTA

"At the beginning of the journey, we had boundless energy and made quick progress. But as we move closer to our core, our hidden beliefs that live in the shadows and secretly call the shots become exposed. They try to convince the ego to bring out the heavy artillery and initiate a take-no-prisoners fight to the finish. What recourse do we have during this dark night of the soul? Let the ego fight. And while it's distracted with its business, let's take every opportunity to go within, to go deeper than ever before, until we're in heaven." Coyne T, Weissman K. The Spiritual Chicks Question Everything: Learn to Risk, Release and Soar. *York Beach, ME: Red Wheel/Weiser; 2002:186.*

Introduction

In 1982, when the *Evaluative Process in Psychiatric Occupational Therapy* was published, the author proposed a method for assessing patients. It was a structure for selecting assessments based on the ability of the therapist to identify patient dysfunction and progress. This structure allowed the therapist to select and use assessments from a broad repertoire to achieve an integrative view of patients with emotional disorders. The integrative view of patients is the *holistic* view. It is the mind, body, and spirit triad. In past publications, the spiritual aspect of this triad was not addressed. The integrative approach to assessment embodies the concept of holism when achieving a profile of the patient.

Holism—An Integrative Approach to the Patient Profile

Assessing the patient's physical and mental functioning can provide valuable information for understanding his or her spiritual functioning. Information about the patient's thought patterns, content of speech, affect, cultural orientation, social relationships, and customs may assist in identifying patient needs.[1]

Practitioners recognize the interdependence of body, mind, emotion, spirit, and environment, and work toward the health of those parts simultaneously with the patient.

The literature mentions holism as a value and a significant concept in the philosophy of occupational therapy.[2-6] Occupational therapists view health as the total condition—one that cannot be divided into physical, mental, or social health—of a biopsychosocial being. If the initial or major health problem occurs in one area, other areas will be impacted as well.[6] In a profession in which therapists believe that major physical health problems impact mental health and social functioning, it seems reasonable to assume that such a belief would be reflected in patient assessment and treatment.

Health care has begun to consider the spiritual aspect of the human health experience, which has been neglected in past publications. Spirituality has been recognized as important in the treatment of alcoholism,[7] depression,[8] and AIDS.[9] "Spirituality deals with the life principles that pervade and animate a person's entire being, including emotional and volitional aspects of life."[9(p187)] It has been stated that spiritual concerns are a part of the concern for health and cannot be ignored by any professional in health care, including occupational therapists. Spirituality, therefore, should be included in the assessment process.

The limitations of spiritual assessments include the use of terms that are broad enough that spirituality can be substituted for the word "God." When the term God is used, it is assumed that the patient is of Christian tradition and other traditions are not included. The therapist must take precautions about assessing individuals who are not of the Christian faith with an assessment that is based on Christian ideology. When integrating spirituality in the assessment process, it must be inter-faith and ecumenical.

Seaward[10] states that there are three components of spirituality: 1) relationships (both intra- and interpersonal), 2) a personal value system, and 3) a purposeful, meaningful life—often referred to as personal well-being. In addition, the concept of motivation is important to consider because without motivation a person does not seek a spiritual life and does not engage in meaningful occupation. Motivation depends on the hopefulness of the individual. Hope is dependent on one's spiritual life. Therefore, motivation is an essential ingredient in patient wellness and spiritual health. It is these general concepts that are addressed in the evaluation process.

Spirituality and the Evaluation Process

In 2002, the Commission on Practice developed the *Occupational Therapy Practice Framework: Domain and Process*[11] (*Framework*), in which the evaluation process was described. The evaluation process includes the occupational profile and states, "the initial step…provides an understanding of the patient's occupational history and experiences, patterns of daily living, interests, values, and needs. The patient's problems and concerns about performing occupations and daily life activities are identified, and the patient's priorities are determined."[11] The context that is described as the "overarching" influence on the treatment process includes the patient's spiritual locus of control and well-being, personal beliefs, level of spiritual maturity, and religious tradition and values.

The *Framework* does not define holism. The term *holistic*, in this context, is used when the focus is on the whole person: "An integration of body, mind, feelings, spirit, and life-styles well as the physical and social environment of the individual—and on the interdependence of these factors in growth and change. The goal of an activity is the positive wellness of the person—senses of heightened well-being and fitness."[12(p99)] The English word *health* is based on the Anglo-Saxon word *hale*, meaning "whole," so to be healthy is to be whole. The word holy comes from the same root.[13] Humans have always considered that wholeness as an absolute necessity to make life worth living.

Spirituality as an Occupation

It is the occupational profile that is pertinent to assessment. Spirituality is considered here an occupation—not as a performance component. Occupations are the ordinary and familiar things that people do every day.[11] Occupations are activities that fulfill time and give life meaning. Occupations involve mental abilities and skills and may or may not be observable. There is a degree of personal meaning having contextual, temporal, psychological, social, symbolic, cultural, ethnic, and/or spiritual dimensions.[14] Information that is gathered about a person's spirituality should describe the patient's spiritual journey and illness experience, and address the here-and-now. The information is gathered formally or informally. There are interview methods and specific application of instruments. The data gathering process is designed to gain an understanding of the patient's illness story, his or her feelings, thoughts, and beliefs. Through telling and reflecting on their spiritual journey, patients can begin to gain meaning and insight into their current life situation. One method of telling their story is through personal journal work. Chapter 5 is devoted to journal writing as an assessment tool. In addition, Chapter 2: Interviewing, Chapter 3: The Client-Centered Assessment, and Chapter 4: Role Change Assessment are presented.

Along with interview methods and application of specific instruments, journal work can assist the patient in gaining insight and understanding into his or her inner and outer worlds. This method of assessment can encourage a holistic view of the patient's motivations, perceptions of his or her world, and a review of his or her life and the relevance that it has on the present situation.

The Integrative Approach—The Patient's Profile

The integrative approach is a concept that assures a holistic approach to patient assessment. The American Occupational Association (AOTA)[11] has various dimensions that are considered in the delivery of health care. These dimensions are cognitive, physical, spiritual, emotional, and contextual. These are occupations that are expressed in a human being's everyday life. Krishnagiri[15] further discusses the biological, temporal-spatial, sociocultural, psychological, and spiritual dimensions in occupations. This author prefers to use the *psychological, behavioral, learning,* and *biological,* because they seem to be closer to the dimensions suggested by AOTA. It has been suggested that the therapist's theory or frame of reference will guide the gathering of patient information that results in the patient's occupational profile. This author further suggests that more than one theory and more than one frame of reference can be used to develop the patient's occupational profile. The use of a variety of assessments when developing a patient profile, based on a variety of theories, is supported in the occupational therapy literature.[3] Educators and clinicians have recognized the need for a system that integrates numerous bodies of knowledge into occupational therapy. This is particularly true when the individual has multiple diagnoses. Whenever possible, standardized tests should be used. Spirituality is an overall occupation and is included in all four dimensions. In the integrative approach to assessing patients, the therapist views assessments according to these four dimensions and then administers the appropriate assessment that will give him or her an occupational profile of the patient. Each dimension is defined in the context of occupational therapy, drawing upon theories and frames of reference.

PSYCHOLOGICAL DIMENSION

The *psychological* dimension "is the ability to process information from past events and information currently available…to view one's self, others, and one's life situation realistically. The psychological dimension is influenced by and derived from the emotions and feelings of the human experience."[15] Krishnagiri would include the cognitive aspects of the human in this dimension, but this author prefers to include it in the learning dimension. This is an arbitrary division and only serves to describe testing procedures. In the psychological dimension, Azima, Fidler, Mosey, and others have proposed testing procedures. To support the assessment tool theoretically, theories of Freud,[16] Jung,[17] Rogers,[18] Maslow,[19] May,[20] and Perls[21] are utilized.

Mosey coined the term *object relations* to describe a person's relationship to people and occupation—the person's ego function. This part of the patient's psyche helps therapists to identify patient needs and body image and to gain insight. Other psychological functions such as reality contact, intrinsic gratification, body concept, decision making, problem solving, and social relationships are evaluated. The most effective methods for evaluating these occupational performances is with projective media such as painting or pencil drawing. The occupational performances in the psychological dimensions can be measured with projective media. The focus is on completion of a task, not on analyzing symbolic content. Although the patient is able to project his or her unconscious needs into symbolic images, it is the responsibility of the therapist to observe the manner in which the task is completed. Viewing the patient in action is valuable when observing how patients express their innermost needs, feelings, and emotions onto the environment. See Chapter 6: Expressive Media as an Assessment Tool.

Projective assessments were developed in the past, but little has been done to advance their use. They are: Azima,[22] Shoemyn,[23] Fidler,[24] and the BH Batteries.[25] Other assessments are the Goodman Battery,[26] Carol Lerner's Collage Scoring System,[27] and Build A City.[28]

Frequently, the use of projective media will facilitate the expression of religious content. Allowing the patient to express his or her faith tradition is a means by which the therapist can assess the patient's level of spiritual development and his or her concerns about the relationship between his or her disability and faith tradition.

In evaluating a mentally ill patient where religious content is presented, it is important for the therapist to distinguish between a mystical experience and religious delusions. Mystics describe their experience as ecstatic and joyful. When they express their experience, the words "serenity," "wholeness," "transcendence," and "love" are used. Psychotics are often confused and frightened by the religious hallucinations, which are distressing and often accompanied by an angry God. Both mystics and psychotics experience what appears to be a break from reality. For mystics, this period of withdraw is welcomed. However, when the period ends, they return to normal activity. For the psychotic, the withdrawal from reality is involuntary. Delusions can last for years and result in driving the individual into deeper distress. Mystics are often respected members of the community.[29]

Another difference is in how each interprets his or her religious experience. Psychotics may have feelings of religious grandiosity and inflated egotistical importance. They may think they have messages from God, or have some spiritual powers. Mystics experience a state of calm, loss of pride, and the emptying of the self.

BEHAVIORAL DIMENSION

The next dimension is the *behavioral*. It draws upon the theories of cognitive, behavioral, social, and learning sciences. Such techniques as reinforcement, modeling, token economies, desensitization, biofeedback, and stress management are used as treatment principles. The body of knowledge from occupational therapy literature comes from the writings of Reilly,[30] Mosey,[24] Fidler,[31] and Kielhofner.[32] In the behavioral dimension, the therapist is concerned with the role the environment plays in the acquisition of behavior for occupational performance. It is important in this dimension to consider the patient's behavior in the context of the environment.

The patient's environment (life space) and the patient's lifestyle are analyzed. The patient's life space includes the expected environment. For example, it is important to know if the patient is homeless, comes from the inner city, lives in a rural area, or comes from a middle-class neighborhood.

The patient's lifestyle (race, ethnic background, value system) influences the assessment process. The patient's lifestyle and life space can influence the acquisition of behavior. For example, an assessment that is culturally biased will not give a true picture of the patient's disabilities or abilities.

Social interaction process, based on the principle that socialization is a developmental process that results from classical conditioning, is assessed in the behavioral dimension. In this dimension, socialization is not a skill, but an occupation that an individual acquires through interaction with the environment. The occupations of communication and group interaction are attributes evaluated in this dimension. It is important to identify any environmental barriers that are prohibiting the performance of the activity.

The assessment is generally done through history taking with the use of interviewing techniques and checklists. Such assessments as the Interest Checklist,[33] Occupational Role History,[34] Life Style Performance Profile,[35] Activity Configuration,[36] Adolescent Role Assessment,[37] History Interview,[38] and The Barth Time Construction[39] are used to assess the behavioral dimension. The assessments based on the Model of Human Occupation (MOHO) are included in this dimension. Included in this text are The Role Checklist (Chapter 16),[40] The Bay Area Functional Performance Evaluation (Chapter 14),[41] The Assessment of Occupational Functioning (Chapter 15),[42] and the Role Activity Performance Scale.[43] There are three summary chapters: Chapter 11: Assessments Used With the Model of Human Occupation, Chapter 12: Work Assessments From the Model of Human Occupation, and Chapter 13: Role Assessments Used in Mental Health.

The behaviors that express the patient's spirituality are included in this dimension. Such occupational performances as religious attendance, praying, reading spiritual material, attending spiritual groups and volunteering, and engaging in activities that have deep spiritual meaning are expressions of a patient's spirituality. Chapter 17: The OT-Quest Assessment assesses the spiritual performance of patients.

LEARNING DIMENSION

There are two differences between the behavioral and the *learning* dimension. The first difference is the method of administration. The behavioral assessments are administered by interview only or by interview and task performance. The therapist is interested in learning what is hindering the patient from performing the activity. Learning assessments are administered by task only. The therapist is interested in the performance of a skill. It is important to actually observe the skill in context and determine what is preventing the patient from performing the skill. The second difference is the method of assessment. Learning assessments use scales or some other form of measurement to compare scores, while behavioral assessments generally do not.

There are two factors that the therapist must be concerned with when using a learning assessment: the patient's cognitive function and the patient's level of skill development. Cognitive functions have a direct bearing on the patient's performance—the ability to learn. However, the therapist is interested in the performance of a skill, not how the patient acquired the skill. Assessments that measure skill do not measure cognitive function. Cognitive function is a biological dimension, not a skill function. Finally, the patient's developmental level must be related to the assessment or the task being performed. The therapist cannot ask a 2-year-old to tie his or her shoe when the child is not developmentally ready.

Functions that are assessed in the learning dimension are work skills, activities of daily living (ADL), leisure, and social skills. It is most important that the assessment involve a task that simulates a life skill. This is what distinguishes a learning assessment from all other occupational therapy assessments. Even though the same functions appear to be assessed in the behavioral dimension, learning assessments are used by actually performing or simulating the skill. The Milwaukee Evaluation of Daily Living Skills,[44] Work Capacity Evaluation,[45] and the Paracheck[46] are examples of learning assessments. The Kohlman Evaluation of Living Skills,[47] the Performance Assessment of Self-Care Skills,[48] the Comprehensive Occupational Therapy Evaluation(revised),[48] and Community Adaptive Planning Assessment are also included in this dimension. A summary chapter (Chapter 10: Vocational Assessments Used in Mental Health) is also included in this text.

In the area of spirituality, the therapist needs to know the patient's faith tradition in order to understand the problems that might arise when teaching an occupational performance such as dressing. For example, in some Amish traditions, buttons are not used on clothing. Teaching a person who does not have buttons on his or her clothing would require some creative maneuvering.

BIOLOGICAL DIMENSION

The fourth dimension is *biological*. This area of assessment has received the most attention and research. Its concepts can easily be observed and measured. In the psychological literature, it is referred to as the *biomedical* model. It asserts that abnormality is an illness of the body. The Allen Cognitive Levels (ACL)[49] is an assessment that examines the level of cognition with the use of a leather-lacing project. It has been rigorously examined to determine its reliability and validity.

There has been a series of research reporting[29] a connection between spirituality and the mind. The brain is a collection of "physical structures that gather and process sensory, cognitive, and emotional data: the mind is the phenomenon of thoughts, memories, and emotions that arise from the perceptual processes of the brain."[29(p33)] The brain makes mind. "Science cannot demonstrate a way for the mind to occur except as a result of the neurological functioning of the brain."[29(p33)] All that is meaningful in human experience and spirituality happens in the mind. Studies have indicated that the limbic system is integral to religious and spiritual experience. It is the association between areas of the brain that is essential if the individual is going to have a meaningful and spiritual life.

The association areas of the brain are structures that gather together or associate neural information from various parts of the brain. The association areas eventually tap into memory and emotional centers to allow the person to organize and respond to the exterior world. For example, it has been suggested that the visual association area is active in individuals who use images to help facilitate meditation or prayer. There are several association areas in the cerebral cortex. They are *visual, orientation, attention,* and *verbal.*

These four association areas are extremely important in patient assessment. They relate to each other and can have an effect on the patient's sense of self, emotional response to activity, and the ability to express religious beliefs. If an area of the brain is affected by trauma, stroke, depression, alcoholism, or drugs, the therapist needs to know the relationship to the patient's faith tradition.

For example, if a patient has a strong religious tradition that believes in using images in worship, such as during communion, and the patient has an injury in the visual association area, he or she will have difficulty relating to these images in recovery. These patients will have trouble praying and using meditation. Damage in the orientation area will cause trouble relating to mystical and religious experiences. The verbal association will make it difficult for the patient to express his or her religious beliefs. The OT-Quest Assessment is in this dimension.

Developing the Patient's Profile

THE EVALUATIVE PROCESS

There are two steps to the evaluative process. The first is the occupational profile. It is the use of assessment procedures to ascertain an holistic view of patients from their occupational history; pattern of ADL; nature of biological, physical, and neurological status; range of interests; cultural values and traditions; and spiritual and emotional needs. This process is for the purpose of obtaining and interpreting data that is pertinent for intervention. The second step is the analysis of occupational performances. The results are analyzed and integrated into the patient's profile and used to develop goals and objectives for the treatment process. Once the patient's profile is developed, the assessments are used for detecting change in function or can be used to adjust treatment goals. It is important that therapists bring to bear their knowledge about diseases and disability, and relate this to their personal skills in clinical reasoning and theoretical perspectives.

The development of the patient profile begins with the data gathering process. This is designed to obtain information relevant to the occupational dimensions—psychological, learning, behavioral, biological. The data gathering process also identifies barriers to occupations. There are a number of resources that the therapist uses: 1) medical sources, 2) interviews, and 3) standardized and unstandardized tests. During the data gathering process, the patient must participate in the identification and development of occupations and activities that would enhance the delivery of health care. When it is impossible to get reliable information from the patient due to dementia or other cognitive problems, significant others or family must be employed.

The development of the patient profile is a dynamic process. During this time, hypotheses are made about the patient's function based on specific theories and frames of reference. Different theories and frames of reference can be used to treat specific occupational dimensions with the same patient. This makes it possible to use more than one instrument to assess patients. This is a holistic approach to obtaining the patient's profile. Even though the therapist is practicing from a specific frame of reference, it is imperative that the patient be assessed from a holistic view and be given assessments from other frames of reference. This approach is not new. The need to integrate numerous bodies of knowledge into occupational therapy practice when treating patients with mental health disorders has long been recognized. Mosey states "in the process of intervention with a patient, more than one frame of reference is often used to guide practice."[3]

Summary

In developing a patient's profile, the therapist gathers information from a wide variety of sources. This includes information obtained from the patient, the family, and past history—medical, spiritual, and cultural. This information can be obtained through standard and nonstandard testing, interviewing the patient, and from the environment. This chapter presented four dimensions that may be used to gather and integrate information about patients in order to develop a profile. The integrative approach to develop a patient's profile is based on a holistic triad—mind, body, and spirit. In an attempt to present a holistic approach to assessments, spirituality was added to the discussion. There is a suggestion that more than one assessment from competing frames of reference can be used to achieve a holistic approach. Therefore, the integrative approach to patient assessment draws upon the concepts and philosophy of occupational therapy. The principles in the *Framework* developed by the AOTA are the guidelines used during the assessment process and the chapter utilizes the *Framework* and integrates the language of applying assessments to the evaluative process. Many of the assessments are currently being developed and it cannot be overemphasized that assessment development in mental health is desirable.

References

1. Rogers C. *Client-Centered Therapy*. Boston, MA: Houghton-Mifflin; 1951.
2. Dunning RE. Philosophy and occupational therapy. *Am J Occup Ther*. 1973;27:18.
3. Mosey AC. *Psychosocial Components of Occupational Therapy. Three Frames of Reference for Mental Health*. New York, NY: Raven Press; 1996:5,12-15.
4. Clark PN. Human development through occupation: theoretical frameworks in contemporary occupational therapy practice. (Pt 1) *Am J Occup Ther*. 1979;33:505.
5. Meyer A. Philosophy of occupation therapy. *Archives of Occupational Therapy*. 1922;1:1-10.
6. Reed K, Sanderson SN. *Concepts of Occupational Therapy*. 14th ed. Baltimore, MD: Lippincott, Williams & Wilkins; 1999.
7. Prezioso F. Spirituality in the recovery process. *J Subst Abuse Treat*. 1987;4:233-238.
8. Sullivan W. The role of spirituality among the mentally challenged. *Psychosocial Rehabilitation Journal*. 1993;16(3):125-134.
9. Dombeck M, Karl J. Spiritual issues in mental health care. *J Relig Health*. 1987;26(3):183-197.
10. Seaward BL. *Managing Stress: Principles and Strategies for Health and Well-Being*. Boston, MA: Jones and Bartlett; 1999.
11. The Commission on Practice. *Occupational Therapy Practice Framework: Domain and Process*. Bethesda, MD: American Occupational Therapy Association.
12. White V. Promoting health and wellness: a theme for the eighties. *Am J Occup Ther*. 1986;40(11):745.
13. Peters T. *The Cosmic Self*. San Francisco, CA: Harper Collins Publishers; 1991.
14. Christiansen, C, Clark F, Kielhofner G, Rober J, Nelson, D. Position paper: occupation. *Am J Occup Ther*. 1995;49:1015-1018.
15. Krishnagiri S. Occupations and their dimensions. In: Hinojosa J, Blount M, eds. *The Texture of Life: Purposeful Activities in Occupational Therapy*. Bethesda, MD: AOTA; 2000.
16. Freud S. Psychical (or mental) treatment. In: Starchey J, ed-trans. *The Complete Psychological Work*. Vol 7. New York, NY: Norton; 1976.
17. Jung C. *Man and His Symbols*. Garden City, NY: Harper and Row; 1954.
18. Rogers C. *Client-Centered Therapy*. Boston, MA: Houghton-Mifflin; 1951.
19. Maslow AH. *Motivation and Personality*. New York, NY: Harper and Row; 1954.

20. May R. *Man's Search for Himself*. New York, NY: Norton; 1954.

21. Perls F. *Gestalt Verbatim*. Moab, UT: Real People Press; 1969.

22. Azima H, Azima F. Outline of a dynamic theory of occupational therapy. *Am J Occup Ther*. 1958;8(5):215.

23. Shoemyen C. The Shoemyen Battery. In: Hemphill B, ed. *The Evaluative Process in Psychiatric Occupational Therapy*. Thorofare, NJ: SLACK Incorporated; 1982.

24. Fidler G. The Lifestyle Performance Profile: an organizational frame. In: Hemphill B, ed. *The Evaluative Process in Psychiatric Occupational Therapy*. Thorofare NJ: SLACK Incorporated; 1982.

25. Hemphill, B. How to use the B.H. Battery. In: Hemphill-Pearson BH, ed. *Assessments in Occupational Therapy Mental Health: An Integrative Approach*. Thorofare, NJ: SLACK Incorporated; 1999.

26. Evaskus M. The Goodman Battery. In: Hemphill B, ed. *The Evaluative Process in Occupational Therapy*. Thorofare, NJ: SLACK Incorporated; 1982.

27. Lerner C. The Magazine Picture Collage. In: Hemphill B, ed. *The Evaluative Process in Occupational Therapy*. Thorofare, NJ: SLACK Incorporated; 1982.

28. Clark, E. Build A City. In: Hemphill-Pearson BH, ed. *Assessments in Occupational Therapy Mental Health: An Integrative Approach*. Thorofare, NJ: SLACK Incorporated; 1999.

29. Newberg A, D'Aquili E, Rause V. *Why God Won't Go Away*. New York, NY: Ballantine Books; 2002.

30. Reilly M. Occupational therapy: a historical perspective: the moderation of occupational therapy. *Am J Occup Ther*. 1971;25(5):243.

31. Fidler G, Velde B. *Activities: Reality and Symbol*. Thorofare, NJ: SLACK Incorporated; 1999.

32. Kielhofner G. *A Model of Human Occupation: Theory and Application*. 2nd ed. Baltimore, MD: Williams and Wilkins; 1999.

33. Matsutsuyu J. The Interest Checklist. *Am J Occup Ther*. 1983;23:323-328.

34. Florey L, Michelman SM. The Occupational Role History: a screening tool for psychiatric occupational therapy. *Am J Occup Ther*. 1982;36(5).

35. Fidler G. The Lifestyle Performance Profile: an organizational frame. In: Hemphill B, ed. *The Evaluative Process in Psychiatric Occupational Therapy*. Thorofare, NJ: SLACK Incorporated; 1982.

36. Spahn R. The Patient Gets Busy: Change or Process. Paper presented at March 1965 meeting of the American Orthopsychiatric Society. New York.

37. Black M. Adolescent Role Assessment. *Am J Occup Ther*. 1976;30:73-79.

38. Henry A, Malinson T. The Occupational Performance History Interview. In: Hemphill-Pearson B, ed. *Assessments in Occupational Therapy Mental Health: An Integrative Approach*. Thorofare, NJ: SLACK Incorporated; 1999.

39. Barth T. The Barth Time Construction. In: Hemphill B, ed. *Mental Health Assessment in Occupational Therapy: An Integrative Approach to the Evaluative Process*. Thorofare, NJ: SLACK Incorporated; 1988.

40. Dickerson AE. The Role Checklist. In: Hemphill-Pearson BH, ed. *Assessments in Occupational Therapy Mental Health: An Integrative Approach*. Thorofare, NJ: SLACK Incorporated; 1999.

41. Bloomer J, Williams S. *The Bay Area Functional Performance Evaluation*. Research ed. Palo Alto, Calf: Consulting Psychologists Press; 1979.

42. Watts JH, Hinson R, Madigan MJ, McGuigan MP, Newman S. The Assessment of Occupational Functioning. In: Hemphill-Pearson BH, ed. *Assessments in Occupational Therapy Mental Health: An Integrative Approach*. Thorofare, NJ: SLACK Incorporated; 1999.

43. Good-Ellis MA. The Role Activity Performance Scale. In: Hemphill-Pearson B, ed. *Assessments in Occupational Therapy Mental Health: An Integrative Approach*. Thorofare, NJ: SLACK Incorporated; 1999.

44. Haertlein CL. The Milwaukee Evaluation of Daily Living Skills. In: Hemphill-Pearson B, ed. *Assessments in Occupational Therapy Mental Health: An Integrative Approach*. Thorofare, NJ: SLACK Incorporated; 1999.

45. Matheson L, Ogden L. *Work Capacity Evaluation*. Anaheim, CA: Employment and Rehabilitation Institute of Southern California; 1987.

46. Parachek J, King L. *Paracheck Geriatric Rating Scale*. 3rd ed. Glendale, AZ: Center for Neurodevelopmental Studies; 1986.

47. Thomson LK. The Kohlman Evaluation of Living Skills. In: Hemphill-Pearson B, ed. *Assessments in Occupational Therapy Mental Health: An Integrative Approach*. Thorofare, NJ: SLACK Incorporated; 1999.

48. Masagatani GN. The Cognitive Adaptive Skills Evaluation. In: Hemphill-Pearson B, ed. *Assessments in Occupational Mental Health: An Integrative Approach*. Thorofare, NJ: SLACK Incorporated; 1999.

49. Allen C, Kehrberg K, Burns T. Evaluation Instruments. In: Allen CK, Earhart C, Blue T, eds. *Occupational Therapy Treatment Goals for the Physically and Cognitively Disabled*. Rockville, MD: The American Occupational Therapy Association Inc; 1992.

PART II:
THE INTERVIEWING PROCESS

2

INTERVIEWING IN OCCUPATIONAL THERAPY

Marilyn S. Page, MA, OTR/L

"Communication is the greatest single factor affecting a person's health and his relationship to others." Satir V. Peoplemaking. *Palo Alto, Calif: Science & Behavior Books, Inc; 1972:30.*

Introduction

"Engagement in occupation to support participation in context is the outcome of occupational therapy intervention."[1(p611)] Therapists within the profession hold the belief that by valuing and considering the patient's desires, choices, and needs, therapists will assist patients to engage in meaningful occupations. Engagement in occupation is an emotional and psychological or subjective experience as well as an objective interaction.[1] To achieve this outcome, occupational therapists are required to perform a comprehensive evaluation for each patient.[1,2] Relying on professional expertise, the therapist must choose the most effective and efficient assessment tools.

Occupational therapists employ what is called the *client-centered approach*.[1-3] This involves the concept that all interventions must be focused on patient priorities. The type of interaction to assure successful outcomes requires the patient to be internally motivated and involved as an active participant in the intervention process.[1] It is the patient who identifies what occupations and activities are important and determines the amount of participation in each occupation. "The patient contains all that needs to be known concerning what is going wrong and what needs to be attended to."[5(p7)] The skills and attitudes of the therapist are required to assist a patient in identifying desired occupations and to develop motivation in the patient when necessary. To accomplish these complex goals, the occupational therapist needs to develop a therapeutic rapport with each patient. Within this rapport, the therapist determines what the patient wishes to accomplish within a given range of abilities and contexts. The interview assessment enables therapists to gather the necessary information and establish a therapeutic relationship.[6]

Even with the development of new standardized and improved assessment tests and techniques, the interview has remained a primary assessment tool.[7,8] This chapter focuses on the use of a nonstandardized, traditional approach to interviewing in occupational therapy. Given that several assessment tools, some standardized, will be used in the total evaluation process, the traditional interview is a valid and essential method of gathering data. Identifying the assumptions underlying interviews shows how the technique is different from objective testing (Table 2-1).

The Power of an Interview

"The purpose of interviews is to find out what is in a person's mind...to access the perspective of the person...to find out things...we cannot directly observe."[9(p32)] An interview focuses on understanding a patient's perspective rather than on checking the accuracy of the information.[9] The interview is a method that allows patients to report the personal, subjective view of their situation and function. Since occupational therapy is based on the patient's needs, goals, and abilities, this is a critical step in the evaluation process. The *Occupational Therapy Practice Framework: Domain and Process* (*Framework*) identifies the data from the evaluation as an occupational profile, which includes the patient's self-reports.[1] The clinical reasoning literature shows that narrative reasoning is an essential aspect of evaluation and intervention.[10] A closed question assessment tool, such as a questionnaire or other short response tool, will not provide the therapist with the patient's total story.

Interviews are also used as an intervention technique. In occupational therapy, the interview sounds more like conversation and accompanies or follows participation in an occupation. Its purpose is to help patients use the knowledge obtained through the occupational process to better understand and increase their level of function. Interviews for change or for motivation to change require a different agenda, contract, and skills.[11]

Interview Defined

There are varied definitions of an interview.[12] For the purposes of this discussion, an *interview* is defined as a planned oral communication that has a clear purpose, specific content, and a format that allows patients to tell their stories.

The interview enables therapists to understand the patient's perspective, the level of the patient's current occupational performance, if further functional assessment is required, and to determine how occupational therapy will benefit the patient.

An interview is an interactive process whereby the patient and the therapist develop a relationship that allows the patient to identify and determine the needed methods and goals. The first part of the word, *inter*, means reciprocal, shared, or between.[7] The therapist needs to share a feeling of understanding and mutual trust with the patient. This outcome depends on the therapist's ability to listen and empathize with the patient.

The *view* aspect of an interview requires the therapist to be competent in observation. Communication has been identified as involving more than words. It also involves the nonverbal elements, including the tone of voice, rate of speech, facial and body expressions, and sensory information.[13] Communication, therefore, requires the therapist to observe and incorporate more than the words. To observe is to use the therapist's senses to attend to the behavior of a patient. Mosey states that to observe is to watch,

Table 2-1
Assumptions Underlying Interviews

- Facts are not actively sought; they emerge from the communication.
- The interview is crucial in setting the stage for future interaction, establishing a relationship, and for gathering relevant information.
- The communication techniques in an interview can function to facilitate or impede the flow of relevant information.
- It is possible to learn a range of interviewing techniques that can enhance the interview process.
- It is important for a practitioner to practice different techniques until a comfortable style of interaction is developed.

to listen carefully with alertness, taking particular note of detail.[14] This includes the odors or aromas that may be present; the temperature, tone, and color of the patient's skin; the patient's posture, gestures, speech patterns, use of eye contact, manner of dress and grooming; and the patient's response to the present situation. Communication factors include the patient's reactions, tone of voice, nonverbal noises, pacing and body movements, and positioning of the patient's arms and legs. Facial expressions are to be observed, to seek out emotions the patient may not be able to label or express. Although observation is identified as a separate type of assessment, it is an integral part of every assessment procedure.[15] It is the decision of the therapist whether or not to reflect on these observations during the interview. For example, a therapist may observe behavior indicating that the patient is hot or cold. Asking the patient if such is true, then acting to make the room more comfortable will increase the patient's belief that the therapist is concerned for his or her well-being. If a therapist sees tears in the patient's eyes and comments that the topic is sad, it helps the patient feel understood and may lead the patient to elaborate on the underlying feelings.

A therapist must know when to respond to a perceived nonverbal behavior. If a therapist chooses to overtly point out a patient's contradiction or limitation too soon in the relationship, the patient may perceive it as confrontation and become defensive. Whether the observations are discussed or not, they need to be understood as part of the total information gained from the interview. Later, when the relationship is more established and an intervention plan is implemented, the therapist may return to these issues for clarification or awareness.

An Unstructured Interview

The purpose of an occupational therapy interview is to discover what the patient is thinking and feeling, and how the patient understands his or her ability to function in a variety of settings and complete a variety of tasks. An unstructured format best meets these goals. Interviews may also be structured or semi-structured.

A structured interview provides a systematic evaluation by *standardizing*. It uses specific language, sequence, and quantification of responses.[16] This process requires a strict adherence to formulated questions.

Sample questions:
Therapist: "Did you finish high school?"
Patient: "Yes."
Therapist: "Do you cook your own meals?"
Patient: "Yes."
Therapist: "Are you responsible for managing your money?"
Patient: "Yes."

This structured approach is most common when using standardized interview tools.

A semi-structured interview uses standard questions, but allows the interviewer to add nonstandardized questions.

For example:
Therapist: "Do you cook your own meals?"
Patient: "Yes."
The therapist might add:
"What type of food do you cook?"
Patient: "Spaghetti and hamburgers."
The therapist will then return to the next structured question.
Therapist: "Are you responsible for managing your money?"

An unstructured interview, also known as a traditional interview, allows the therapist to develop questions in response to the patient's information. This chapter focuses on unstructured occupational therapy interviews. Unstructured does not mean unplanned. Therapists are strongly encouraged to develop a list of topics with open questions that will form the basis of each interview. This is to ensure that the therapist will be comfortable and familiar with the required content to be covered with each patient and will cover the full range of performance areas.

With experience, the therapist will learn typical responses to the questions. Although a pattern and repetition may develop this does not constitute a standardized interview.

Clinical Reasoning

As has been discussed in the literature, an essential part of clinical reasoning is the patient's narrative story, in which a patient can share personal perceptions, history, and understanding of his or her own life and function.[10] It is assumed that the results of an unstructured but planned occupational therapy interview will be combined with the results of standardized and other needed assessments. The therapist will then blend scientific, narrative, and pragmatic reasoning in analyzing the person's occupational profile, in order to develop an effective intervention plan.

Professional Boundaries

It is important to know the difference between a professional, friendly, supportive interview and a social exchange. Novices may mistake the methods used to establish rapport in an interview as a typical social exchange. A *social interchange* involves a give and take of information and concerns between the participants. The needs of both participants are a valid part of the content. A social interchange may develop a social relationship that establishes boundaries, mores, and ethics that then establishes a friendship. "In a clinical interview, however, most rules of social etiquette do not apply."[7(p21)]

A *professional interchange* and relationship has set boundaries, time limits, and content, and the needs of the patient are the total focus of the interchange. The therapist's statements have a larger purpose than in a social interaction. The therapist has specific goals and expected outcomes as a result of the interaction.[7] It requires skill and experience to develop an interview technique that establishes a friendly, comfortable, and trusting personal environment that allows the patient to express and share the needed information. When a patient responds in a social manner, asking personal questions of the therapist, the response given by the therapist will depend on what is best for the patient. The response may be a simple yes or no or a brief answer with limited information. The interview is not about the therapist. If the topic is on the therapist, then the focus of the interview is not on the patient.

The Therapist's Theoretical Orientation

A major influence on an interview is the theoretical orientation used by the therapist. As interviews are planned, occupational therapists are expected to include the domains included in the *Framework*. This includes the performance areas, skills, patterns, and the context, activity domains, and client factors. The theoretical orientation will determine how the interview data is analyzed, what other assessments will be used, what the total evaluation data indicates as baseline function, and what intervention methods will be used. For instance, the use of the Cognitive Disabilities Frame of Reference by Allen will analyze data to determine a patient's cognitive level and requirements needed for safe placement.[4] A sensory approach will focus on adaptations in the sensory environment to enhance performance, or a Model of Human Occupation (MOHO) approach will focus on what volition, routines, and skills are needed.[4] Using an integrated approach will blend these concepts and develop a comprehensive plan. Whichever approach is used, it is critical that the theoretical orientation be clear, consistent, based on scientific concepts, and well understood by the therapist. Only when therapists know a theoretical approach in depth will a consistent and comprehensive interview plan be developed. It is not enough to ask questions regarding the content of occupational performances; the therapist must know the meaning and significance of the data accumulated.

Another influence on the data that the occupational therapist plans to collect is the therapeutic approach used by the treatment team. All team members will be collecting data. To develop a successful, coordinated intervention plan, the data collected by the team needs to be theoretically consistent and compatible. The occupational therapist must use a compatible occupational therapy approach so that the interview data will be integrated in the team plan. All of this must be known before the therapist plans an interview.

Screening

The first step of an evaluation process is called *screening*. This is the first meeting with the patient after the therapist has received a referral. The therapist sees the patient to learn whether intervention or further evaluation is necessary and to identify dysfunctions in the patient's occupational performance. The interview is often the method selected to gather this information. It is the one tool occupational therapists use that is based on oral interaction and does not require that the person engage in a doing process. To talk about one's performance is often less threatening than demonstrating what one can do. Thus, many patients respond favorably to an initial interview. To use an interview, the therapist must know how to engage the patient to establish rapport and trust enough to discuss topics that will reveal the patient's assets and limitations in occupational performance behavior.

During the screening process, it is not just the therapist who is making an initial assessment; the patient is gaining an impression of the therapist. If intervention is warranted, this interaction is the beginning of the therapeutic relationship. The quality of this brief interaction can make a difference in the patient's cooperation or resistance.

The screening process allows the therapist to meet briefly with the patient to provide information about occupational therapy and the need for an interview.

The therapist needs to explain the interview by giving an idea of the content to be covered, the length of time needed, clarifying that the interview is only the beginning of the evaluation process, and then making an appointment to actually do the interview. This sequence allows patients to feel a sense of control and to think about what they might wish to share. When patients feel this level of respect, it will be easier for them to trust the therapist and provide needed information.

"Hello, Mr. Bluefeather. I'm Ricky Eagle, an occupational therapist here in the program. Occupational therapists work with people on how to accomplish everyday activities, such as shopping and cooking, getting around town, and scheduling time for relaxation techniques. We can focus on job or social needs. I'd like to talk with you later about what you wish to accomplish and how we can help you. This will assist me in knowing the specific activities that would be helpful to you. It may require some other evaluations depending on your needs. It will take about 10 minutes. I'd like to meet with you at 11:00 am if that fits your schedule."

Refusals

It is always the right of a patient to refuse any part of the evaluation or intervention. It is the responsibility of the therapist to assess the patient's reasons for refusing an interview. Often, a refusal is based on the patient's emotional perceptions of the situation. The person feels fearful, suspicious, does not know what will happen with personal information, does not understand or trust the statement of confidentiality, is too depressed or fatigued to make a decision or to talk, or is incoherent in thought. The patient may state that he is leaving the setting soon so an interview is not needed or may give some other reason for the refusal. It requires the art and skill of the therapist to explore the reasons for refusals. By working with the emotional content of the patient, a therapist can often motivate participation in a brief interview. The therapist needs to demonstrate respect for the patient's needs while encouraging the patient's participation. The focus is for a therapist to establish a sense of trust and cooperation. It can be helpful for the therapist to return two or three times to the patient, indicating patience, understanding, and concern. The patient often responds by slowly cooperating with the requests. When a therapist meets a patient and gives the impression of being in a hurry or just doing a job, the result is apt to be a refusal. It takes skill and art, not coercion or manipulation, for a therapist to help a patient understand the benefits of engaging in the assessment process.

I worked with a 15-year-old boy who had been admitted to an adult mental health unit. He stayed under the covers and refused to give more than yes and no responses. The first time I talked to the back of his head under the covers. I told him who I was, that I would be with him for 5 minutes, and that it seemed he was frightened of the unfamiliar place. I provided a verbal description of the unit, the resources, and the expectations of the unit program. After stating that I would sit with him for 2 more minutes, I was quiet. I did not read or talk with others in the room. At 5 minutes I told him it was nice to be with him and I would return at 2:00 pm that day. At 2:00 pm, I repeated the process. This time, he turned and looked at me before I left. The next day the process was repeated, and in the afternoon he began to talk. Later that day, he walked around the unit and became involved in his treatment. I realize that with today's in-and-out demands, this seems impossible. Yet coercing, rushing, or accepting refusals does not allow the person to be treated.

Preparing an Interview

The success of any interview is directly related to the therapist's attitudes, knowledge, and skills. It is not the responsibility of the patient to act or do as the therapist requests. Patients may be hostile, uncooperative, nonresponsive, have incoherent speech, or other patterns of behavior that make it difficult for them to communicate.[12]

The Therapist's Attitudes

RESPECT

A deep and abiding respect for people is the basis for success in the interview and intervention process. This is a therapist's ethical responsibility.[17] This requires that therapists emphasize the dignity of patients, believing that all people have inherent worth, value, and uniqueness. The therapist believes in nurturing the health that enables patients to change. As therapists, we may assume a belief in respecting different patients until we meet someone who believes or behaves in ways that challenge our values. At these times, therapists may make judgmental comments that show disrespect. It is at such times that therapists must be self-aware and search their value system so that true respect for all patients is developed.

EMPATHY

To understand a person's life story requires therapists to put their own perspective aside and take on the patient's perspective. This is what is meant by the Native American saying, "to walk a mile in another person's shoes." It is to feel the stones beneath the feet, to feel the aches and pains of the body, to view the world from that person's perspective. Continual self-management is required by the therapist to experience what a patient experiences about a situation without losing a sense of self. Carl Rogers wrote of the fear therapists have about not being able to remove themselves from the experiences of others. He discusses how therapists often want to demonstrate their own abilities rather than focus on the patient for guidance. This reaction protects the therapist from feeling the emotions of the patient and controls the content of the interview. Rogers implores therapists to permit themselves to understand the patient. When therapists understand the patient's perspective, it enables them to experience hope and belief in the patient's recovery. To become overwhelmed with the patient's pain is not empathy but sympathy or pity. Therapists who feel sympathy know the feelings of pain rather than the comfort that is given by being present.[6] To have empathy means saying, "That must have been a very difficult time for you," rather than, "I'm sorry."

SELF-AWARENESS

Therapists need to be willing to seek self-awareness. They need to know the thoughts and feelings that their culture and experiences have developed in them. Therapists may need to examine their assumptions about a patient's ethnicity, age, diagnosis, language, cognition, size, religion, clothing, or any other difference. Therapists need to acknowledge that they, like other people, are reared within a cultural context that may include stereotypes and misinformation about other groups. Therapists are responsible for monitoring their own personal reactions and any influence those responses may have on clinical judgments. Therapists need to continually strive to keep assumptions about people from skewing their understanding of patients.

CULTURAL AWARENESS

As therapists listen to patients sharing life stories, they need to be aware of cultural differences and biases. As therapists become aware of and identify their own cultural values and beliefs, they will be able to separate those from the values and beliefs of other cultures. Only with this knowledge will therapists be able to hear and understand the differences that patients share with them. It is significant for therapists to know that they cannot be totally objective or neutral as they explore the patient's value patterns. Therapists must constantly question their conclusions and, perhaps, talk them over with members of the intervention team. A person's behavioral health is intimately tied to culture. Therapists need to know how patients' cultures influence the choice of occupations and goals and mental health perceptions.

A team of occupational therapists working at a private psychiatric hospital were planning intervention groups. The objectives were to foster structure, independence, and productive behavior. They set up an IADL group in which people could focus on occupations such as making beds, washing clothes, or cooking a small meal. Another group was to focus on transportation, budgeting, and shopping skills. The patients reacted with incredulity when hearing of the planned interventions. They had maids to do the cooking, cleaning, and bed making. If they didn't travel in a limousine, they used taxis. Budgets were of little importance, as others kept track of the money, and clothes buyers from specific stores helped them shop. The patients saw no need to learn any of the proposed skills. When working closely with the patients, the therapists were able to identify several occupations, primarily leisure ones that met the same therapeutic objectives and still fit the patients' culture.

The Therapist's Skills

OPEN AND CLOSED QUESTIONS

Open questions are those that encourage patients to describe, report, or discuss a subject. *Closed* questions ask only for a yes or no response. There is a time and situation to use either type of question. When therapists use open questions, the focus is on knowing the patient's personal story.

Example:
Therapist: "What would you like to accomplish in occupational therapy?"

More examples of open questions on multiple topics are available in Zuckerman.[19]

One word of caution: When designing the open questions, it is best to avoid asking why. To ask people the "why" of behavior tends to elicit rationalizations. People feel asked to explain rather than describe or recall perceptions of their function.

Open statements are similar to open questions and can decrease the stress for the patient to respond. Open statements request or make a statement but do not demand a response. The patient may choose to respond to the statement or may choose to change the topic.

Example:
Therapist: "I'd like you to tell me about your work experience."

Closed questions are best used to narrow a topic, to clarify a statement, or can be used if the person cannot respond with more than one-word answers.

Example:
Therapist: "Please tell me about your last job."
Patient: "I worked in a gas station."
Therapist: "When did you work at the gas station?"
Patient: "In 2005."
Therapist: "Did you like working there?"
Patient: "Yes."
Therapist: "What parts of the job did you like?"

The therapist has now gone back to the use of open questions so the patient's perspective of the job is understood.

To use closed questions too early or too often can focus on the therapist's perceptions and not give the patient time to share his or her opinion. A series of closed questions can feel like being interrogated or getting the third degree. Patients will resign themselves to meeting the expectations of the therapist and will give up on sharing their own ideas.

LISTENING

To listen is to understand. A critical skill in the art of communication is to focus only on the verbal and nonverbal messages of the sender. Listening is an active rather than passive skill. The interviewer focuses all attention and energy into receiving the message. When using this skill, therapists put aside their personal concerns and clinical assumptions, or anticipation of what the patient will say. To listen means that therapists are not interpreting or thinking of questions while patients are speaking. The focus is on understanding the patient's unique responses to the topics. After the patient has finished a response, the therapist silently analyzes the information and forms the next step of the interview. A therapist does not agree or disagree with a patient during an assessment interview. The skill is to receive and understand a message, not to provide a critique or judgment of its value. The primary aim of listening is to understand the patient's message and demonstrate that the intended message was received. To listen and to understand enables the therapist to have empathy for the patient.

SILENCE

Silence is a part of communication, not the absence of communication. Silence may express reflection, resistance, anger, fear, discouragement, or completion. As in the previous technique, the therapist listens to the patient, totally focusing on the incoming message. When the patient has completed the response to a request, silence occurs. This pause allows time for the therapist to reflect, assimilate, and analyze the message, and then continue guiding the interview. A *reflective* silence may encourage the patient to add more information after thinking about what has been said. An *angry* or *hostile* silence may occur when patients believe a topic is irrelevant to their needs or believe that the interviewer is not listening, is uninterested, or is misunderstanding. A fear of being judged as inadequate or as ill may motivate patients to become silent. When patients feel they have revealed too much of their personal concerns or have shared embarrassing or difficult information, a silence often occurs. When patients are disoriented, forgetful, unable to remember the topic or to sort out the jumbled thoughts or voices in their heads, they often end a topic abruptly and sit in silence. A more comfortable silence of completion occurs when both the patient and the therapist sense that a given topic has been covered and that a new topic is needed.

One of the most difficult aspects of silence for new therapists is avoiding the tendency to fill silence with talk. Therapists who are uncomfortable with silence often feel an immediate response is required. The anxious comments are often irrelevant or not well thought out. In this situation, the lack of comfort in the therapist is what is driving the interview, rather than the need for assessment of the patient's needs. A therapist needs to learn to be silent, to listen, and to value the silence.

IDENTIFYING THOUGHTS AND FEELINGS

Feelings are a person's responses to his or her experiences in the world. Thoughts are a person's interpretation of the responses and the experiences. To identify feelings means to be sensitive to the underlying emotion behind the person's content. According to Egan, every core message has an experience (what happened to the person) or behavior (what action the person feels like taking), and an affect (the emotional response that accompanies the experience or behavior).[20] Egan developed a guide to help therapists respond to a core message: "You feel (affect) because of (experience/behavior)."[20] This wording is not to be used verbatim, but as a guide to identify a person's emotional response to a situation.

Example:
Patient: "I'm getting a raw deal. They say I will be going home soon, but they have not told me my diagnosis."

Therapist: "You're feeling frightened that you will be sent home without treatment."
Patient: "I'm angry."

The person can validate or correct the statement. A therapist need not be overly concerned with identifying the precise feeling, as the process expresses concern for the patient's well-being and encourages the more precise clarification of one's feelings.

The Use of Reflection

The art of reflection is stating the essence of the message in a few words and in a format different from the patient's. The sender can then hear the message from a different perspective. Reflection may help the patient validate, clarify, elaborate, or refute the therapist's understanding. It is helpful to be succinct and use key words stated by the patient. The temptation may be to parrot what patients have said, rather than to use reflection. If patients' words are repeated back to them, it often leads to anger and causes patients to question the therapist's competence. When the therapist reflects so that the patient can hear the message in different words, the technique can help the patient sort out feelings and thoughts. It may take several interactions of reflection before the specific message is understood by both the patient and the therapist.

Clarifying a Message

When patients are relating difficult information, several messages may be lumped together, either because the patient has not been able to sort them out or because they cannot identify which one is the most important. Clarification is the process of making a message clear. The therapist can identify two or three primary messages and ask the patient to elaborate on one or more of them.

Example:
Therapist: "It sounds as though you are concerned about your job, the welfare of your family, the reason you are here, and how you will pay for it."
Patient: "If I don't have my job, I won't be able to care for my family."
Therapist. "Please tell me about your job and what worries you."

When asking for clarification, it may help if the therapist states why the information is important to the evaluation process. It is helpful if the request is as open-ended as possible, although closed questions may be used for specific details.

Example:
Therapist: "I am not sure I understand. Please tell me more about how you quit your job last week."

Using Prompts

At times, patients need assistance to continue discussing their thought or topic. Therapists can encourage communication by using a manner, gesture, or words that do not specify the kind of information sought. Techniques that facilitate communication are called *prompts*. Prompts can be verbal or nonverbal. A common verbal prompt is to highlight a word.

Example:
Patient: "Last week when I lost my job I went shopping. I bought new shoes."
Therapist: "Lost?"

This will focus the patient on that part of the statement. If one word does not seem effective, then the therapist may highlight a phrase. This again encourages the patient to say more about the job loss. Other verbal prompts include "Please go on," "Yes, I'm listening," "I see," or "Um-hm."

One of the most common nonverbal prompts is a *positive nod of the head*. This encourages patients to continue their train of thought. However, a nod of the head can also express agreement and a therapist needs to avoid giving incorrect messages. In some cultures, the up and down movement of the head means "no." Again, therapists have to be aware of the patient's cultural context. A gentle touch is used when a person is feeling sad. The therapist may put a hand on the back of the patient's hand, forearm, or at times, a shoulder. The touch must be strong enough to show caring. A light touch may trigger the autonomic system's flight or fight response, causing the patient to hit out in reflex. To pat a person is often perceived as a belittling or paternalistic expression, especially in the larger American culture. All nonverbal gestures exist within a cultural context. The therapist needs to be aware of other meanings for commonly used gestures and be alert to possible misunderstandings.

SHIFT IN TOPIC

When a patient wants to stay on a topic that has been covered and is repeating him- or herself or if time is getting short, the therapist may have to move the patient off the topic and onto another one. This is a time of transition in conversation. The therapist needs to summarize the first topic, thank the person for sharing the information, then start with another open question. Some patients will continue on the old topic. When this occurs, the therapist needs to ask more questions to discover why the topic is so important to the patient. The therapist can ask some closed questions to take the topic further or in a slightly different direction. This technique may help the patient say something he or she wanted to say, but didn't know how, or the therapist may find that the patient didn't know how to get off the topic. When the result is known, the therapist can explore what the patient wanted to say or transition to a new topic. This is a time when the therapist guides the interview with more structure than when all is going in a typical manner.

Example:
Therapist: "We have talked about the concerns you have about your family and living situation. I appreciated you sharing that information. This is an area we can return to later. Now I would like you to tell me how you spend a typical day. When do you get up and what is the routine pattern of your day?"

The Physical Setting

The setting in which the interview occurs often influences the quality of the interview. It is important that the place allows privacy, is free of interruptions or distractions, and has a comfortable temperature and furniture. All cell phones, telephones, beepers, and other electronic devices need to be turned off. If interruptions cannot be controlled, the therapist should tell the patient that an interruption is possible. Enough time should be scheduled to complete an interview in one setting. There may sometimes be exceptions to this rule, but the majority of interviews need to be completed in one setting.[7]

A young woman who was frightened and suspicious was admitted to the mental health unit. When the therapist went to do the interview, the scheduled room was not available. The only room available was a stark white 8' by 5' room with a table and two chairs. There were no pictures or other warming features. Even though the room was private and free of distractions, its smallness and starkness frightened the young woman, increasing her attention to her suspiciousness, and an interview was not possible.

Planning

To complete a successful interview in an efficient timeframe, a therapist must be prepared by knowing the purpose and agenda for the interview. An experienced therapist often has to just take time to know who the patient is, the reason for the referral to occupational therapy, and what outcomes are expected. For the seasoned therapist, the agenda and content will be familiar and easily accessible from the many interviews already given. Yet even an experienced therapist will give a better interview by taking time to think about the specific patient's situation, needs, and goals.

A novice therapist or a therapist new to a given setting must take the time to plan an interview agenda and outcomes. It can be helpful to review the steps and skills involved in an interview. Only in this manner will all significant topics be covered with skill and ease.

Another aspect of planning an interview requires the skills of establishing a series of open questions that will cover the domains of occupational therapy and the focus of the theoretical orientation. Other suggested questions with specific theoretical formats can be found in the literature.[4] Table 2-2 identifies content from the *Framework* that can be covered in an interview.

Patient Factors

Physical, cognitive, and psychosocial factors influence a person's performance and how it is affected by conditions or illness. Some patient factors that can be assessed by an interview include the global mental functions such as the person's level of arousal, level of consciousness, and orientation to person, place, time, self, and others.[1] Others factors include the patient's ability to recognize familiar images, to categorize and generalize material, to be aware of reality, and the ability to think and speak in a coherent manner.

Sequence of an Interview

OPENING PHASE

If a screening meeting has occurred, the therapist still begins by establishing eye contact and giving his or her name, discipline, and the purpose of the interview.[19] It is

Table 2-2
Performance Areas Assessed in an Interview

Collaborative relationship

- Establish rapport
- Professional interactions

Client mental factors

- Orientation to person, place, time, self, and others
- Level of arousal and consciousness
- Emotional stability
- Level of coherent and logical thought
- Level of cognitive organization
- Level of reality-based thought
- Appropriate content of thought
- Past and immediate memory
- Level of concrete or conceptual thought
- Ability or willingness to express

Mental factors that can be partly assessed in an interview then, if needed, further assessed by additional tools

- Past and current values and interests
- Past and current roles
- Motivation to engage in intervention and goals.
- Self-concept, body image, and self-esteem.
- Decision making and problem solving
- Availability and expression of emotions
- Daily performance patterns
- Specific customs, beliefs, behavior standards, and expectations
- Specific instrumental activities of daily living.

Together, the information will determine what other assessment tools are needed for a complete evaluation.

important for the therapist to identify the patient as the correct person, and thank the patient for the agreed upon time and for the patient's cooperation. The therapist then restates the needed content and procedure. The therapist asks for a specific amount of time and whether this is acceptable for the patient. Providing a time limit shows respect and lets the patient know what to expect. With time limits, patients can determine how much information to reveal. The longer the timeframe, the more personal revelations may occur. The therapist then needs to take a few minutes to personalize the interview, which means that the therapist will call attention to something personal about the patient and comment on it. It might be flowers in the room, the color or selection of clothing, a card nearby, or a book the patient is reading. This technique begins to establish rapport, sets the focus on the patient, and may relax the patient, thereby increasing the focus on the interview material.

BODY OF THE INTERVIEW

The data gathering phase is the body of the interview. It is not more important than the opening or closing phases, but it is longer and more detailed. Here, the focus is for the therapist to elicit subjective material so the patient's narrative story can be known. The therapist will begin with the planned open questions.

As the patient shares information, the therapist will use his or her communication skills to encourage accurate, detailed, clear, and relevant information. The therapist encourages the patient to discuss what is important while still maintaining control of the interview. Control of an interview is like being a guide. The therapist guides the patient through the needed topics while letting the patient state the information in his or her own language, pacing, and at times, sequence. The therapeutic use of self and the skillful use of therapeutic communication techniques by the therapist will determine how well this phase of the interview is accomplished.

CLOSING

The closing is as important to a successful interview as the opening. The therapist's first task in closing is to give a timing reminder. In the opening phase, the therapist and patient agreed on a set time for the interview. The closing phase begins as the therapist reminds the patient of this by stating that a given number of minutes remain. Depending on the length of the interview, 3 to 5 minutes works to indicate that the end of the interview is near. The therapist is to give another timing reminder at 2 minutes before the end. In this timeframe, the therapist stops asking questions or seeking information. The second task of the closing phase is for the therapist to summarize what the patient has shared. The therapist needs to briefly summarize the most significant information. This technique allows the patient to correct or clarify any comments made. The therapist then tells the patient the next step of the evaluation procedure, the next meeting time, and what will be done with the gathered information. The therapist then asks if the patient has questions, wants clarification on any of the procedures, or wishes to add new information. The therapist needs to be careful during this step that the patient does not open a new topic or get into new details. If the patient continues sharing information, the therapist needs to gently let the patient know that not all important information could be covered in the limited time. The therapist states that the patient shared important information that will give the therapist and the treatment team a sufficient base for further planning or intervention. The therapist then thanks the patient for his or her time and cooperation.

Example:
Therapist: "I appreciate what you have shared with me. We have covered significant information and have about 3 minutes left. I'd like to summarize what I understand as the main points of your comments."

Examples of lead-ins to stating the essence of what the patient has said:
"Let's see if I have the whole picture…."
" So far I understand this….."
"Let's review what you have told me."
"Have I missed anything?"

Patient: "Did I tell you that I want to get an apartment of my own?"

Therapist: "Yes, you mentioned you would like to leave your mother's house and live on your own. I realize there is more to your story that we could not cover today. You have given the team and me enough to plan the next steps of your care plan. Is there anything else you believe we must know now?"

Patient: "No. What happens next?"

Therapist: "I will review this information and determine what other assessments will help to understand your specific needs and how we can help you. I will also be talking with the team members so we all know your total treatment needs. I will get back to you tomorrow at 9:00. Thank you again."

Patient: "Thank you."

Documentation

Taking accurate and precise notes is a professional responsibility. The art is to be able to record information from the patient during an interview without interfering with the emotional and physical setting. Most patients expect a therapist to take notes. In fact, they may be upset if notes are not taken, believing the therapist will forget important information. If a therapist has pen and paper and records the significant points verbatim, it will enhance the interview, not detract. It is important that therapists tell patients that, if they wish, they may look at the notes anytime throughout the interview. This discourages patients from believing therapists are writing judgmental statements, as so many of them fear. It behooves the therapist to record only the facts and to not write conclusions, assumptions, or judgments.

The use of electronic devices has to be weighed carefully. No matter what equipment is used, malfunctions can happen. When they do, the focus is on the device and not on the patient. An electronic device can be intimidating, and interfere with the patient sharing important information. Patients may feel that the recorded material will be replayed for others or be put in the chart, and be concerned if they are using the "right" words. Therapist usually use electronic devices in the hopes of saving time when, in fact, it does not take much more time for the therapist to record notes and later compose the formal note or report on a computer.

Initial Evaluation Summary

The *Framework* suggests that data in an initial evaluation summary be organized in categories of the Occupational Profile and Analysis of Performance[1] (Table 2-3).

OCCUPATIONAL PROFILE

This is the data that presents the patient's occupational history and experiences, such as patterns of daily living, interest, values, and needs. The patient's problems and concerns about performing occupations and daily life activities are stated and priorities are determined.[1] An occupational profile describes all the significant data from all of the assessments used in the evaluation. All the tools used need to be identified by name and stated as standardized or not. The data needs to be grouped and reported according to performance areas, patterns, and skills. Specific patient factors need to be included and

Table 2-3
Occupational Therapy Initial Evaluation Report

Identification and background information:

- Name, age, sex, date of admission, treatment diagnosis, date of onset of current diagnosis.

Occupational profile:

- Name and type of assessment with results. State if procedure is standardized. Source of referral and why person is seeking services.
- What areas of occupation are successful, which ones cause problems (education, work, play, leisure, social participation, motor skills; process skills; communication/interaction skills; habits; routines).
- What contexts support or hinder performance? What is the person's occupational performance history? What are the person's priorities and targeted outcomes?

Analysis of occupational performance:

- Synthesize information from the occupational profile.
- State effectiveness and identify factors that are influencing client's performance skills and patterns.
- Identify factors and contexts that facilitate or hinder performance.
- Develop and refine hypotheses about person's occupational performances, strengths, and weaknesses.
- State the type and severity of impairments identified and the functional limitations caused by the impairments.
- Indicate functional outcomes: an anticipated level of performance the client will be able to achieve as a result of occupational therapy intervention.
- Use objective, functional, and measurable terms.

Signature

Printed name

Date

described when describing the level of the patient's function. If some of the data is contradictory, both versions are to be described along with the context in which each occurred. In total, the occupational profile needs to describe the patient's perspective along with the objective results of all assessments tools.

ANALYSIS OF OCCUPATIONAL PERFORMANCE

An accurate and professional analysis of the occupational profile requires the therapist to make clinical judgments about the patient's functional abilities and expected benefits of occupational therapy services. In the analysis of the occupational profile, the therapist applies clinical reasoning using the his or her theoretic orientation and the relationship of performance patterns to function as identified in the *Framework*. The therapist needs to determine the patient's specific functional assets, limitations, and goals, with a plan for intervention. The plan specifies a timeframe and intervention methods, and identifies behavioral outcomes expected from the intervention.

Summary

This chapter discussed the content, process, and techniques needed to accomplish an interview as an initial assessment in occupational therapy. To give effective interviews, therapists need to engage in therapeutic professional relationships, have constructive attitudes, and effective communication skills. Interviews need to be carefully planned, including content according to an occupational performance and a theoretical orientation, an organized sequence, and a comfortable physical setting. Even with an increasing number of standardized assessments available, the interview has remained a technique basic to the evaluation process in occupational therapy.

References

1. American Occupational Therapy Association. Occupational therapy practice framework: domain and process. *Amer J Occup Ther.* 2002;56:609-639.
2. American Occupational Therapy Association. Delineation of the AOTA standards of practice for occupational therapy. In: Crepeau E, Cohn E, Schell B, eds. *Willard and Spackman's Occupational Therapy.* 10th ed. Philadelphia: Lippincott Williams & Wilkins; 2003:1015-1017.
3. Crepeau E, Cohn E, Schell BB. Occupational therapy practice. In: Crepeau E, Cohn E, Schell B, eds. *Willard and Spackman's Occupational Therapy.* 10th ed. Philadelphia: Lippincott Williams & Wilkins; 2003:27-30.
4. Bruce M, Borg B. *Psychosocial Frames of Reference: Core for Occupation-Based Practice.* 3rd ed. Thorofare, NJ: SLACK Incorporated; 2002.
5. Greenberg M, Shergill S, Szmukler G, Tantam D, eds. *Narratives in Psychiatry.* Philadelphia: Athenaeum Press; 2003.
6. Peloquin S. The therapeutic relationship: manifestations and challenges in occupational therapy. In: Crepeau E, Cohn E, Schell B, eds. *Willard and Spackman's Occupational Therapy.* 10th ed. Philadelphia: Lippincott Williams & Wilkins;2003:157-170.
7. Craig, R. *Clinical and Diagnostic Interviewing.* 2nd ed. Oxford: Aronson; 2005.
8. Henry, A. The interviewing process in occupational therapy In: Crepeau E, Cohn E, Schell B, eds. *Willard and Spackman's Occupational Therapy.* 10th ed. Philadelphia: Lippincott Williams & Wilkins; 2003:285-297.
9. Arskey H, Knight P. *Interviewing for Social Scientists.* London: Sage Pub. Ltd; 1999:32.
10. Schell BB. Clinical reasoning: the bases of practice. In: Crepeau E, Cohn E, Schell B, eds. *Willard and Spackman's Occupational Therapy.* 10th ed. Philadelphia: Lippincott Williams & Wilkins; 2003:129-139.
11. Miller W, Rollnick S. *Motivational Interviewing: Preparing People for Change.* 2nd ed. New York, NY: Guilford Press; 2002:7.
12. Page M. Interviewing as an assessment tool in occupational therapy. In: Hemphill-Pearson B, ed. *Assessments in Occupational Therapy Mental Health: An Integrative Approach.* Thorofare, NJ: SLACK Incorporated; 1999:19-39.
13. Satir V. *Peoplemaking.* Palo Alto, CA: Science & Behavior Books, Inc; 1972:30.
14. Mosey A. *Psychosocial Components of Occupational Therapy.* New York, NY: Raven; 1986:307-308.

15. Denton P. *Psychiatric Occupational Therapy: A Workbook of Practical Skills.* Boston, MA: Little, Brown and Company; 1987:29.

16. Rogers R. *Handbook of Diagnostic and Structured Interviewing.* New York, NY: Guilford Press; 2005:3.

17. Hansen R. Ethics in occupational therapy. In: Crepeau E, Cohn E, Schell B, eds. *Willard and Spackman's Occupational Therapy.* 10th ed. Philadelphia, PA: Lippincott Williams & Wilkins; 2003:953-961.

18. Rogers C. Empathetic: an unappreciated way of being. *Couns Psychol.* 1975;5(2):2-10.

19. Zuckerman E. *Clinician's Thesaurus: The Guide to Conducting Interviews and Writing Psychological Reports.* 6th ed. New York, NY: Guilford Press; 2005:21.

20. Egan G. *You and Me: The Skills of Communication and Relating to Others.* Monterey, CA: Brooks/Cole Publishing Co; 1977:87-88.

21. Cohn E, Schell B, Neistadt M. Introduction to evaluation and interviewing. In: Crepeau E, Cohn E, Schell B, eds. *Willard and Spackman's Occupational Therapy.* 10th ed. Philadelphia, PA: Lippincott Williams & Wilkins; 2003:28-29.

3

CLIENT-CENTERED ASSESSMENT: THE CANADIAN OCCUPATIONAL PERFORMANCE MEASURE

Susan Baptiste, MHSc, OTReg (Ont)

"...human beings become increasingly trustworthy once they feel at a deep level that their subjective experience is both respected and progressively understood." Thorne B. Carl Rogers. *London: Sage Publications Ltd; 1992:26.*

Introduction

In the years since the first edition of *Assessments in Occupational Therapy Mental Health,*[1] there have been pervasive and rich developments across the professional and theoretical landscape within which occupational therapy lives as a discipline. At the time of that first edition, the notion of client-centered practice was relatively new, as was the intention to frame our overall practice in an occupation-centered manner, using the impairment lens as one element of a more detailed approach to assessment and intervention. So, it is a refreshing task to take the opportunity offered in writing this second iteration of client-centered assessment. This chapter will take the approach of revisiting the assumptions underlying client-centeredness as a construct; this will be approached through a high-level reflection on the theoretical literature. This picture will be further informed by a look at the development of the *Occupational Therapy Practice Framework* (*Framework*) from the perspective of a Canadian therapist relating this to Canadian practice models and the Canadian Occupational Performance Measure (COPM).[2] The COPM will be explored in more detail. Some discussion will be provided of the evidence that has emerged over the past few years regarding its utilization in practice, with specific reference to practice in the mental health and mental illness arena.

By way of summary, case studies will be provided that illustrate the broad approach possible in the implementation of the COPM as a gateway step in determining the patient's perspective upon which to build a therapeutic relationship and process.

The Practice Context

Over the past 5 to 10 years, occupational therapy practice has undergone radical shifts related to the application of theory to practice and integration of evidence in the choices of assessments and interventions. While there is still a relatively long way to go before all practice is so guided, there has been enough of a change that many therapists have loudly declared their need for a clearer understanding of how evidence can steer and enrich practice, and, similarly, how practice frameworks can provide additional clarity and security when pursuing the therapeutic mission. From these pervasive trends have emerged frameworks to provide the busy practitioners with a sense of logical order to their clinical reasoning, in a culture of overwhelming resources and change.[3-5] Two frameworks that will be used to inform our discussion here are the Canadian Model of Occupational Performance (CMOP)[4] and the *Occupational Therapy Practice Framework*.[5] Both of these frameworks declare as one of their foundational values the belief in a client-centered approach to an occupation-centered professional practice. For the purposes of this chapter, the term *client* will be employed rather than *patient*, since this is congruent with the foundational beliefs, theories, and models upon which the CMOP was developed. The term *patient* will be used when referring to the *Framework*.

THE CANADIAN MODEL OF OCCUPATIONAL PERFORMANCE

The CMOP was one of the outputs of a consensus process undertaken in the mid-1990s by the Canadian Association of Occupational Therapists (CAOT).[6] The process was another link in the chain that commenced a decade earlier with the development of guidelines for Canadian occupational therapy practice, jointly supported by the CAOT and the Department of Health and Welfare of the federal government of Canada. The book, *Enabling Occupation: A Canadian Perspective*, was the overall outcome of the consensus process within which the CMOP was a central innovation. The CMOP (Figure 3-1) has become one of the core elements of contemporary occupational therapy practice in Canada and beyond since the book's first edition in 1997.

As can be seen when examining the CMOP, there are distinct domains illustrated within it. In essence, it provides a graphic depiction of the three central elements of practice in occupational therapy: the *person*, the *environment*, and the *occupation*. The person element includes affective, cognitive, and physical components; the occupation element encompasses components of productivity, self-care, and leisure; and the environment element includes components of the physical, social, cultural, and institutional environments. Its sister model, the Person-Environment-Occupation model (PEO),[7] introduces another way in which these elements can be viewed with the addition of the overlapping central element that is *occupational performance*—the central focus and purpose of occupational therapy practice.

In both manifestations of the occupational therapy philosophy, there is a clear commitment to the centrality of the person, the patient, in the partnership of therapeutic engagement. The COPM is the outcome measurement tool developed in concordance with the conceptualization and formation of the CMOP and the PEO, and will form a major part of our discussion in this chapter.

THE OCCUPATIONAL THERAPY PRACTICE FRAMEWORK

By the fall of 2002, a Practice Framework had been adopted by the Representative Assembly of the American Occupational Therapy Association (AOTA) and published in

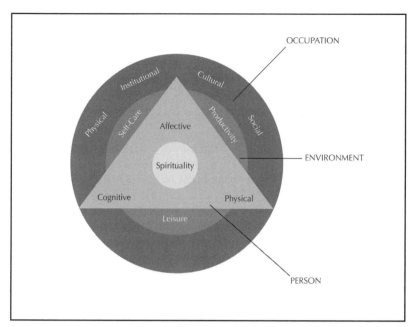

Figure 3-1. Canadian Model of Occupational Performance. Copyright Canadian Association of Occupational Therapists. Reprinted with permission.

the American Journal of Occupational Therapy (AJOT).[5] This text is using this *Framework* as a specific anchor for the discussions across the entirety of its content; therefore, my discussion of it here will be cursory at best, and will reflect specifically the points at which there is a particular connection with the CMOP and the COPM. Overall, the *Framework* celebrates the concept of client-centeredness throughout, culminating in a specific client-centered focus within the center of the Collaborative Process Model.[5]

The *Framework* was developed, as stated earlier, to assist practitioners in the ever-emerging complexity of everyday practice. Its main intention was to combine the essential and foundational concepts of occupational therapy practice together with the practice process from assessment to intervention and thence to evaluation, always mediated within the understanding that occupation is the profession's central belief and value.[5] This *Framework* is premised upon an understanding that the domain of occupational therapy is best articulated through the concepts of performance in areas of occupation, performance skills, performance patterns, context, activity demands, and specific client factors. In many ways, the formulation of the overarching concepts and constructs here are similar and reaffirming of those expressed and illustrated within the CMOP.

The performance areas of occupation as stated within the *Framework* provide a detailed menu of domains of occupation, including specific reference to education, play, and social participation. In addition, the performance skills and patterns, another component of the *Framework*, are well-articulated elements that often remain as more covert components of clinical reasoning for those practitioners not adopting the *Framework* for their practice.

Within the area of context, the inclusion of the temporal and virtual environments is invaluable. The detailed level of interpretation of the activity demands and client factors within the *Framework* also provides a clear and exhaustive list of areas to which any practitioner should attend when entering into a new patient-therapist relationship.

All domains that are identified within the *Framework* bear relevance and importance in the application of a client-centered approach to practice. With specific reference to the connection with the CMOP and COPM, however, it is in the process application of the *Framework* that the closest ties and relationship are revealed. In the detailed description of the *Framework* published in AJOT,[5] a graphic depiction is given of the Framework Collaborative Process Model, at the center of which is the collaborative process between practitioner and patient. This is where the direct application of the COPM can best be envisioned.

The overall context of the Collaborative Process Model reflects the integrated nature of occupational therapy practice, involving the analysis of occupational performance and development of an intervention plan centered upon outcomes that reflect engagement in occupation that supports participation.

Client-Centered Practice

Several texts have been written that explore in specific detail the complexities and central tenets of client-centeredness. All agree that the approach and belief system owes its origins to Carl Rogers,[8] who described the importance of developing an open relationship between patient and therapist that is driven by elements of partnership rather than an obvious differential in power between the two participants. A client-centered approach can be employed between any therapist and any patient, regardless of clinical circumstances and conditions. However, undoubtedly, the temporal component of any practice framework is critical to engage when deciding when to begin the partnership development process. There are challenges inherent within the utilization of a partnership model with patients of any patient group. Gage[9] explores the challenges of applying this approach when working with patients with physical disabilities. Similarly, Hobson[10] addresses its use with the elderly and persons who have cognitive impairment. Of particular interest to this chapter, Kuznir and colleagues[11] discuss the challenges of client-centered practice in mental health settings.

Foundational principles of client-centeredness are clear and well-articulated throughout the literature.[12-14] The following are the most commonly defined components of a client-centered practice approach:

- It is flexible and open to the specific needs of the patient and family
- It embraces the belief that everyone is capable of choice
- It centers upon the needs of each individual, as expressed by them
- It is a partnership within which the therapist assumes the role of enabler
- It measures its success by the accomplishment of outcomes as defined originally by the patient and negotiated through the interview process with the therapist
- It is essentially connected and congruent with the patient's context and environmental niche
- It is an open and honest process with nothing covert or undeclared between the partners
- It is supportive of patient autonomy
- It enhances the collaborative nature of the therapeutic partnership between patient and therapist.

The development of a client-centered approach to occupational therapy mental health practice has been emerging over the past 20 years. This specific practice field was not isolated from the general discussions that underpin the development of the CMOP, the PEO, and the COPM. However, additional attention was paid to occupational therapy practice in mental health and mental illness settings through the development of a revised Model of Occupational Performance[4] included within the *Occupational Therapy Guidelines for Client-Centered Mental Health Practice*.[15] This model identifies the performance components of the person as physical, mental, sociocultural, and spiritual, with the model element being illustrated as the center of a flower. The second layer of the model, the petals, are illustrative of the areas of occupational performance (self-care, productivity, and leisure) intermingled with the environmental elements (social, cultural, physical, legal, economic, and political).

In summary, client-centered practice is deemed to be a partnership approach that enables "occupation with clients, who may be individuals, groups, agencies, governments, corporations, or others" with central tenets that reflect respect for patients by appreciating and honoring their knowledge and expertise within their own life experience, their involvement in decision-making, and advocacy for and with patients to meet their identified needs.[4]

Specific Challenges for Therapist–Client Partnerships in Mental Health Practice

While the field of mental health practice is one of the historical bases from which occupational therapy grew, and therefore is rich with parallel and similar processes to those experienced in other practice fields, specific challenges remain that are important to identify here.

The existence of often very active pathological conditions influence clients' abilities to negotiate and manage their environment in ways that can be very different from those problems and barriers experienced by individuals learning to cope with problems arising from physical conditions. Kuznir and colleagues[11] discuss the results of a research project within which occupational therapists were asked to consider their mental health practice, and to reflect on when maintaining a client-centered approach became challenging or impossible. The results of their qualitative analysis revealed five emerging themes:

1. Patient reluctance to become involved in the occupational therapy process
2. Dissonance between opinions or expectations of patients and therapists
3. Difficulty in patients making decisions
4. Lack of fit between the patient decision and skill level
5. Difficulties in modifying the patient environment

Again, these statements in and of themselves may not appear that different from those that could be made by therapists working within other practice settings; however, they do invite a closer examination.

The willingness of a patient to get involved in occupational therapy when coming from the perspective of coping with an episode of mental illness is often clouded by a lack of awareness of how the pathology may be affecting abilities to synthesize and integrate new knowledge and information. Also, the patient may not be aware of timelines for hospitalization and a potentially quick discharge, which impacts his or her ability to engage in a timely manner. It is at this stage when the role of the therapist as an active partner and as an enabler of change should come to the fore. Being client-centered does not mean that the therapist should wait for the patient to articulate concerns with occupational performance before starting to build the relationship. At times like this, the therapist has the responsibility to be the stronger and more focused one in the partnership by providing suggestions, but listening with care and attention to how those suggestions are received.

The Canadian Occupational Performance Measure

The COPM was developed approximately 15 years ago in response to a call from the CAOT and Health Canada. The intention was to explore existing outcome measures and determine whether there was something "out there" that would assist occupational therapists in evaluating their interventions. In the event that no tool was identified, the development of such a measurement tool was mandated. The COPM was the result of this process.[14] Over the past decade, the measure has garnered widespread interest, is used around the world in over 35 countries, and has been officially translated into 21 different languages.

The COPM is a semi-structured interview designed to identify problems in occupational performance as articulated by the patient in partnership with the therapist. It is designed to interdigitate with the CMOP.[4] The COPM has three distinct sections:

1. Self-care: Activities of daily living and instrumental activities of daily living

2. Productivity: Education and work

3. Leisure: Play, leisure, and social participation

Two scores are provided following completion of the interview process: performance and satisfaction. These are both self-rated by the client. The occupational performance problems identified in this process may also be weighted in terms of importance to assist in establishing the client's priorities, thus providing information and clearer direction for the additional components of the therapeutic interchange of setting goals and planning interventions.

The COPM was designed to apply equally to all clients. This includes all ages, developmental stages, disabilities, conditions, and cultural backgrounds. In addition, the COPM can be used with clients that are not necessarily the designated client. For example, the tool can be very useful in guiding conversations with clients such as government agencies, business and industry partners, and other community groups that are engaging in an occupational therapy intervention process. The only real requirements to using the COPM are that the client-therapist relationship be built in a manner that supports and illustrates the core values and expectations of client-centeredness, and that the therapist practices in an occupation-centered manner, therefore focusing upon the assessment of occupational performance and satisfaction with occupation.[16-18] It is becoming increasingly clear, however, that using the COPM is more complex in some situations than others. The practice of occupational therapy with clients with mental illness and mental health issues is one of those particular circumstances.

Maintaining a Client-Centered Approach While Using the COPM

McColl et al[19] addressed the particular nature of special applications in using the COPM, including special clinical circumstances. Seven discrete areas were identified and will be addressed here with illustrations from mental health practice.

1. *Legitimacy of the client's point of view*: In many clinical situations, there is concern expressed as to whether the client is a reliable source of information about his or her own experience, thus potentially compromising the relevance and quality to the client of the emerging therapeutic plan. It is always difficult to allow the client's priorities to shine through, thus relegating the therapist's goals to the back burner. However, it is critical, if practicing in a truly client-centered fashion, to strive for this in every client encounter. This is of particular difficulty when working with clients who are contending with pervasive mental illness and whose form of communication is unfamiliar.

2. *Inclusion of other stakeholders*: Other members or participants in the client's support system are frequently needed as central players in the development and execution of a client-centered treatment plan. While there may be many participants in the process, from the perspective of using the COPM, the core client is the individual or group who seeks to address perceived concerns around occupational performance.

3. *Modifications to the approach*: While the COPM has been developed as a semi-structured tool, thus implying the use of a standardized approach to the interview and information collection, there are undoubtedly many situations during which adapting the model may be helpful while staying true to the process overall. For example, there may be a need to communicate the message in a way more suited to the cognitive or language skills of the client. Also, the scoring scheme can appear confusing to some people, and a creative approach to the measurement of performance, importance, and satisfaction can be applied. Examples of this include the use of a happy face to illustrate the number 10 and a sad face to illustrate number 1.

4. *Use of another person to act as a communication proxy for the client*: Interpreters can be an invaluable resource, but should be selected based on their ability to retain an objective position, thus reporting the client's information, opinions, and feelings in an unbiased manner. Another situation where a proxy respondent may be used is when the client is noncommunicative. This is a very difficult situation for everyone involved and the respondent must be clearly advised to try to represent the client's viewpoints—putting his or her own wishes to the side and trying to represent what he or she believes the client would wish to impart.

5. *Ability to identify problems*: With many clients, it is necessary to engage in a therapeutic process ahead of the experience of identifying central occupational performance issues. Thus, the timing of the application of the COPM can be critical. Proceeding with the COPM interview too early can suggest that the client is unable to engage; while completing the process at a later time can be hampered by decisions and experiences that impact on the client's ability to understand his or her own priorities.

6. *Problems with memory and attention*: If clients exhibit problems with concentration or particular signs of tiredness, it is important to consider using the COPM across several occasions, rather than trying to complete the whole process at once.

7. *Cultural differences*: In this example, the word *culture* is used broadly, and embraces not only ethnic groups, but also all other potential cultural filters such as age and stage, socioeconomic status, and rural-urban lifestyle expectations. Awareness and respect for cultural diversity is a critical component of the application of the COPM and for a client-centered practice approach overall. Considerations of cultural elements include the following: a client's comfort with roles within his or her own life and also within the health care system, expectations of experts, understanding of power in a therapeutic relationship, and comfort with standing up for his or her own needs and expressing views and opinions.

Case Scenarios

In order to help in understanding the potential for applying the COPM within an occupation- and client-centered practice model, the following case scenarios are offered. Following each patient story, there are some guiding questions to assist the therapist in considering how the client-centered principles were applied in the case examples and also how the COPM assisted in determining the direction for the ongoing therapeutic engagement.

OLIVIA

Olivia is 16 years old and has a 4-year history of anorexia nervosa. Olivia completed an intensive inpatient eating disorders program where her weight was restored to within 80% of typical weight, and she began to participate in group therapy to address the underlying causes of her eating disorder. Olivia spent 4 months in the hospital. She was discharged to a Department of Psychiatry outpatient program at a community hospital close to her home. The occupational therapist at the outpatient program is working with Olivia and her family to help Olivia maintain the medical improvements achieved in the hospital and to continue to address the underlying psychosocial issues related to her eating disorder. The occupational therapist used the COPM in the initial interview, with the main goal to identify occupational performance issues with Olivia and to engage Olivia in the goal-setting process. Olivia responded to the interview well and was active in setting her goals. Olivia stated that she was happy to see the occupational therapist was listening to her goals and not dictating to her what goals she should be working on in therapy. The occupational performance issues (OPIs) identified are summarized in Table 3-1. Olivia met with the occupational therapist weekly for 3 months. Session content focused on the skills and resources needed to meet her identified OPIs. Olivia completed a second COPM at the end of 3 months to identify her performance and satisfaction on the original OPIs. Performance and satisfaction ratings at the second COPM are found in Table 3-1. It is apparent that Olivia identified a significant improvement in the performance and satisfaction with each OPI. Olivia remained committed to improving her performance in areas that were important and therefore meaningful for her. Olivia was able to remain out of the hospital and continued to improve with respect to her eating disorder. At the time of discharge from the outpatient program, Olivia was integrated back into her school environment, was becoming more responsible for her meal planning, and was thriving in her social environment (Table 3-2).

Table 3-1
The Occupational Performance Issues For Olivia

OPI	Interest	Performance(1)	Satisfaction(1)	Performance(2)	Satisfaction(2)
Plan my own meals	10	3	2	8	9
Increase tolerance for walking	7	5	4	9	10
Increase attention span at school in classes	9	2	1	8	8
Feel more confident in social situations outside of classes	10	2	1	7	9

Table 3-2
Guiding Questions to Assist Clinical Reasoning (Olivia)

- Were the principles of client-centered practice realized in this particular case scenario?

- If so, at which junctures were they most apparent?

- What were the most useful outcomes of using the COPM with this client?

- What elements of your practice are reflected in this scenario?

- Are there components of this process that are familiar?

- Are there components of this process that are new to you?

- If so, are those components something that you feel have value for your practice?

- If so, how can you integrate them into your work?

Andrew

Andrew, a 27-year-old man, was seen by an occupational therapist at a private clinic that focused on weight management through lifestyle changes. Andrew was referred to the program by his family physician who was concerned about Andrew's significant weight gain since he started taking an atypical antipsychotic medication. Andrew was diagnosed with schizophrenia at the age of 23, after traveling and experiencing a psychotic break leading to hospitalization. He had completed a community college program in business administration the year before. Andrew had attended a psychiatric day program to learn more about his illness and coping strategies. He started a sedentary job in an office and reported feeling uncomfortable at his current weight, which is 65 pounds above his typical weight. He reported being short of breath and tired all of the time. He reported suffering from sleep apnea and had recently started using a CPAP machine. Andrew was once active in recreational sports but did not feel physically able to participate at the time of meeting with the therapist. He was also concerned about an increase in his blood pressure and a family history of diabetes. Andrew was aware that he needed to stay on his medications to manage his illness and to continue to function at his job. The occupational therapist met with Andrew at the clinic and together they completed the COPM as part of the initial interview. Andrew stated that he enjoyed participating in the goal-setting process and often referred to the copy of the COPM that he took away from his assessment on that first visit. Andrew also shared the COPM with his family to help them better understand his goals. Table 3-3 summarizes the results of the COPM completed at two points in time (Table 3-4).

Lessons Learned

Recently, the authors of the COPM undertook the task of completing an annotated bibliography of the literature, illustrating articles that have explored the relative merits of the tool.[20]

Research on the COPM

Reliability

Test-retest reliability is the only type of reliability that is relevant for the COPM. Within the studies reviewed, one has specific relevance for mental health practice and shows that the reliability was well above an acceptable range (over 0.80). This study was completed with a population of patients living with schizophrenia in Taiwan.[21] The overall sense is that the COPM can be repeated at different points in time to produce consistent results.

Validity

Three types of validity have been evaluated in relation to the COPM: content, criterion, and construct validity.

In general, the studies examined support the notion that the COPM is a measure of occupational performance. Boyer et al[22] worked with a group of people living with schizophrenia and illustrated that the COPM was a helpful addition to their planning and intervention with these patients.

Table 3-3
Canadian Occupational Performance Measure for Andrew

OPI	Interest	Performance(1)	Satisfaction(1)	Performance(2)	Satisfaction(2)
To improve sleep and hygiene	8	3	4	7	7
To plan meals that fit my budget and nutritional needs	9	2	2	9	10
To have more energy to attend work	9	3	3	9	9
To participate in recreational ice hockey twice a week	10	1	1	9	9

Table 3-4
Guiding Questions To Assist Clinical Reasoning (Andrew)

- Were the principles of client-centered practice realized in this particular case scenario?

- If so, at which junctures were they most apparent?

- What were the most useful outcomes of using the COPM with this client?

- What elements of your practice are reflected in this scenario?

- Are there components of this process that are familiar?

- Are there components of this process that are new to you?

- If so, are those components something that you feel have value for your practice?

- If so, how can you integrate them into your work?

Utility

Within the literature, there are many references to the usefulness of the COPM, including responsiveness to change, ease of administration, and how well it adapts across practice settings, patient/client populations, cultural environments, and languages. Some therapists report that the COPM takes too long, but this seems to relate to the comfort of the practitioner in spending time to engage in conversation rather than simply "getting on" with therapy. It is possible to complete the COPM process within 15 minutes if no extra conversation occurs, ie, if therapists are not enticed into the process of doing therapy prior to completing an exploration of a client-centered assessment of priority issues.[23]

In essence, it would seem that it is indeed not only possible but also desirable to approach occupational therapy practice in mental health and mental illness settings in a client-centered manner. Also, it would seem to be helpful to utilize an outcome measure like the COPM to provide a framework and process model to guide the identification of patient-priority OPIs, despite some of the potential pitfalls inherent in working with such a patient population. Reflecting upon the examples provided within the case scenarios should provide opportunities for thinking about personal practice and determining ways in which client-centered principles can be best applied.

References

1. Hemphill-Pearson BJ. *Assessments in Occupational Therapy Mental Health: An Integrative Approach.* Thorofare, NJ: SLACK Incorporated; 1999.
2. Law M, Baptiste S, Carswell A, McColl MA, Polatajko H, Pollack N. *Canadian Occupational Performance Measure (COPM).* 4th ed. Ottawa, ON: CAOT Publications ACE; 2005.
3. Jenkins M, Brotherton C. In search of a theoretical framework for practice, part 1. *Br J Occup Ther.* 1995;58;7:280.
4. Stanton S, Law M, Polatajko H, et al., eds. *Enabling Occupation: An Occupational Therapy Perspective.* Ottawa, ON: CAOT Publications ACE; 1997.
5. Youngstrom MJ. The Occupational Therapy Practice Framework: the evolution of our professional language. *Am J Occup Ther.* 2002;56(6):609-39.
6. Townsend E, Brintnell S, Staisey N. Developing guidelines for client-centred occupational therapy practice. *Can J Occup Ther.* 1990;57(2):69-76.
7. Law M, Cooper BA, Strong S, Stewart D, Rigby P, Letts L. The Person-Occupation-Environment Model: a transactive approach to occupational performance. *Can J Occup Ther.* 1996;63:9-12.
8. Rogers CR. *Client-Centred Therapy: Its Current Practices, Implications, and Theory.* Boston, MA: Mills;1951.
9. Gage M. In: Sumsion T, ed. *Client-Centred Practice in Occupational Therapy: A Guide to Implementation.* 2nd ed. Amsterdam: Elsevier; 2007.
10. Hobson S. In: Sumsion T, ed. *Client-Centred Practice in Occupational Therapy: A Guide to Implementation.* 2nd ed. Amsterdam: Elsevier; 2007.
11. Kusznir A, Scott E, Cooke R, Young LT. Functional consequences of bipolar affective disorder: an occupational therapy perspective. *Can J Occup Ther.* 1996;63(5):313-322.
12. Law M, Baptiste S, Mills J. Client-centred practice: what does it mean and does it make a difference? *Can J Occup Ther.* 1995;62(5):250-257.
13. Sumsion T. *Client-Centred Practice in Occupational Therapy: A Guide to Implementation.* 2nd ed. Amsterdam: Elsevier; 2007.
14. Law M. *Client-Centred Occupational Therapy.* Thorofare, NJ: SLACK Incorporated; 1998.
15. Health Canada. *Occupational Therapy Guidelines for Client-Centred Mental Health Practice.* Ottawa, ON; 1997.
16. Pollock N, McColl M, Carswell A, Sumsion T, eds. *Canadian Occupational Performance Measure in Client-Centred Occupational Therapy.* London: Churchill Livingstone; 1999.
17. Pollock N, McColl M. Assessment in client-centred occupational therapy. In: Law M, ed. *Client-Centered Occupational Therapy.* Thorofare, NJ: SLACK Incorporated; 1998.

18. McColl M, Pollock N, Law M, Baum C. Measuring occupational performance using a client-centred perspective In: Law M, Baum C, Dunn W, eds. *Measuring Occupational Performance: Supporting Best Practice in Occupational Therapy*. Thorofare, NJ. SLACK Incorporated; 2005.

19. McColl MA, Law M, Baptiste S, Pollock N, Carswell A, Polatajko H. Targeted applications of the Canadian Occupational Performance Measure. *CJOT Abstracts*. 2005;72(5).

20. McColl MA, Carswell A, Law M, Pollock N, Baptiste S, Polatajko H. *Research on the Canadian Occupational Performance Measure: An Annotated Resource*. Ottawa, ON: CAOT Publications ACE; 2006.

21. Pan AW, Chung L, Hsin-Hwei G. Reliability and validity of the Canadian Occupational Performance Measure for clients with psychiatric disorders in Taiwan. *Occup Ther Int*. 2003;10(4):269-277.

22. Boyer G, Hachey R, Mercier C. Perceptions of occupational performance and subjective quality of life in person with severe mental illness. *Occupational Therapy in Mental Health*. 2000;15(2):1-15.

23. Chen YH, Roder S, Polatajko H. Experiences with the COMP and client-centred practice in adult neurorehabilitation in Taiwan. *Occup Ther Int*. 2002;9(3):167-184.

4

ROLE CHANGE ASSESSMENT: AN INTERVIEW TOOL FOR OLDER ADULTS

Joan C. Rogers, PhD, OTR/L, FAOTA
Margo B. Holm, PhD, OTR/L, FAOTA, ABDA

"There comes a point in many people's lives when they can no longer play the role they have chosen for themselves. When that happens, we are like actors finding that someone has changed the play." Moore B. Thinkexist.com Web Site. Available at: http://en.thinkexist.com/quotation/there_comes_a_ point_in_many_people_s_lives_when/324225.html. Accessed March 18, 2006.

Introduction

The Role Change Assessment (RCA) is a client-centered, semi-structured interview tool developed by Jackoway, Rogers, and Snow in 1987[1] to describe the perceived role participation of older adults. It examines past and current role participation, changes in role participation, and the relative value or importance of various social roles to a patient. It was revised by Rogers and Holm in 1995[2] to simplify the format for use by clinicians and researchers.

This chapter begins with a brief explanation of the conceptual basis of the RCA, including the significance of the concept of role for participation, particularly as this relates to practice with older adults. Then, in sequence, the RCA is described, its user's manual is presented, its psychometric properties are delineated, and its research applications are discussed.

Conceptual Basis

Role is a fundamental concept in the social sciences. Roles are socially defined units of behavior enacted by individuals. Roles have a societal component that defines role expectations, as well as a personal component that relates to the manner in which individuals fulfill roles.[3] For example, society expects adults to provide for their financial needs through work. However, the work of an occupational therapist differs from that of a social worker, and furthermore no two occupational therapists enact the role of an occupational therapist in exactly the same way. Over the course of young adulthood, individuals accumulate roles as they marry, have children, initiate their careers, and engage in volunteer and leisure activities. The number of roles individuals engage in and the intensity of engagement are markers of social participation.

In later maturity, role participation is characterized by multiple role transitions. Older adults may move from being full-time, paid workers to being retirees, part-time workers, or volunteer workers. Release from work frees time for increased leisure. The parent role may be exchanged for the grandparent role. With the loss of a spouse, sibling, or confidant, an individual's social connectedness may be disrupted. The emergence of frailty or ill health may decrease the intensity of role involvement or may signal a gradual transition from independent to dependent role functioning. These changes vary in the extent to which they are scheduled and voluntary or unscheduled and imposed. They may be perceived as positive, neutral, or negative. Common to all role changes, however, is the need to adapt to change. Change disrupts the present dynamic and adaptive processes are needed to restore equilibrium.[4,5]

Although role change is characteristic of late life, this change is more frequently of loss and decreased intensity than of replacement, gain, or increased involvement.[6] When frailty develops, due to the accumulation of disease-associated or age-related impairments, performing the activities that make up roles becomes difficult or impossible, and role performance is disrupted or terminated. Role loss implies the loss of rewards and expectations associated with a position, including social status, contacts, and expectations. Loss of any role, but particularly one that is highly valued, may pose a severe threat to an individual's self-identify and self-worth. Thus, role loss has the potential for exerting wide-ranging effects on well-being and life satisfaction.

The domain of occupational therapy encompasses role function in seven occupational areas: activities of daily living (ADL), instrumental activities of daily living (IADL), education, work, play, leisure, and social participation.[7] The specific occupations subsumed under each occupational area are aggregated and integrated into roles. The RCA was devised to provide insight into the number of roles occupied by patients, the way in which roles are enacted, the changes that occur in roles following injury or illness and with age, and the relative value that patients place on the various roles they enact. Hence, the RCA provides the practitioner with critical information about patients' perceptions of their social participation for use in planning interventions. For example, if the homemaker role is essential to a person's self-worth, and critical occupations such as cooking and food shopping are threatened by depression, dementia, or other pathologies, these occupations must be addressed in occupational therapy.

The Role Change Assessment (Version 2.0)

The RCA consists of six data grids, one grid for each role category, with two columns for role items and six columns for response options. A comparable summary table appears at the end of the instrument.

Role Categories, Roles, and Definitions

The RCA (Version 2.0) consists of 43 specific roles classified under 6 role categories: relationship (9 items), self-care/home maintainer (9 items), productive (3 items), leisure (11 items), organizational (8 items), and health and wellness (3 items). Each role is named and descriptively defined. For example, the role of shopper is descriptively defined as

---

Table 4-1

Examples of Role Items

Productivity Roles

Role	Role Definition
Worker for pay	Works for pay, full-time, or part-time (includes relief or seasonal work)
Caregiver	Provides unpaid assistance to another person
Student	Takes one or more classes where regular attendance is expected

---

shops for food, clothing, and household items. Rogers and Holm[8] should be consulted for a discussion of the revisions resulting in Version 2.0 (category renaming; item retention, consolidation and deletion). The Version 2.0 role categories and items are listed below.

1. *Relationship* roles are identified as spouse, parent, grandparent, son/daughter, sibling, other relatives, friend, neighbor, and pet owner.

2. *Self-care/home maintainer* roles are defined as self-carer, cook, housekeeper (light), housekeeper (heavy), launderer, shopper, driver, gardener, and repairer.

3. *Productive* roles are described as worker for pay, caregiver, and student.

4. *Leisure* roles are identified as hobbyist/craftsperson, musician/artist, sports participant, dancer, collector, aerobics participant, game player, traveler/tourist, observer/reflector, reader, and event attender.

5. *Organizational* roles are listed as religious, civic, political, senior citizens, social, support/self-help, educational, and professional.

6. *Health and wellness* roles are designated as recipient of health care, recipient of therapy care, or therapy/wellness participant.

The format and the content of one item, productivity roles, are illustrated in Table 4-1.

RESPONSE FORMAT

Following a thorough discussion of each role item, patients rate or describe their role participation in several ways.

1. Using a 5-point ordinal scale, patients rate the frequency of their role participation. Present or current participation in a role item is rated as: 0 = no contact/not appropriate, 1 = at least 1/month, 2 = at least 1/every 2 weeks, 3 = at least 1/week, and 4 = daily.

2. The frequency of past participation in a role item is rated on the same ordinal scale as present participation.

3. Present participation is compared to past participation and rated as being stable (ie, no change) or as having changed. Changes in role participation are further identified as reflecting an absolute gain or loss of a role, or a relative increase or decrease in participation. Role gain is indicated if there was no participation in

a role in the past, but there is current participation. Role loss is indicated if there was participation in a role in the past, but there is no current participation. Role increase and decrease occur when there is a change in the intensity of participation, as opposed to the addition or loss of a role. Role increase occurs when the time or energy devoted to a role has increased. Conversely, role decrease occurs when the time or energy devoted to a role has decreased.

4. Perceived role changes are recorded as having positive (+), neutral (0), or negative (-) value or sentiment attached to them.

5. Respondents also rank the three role items in each role category that: (1) provide a focal point for managing their time (1 = the most time consuming), and (2) are the most valued (1 = the most valued). Taken together, these two rankings indicate the extent to which patients are investing their time in the roles that they most value. These data suggest roles and activities to be targeted for intervention.

6. The interviewer takes notes throughout the interview to record the respondent's perceptions.

The format of the responses for the role items is illustrated in Table 4-2.

DATA SUMMARY TABLE

An overall profile of role participation is created in the summary table at the end of the RCA. This summarizes role gains, losses, increases, and decreases in each of the six role categories, the three roles that consume most of the respondent's time, and the three roles that are most valued by the respondent. The summary facilitates an overall judgment of role participation in terms of stability, change, and value.

The Role Change Assessment Manual

The Role Change Assessment Manual describes the interviewing process.

DEFINING THE TIMEFRAME

During administration of the RCA, respondents are asked to compare their present or current role participation with their past role participation. The past, or the time interval to be compared, is unique for each administration of the interview, and is established at the beginning of the interview. Depending on the purpose of the evaluation and the health or disability status of the respondent, different timeframes may be appropriate. For example, for traumatic conditions (eg, car accident) where change is precipitous, the past may be defined as preinjury or pre-episode. This would facilitate understanding how and to what extent trauma disrupted a respondent's life because postnjury role participation would be compared to preinjury role participation. For chronic conditions (eg, rheumatoid arthritis) that progress more slowly and subtly, a longer retrospective interval might be required for respondents to perceive change. Thus, the interviewer is free to establish the retrospective interval to meet the purpose of the evaluation or the research study.

Table 4-2
Example of Response Format for the Role Items

Role	A #Past	B #Present	A:B = C (+, =, -)	D Change Value	Value (Time) Ranks 1 - 3	Value (Meaning) Ranks 1 - 3
Caregiver	2	4	+2	+ 0 -	1	1

INTERVIEWING STRATEGY

The RCA involves a semi-structured interview. Guiding questions for each role are given in the Role Change Assessment Manual; however, these questions can be rephrased as necessary to facilitate clarity. For example, inquiry about self-care and home maintenance roles begins with, "Now, I will ask you about the roles in which you take care of yourself and your home. How often do you (did you) participate in the following roles?" Following the introductory question, the interviewer is expected to add probing questions so that the respondent and the interviewer collaboratively construct an accurate picture of the respondent's role participation.

The interviewing strategy should foster inquiry about role stability as well as change. Inquiry about participation is to highlight role stability or continuity, role addition or loss, increased intensity or decreased intensity of participation in a role, the positive or negative sentiment attached to role changes, the most valued roles, and the time devoted to the most valued roles. The interviewer's responsibility is to keep the interview focused on eliciting and validating the patient's perceptions.

ORDER OF QUESTIONING

Role categories are to be examined in the order in which the categories are presented on the interview protocol, with relationship roles discussed first and health and wellness roles discussed last. The following principles are followed in guiding the interview:

1. Examine the *first* role listed in each category.

2. Examine *present* status in the first role. After a general discussion of participation in the role, the frequency of contact scale is presented on a 5-inch x 8-inch index card to help respondents rate their participation.

3. Proceed to the *second* role listed in each category or to *other roles within the same category* as directed by respondent comments.

4. Examine *present* status in each role, until all roles within a category are covered.

5. Define the *past*, as it is to be interpreted during the interview.

6. Using the same order of roles followed for inquiry about present status, respondent and interviewer collaboratively relate *present* status to *past* status in a role; for identified role changes, ascertain respondent's perceptions of change as positive, neutral, or negative.

7. Before concluding a role category, examine the relative value of roles in terms of time spent and meaning or importance.
8. Proceed to the *next* role category, until all role categories are covered.
9. Complete the summary table and verify impressions with the respondent.

DURATION

An interview of 1-hour duration is recommended but not mandated. Within a 60-minute timeframe, approximately 9 minutes can be devoted to each of the six role categories, allowing 6 minutes for patients to summarize their perceptions.

Psychometrics

RELIABILITY

Reliability refers to the accuracy of test results. The goal of the interview schedule is to assist the interviewer and the respondent to understand the influence that role stability and change have on a respondent's life situation. As a structured interview, the RCA yields both qualitative and quantitative findings. Reliability of the qualitative data, ie, the descriptive information respondents share about their role participation, is ascertained through *member checking*. In member checking, the interviewer obtains respondent verification that the data collected and the interpretation of data are accurate.[9,10] Member checking is accomplished throughout the interview, in an iterative process whereby the interviewer asks questions, probes for detail, synthesizes the information, and states interpretations in collaboration with the respondent, verifying interpretations or rephrasing them to match the respondent's intent. Member checking thus ensures reliability.

The interpretations of participation, in terms of role stability or change, are quantifiable. Test-retest reliability of the RCA (Version 2.0) was determined on a convenience sample of 11 retirees (6 women) having a mean age of 67 years.[8] The test-retest interval was 1 day. Past was defined as 1 year ago. Reliability was calculated with percent agreement, defined as the percentage of scores that were identical in the test and retest administrations, divided by the total number of relevant items for which there was a response on either administration. Percent agreement for past roles ranged from 84% (relationships) to 97% (health/wellness), and for present roles from 88% (relationships, productivity, and organizations) to 97% (health/wellness). For nomination of valued roles, percent agreement ranged from 86% (leisure) to 95% (relationships), while for time spent in valued roles it ranged from 90% (self-care/home maintenance) to 95% (relationships). Percent agreement for changes perceived to have a positive value was 97%; for those perceived to be neutral, 95%; and for those perceived to be negative, 65%. Changes from negative to positive sentiment were common from testing to retesting. Thus, test-retest reliability of the RCA, except for the negative value item, is substantial.

VALIDITY

Content validity of the RCA is based on a review of the relevant literature, logical analysis of clinical experts, and feedback from pilot subjects. The literature review on roles of adulthood and later maturity and role instruments yielded six role categories and a master list of specific roles.[6,11-19] The master role list was shortened by consolidating functionally-related or similar role descriptions into broader role categories. Thus, sports participant is listed as a role in preference to hunter or golfer. The role categories were critically analyzed by four experts in geriatrics (a physician, a nurse, and two occupational therapists) for their logical coherence. The expert reviewers were instructed to critique the comprehensiveness of the role categories, the assignment of roles to the categories, the role definitions, and the sequencing of role categories and roles within each category. A beta version of the instrument was constructed and pilot tested. Pilot respondents were asked to identity roles they currently held that they felt were not adequately covered on the RCA (Beta Version). Pilot testing resulted in the addition of four roles: contact with other relatives to the relationship category, musician to the leisure category, trustee/director to the productive category, and professional and special interest organization to the organizational category. No substantive changes were made in item content between Versions 1.0 and 2.0.

Criterion validity was examined by Jackoway[20] in conjunction with the development of the RCA. In 25 (15 women) healthy, community-dwelling older adults, role loss correlated with change in life satisfaction ($r = .43$, $P < .05$), as measured on Cantril ladders,[21] with loss of roles over 12 months contributing to increases in life satisfaction. The association between role loss and increased life satisfaction is consistent with the concept of selective optimization,[22] whereby older adults reduce their participation in some roles to enable more effective participation in other roles.

Research Using the Role Change Assessment

Hogan and colleagues[23] used the RCA (Version 2.0) in a qualitative study exploring role changes of in-home caregivers (n = 8) of individuals with Alzheimer's disease. Significant role changes were experienced in four of the six role categories: leisure, relationship, self-care/home maintenance, and health and wellness. Reductions in leisure occurred because time previously available for leisure was now consumed by caregiving activities. Interestingly, although caregivers recognized that asking for assistance was a useful strategy for maintaining their well-being, they felt guilty about asking for help so that they could engage in leisure! In the relationship category, disruptions attributable to caregiving were most often marked for the roles of spouse and son/daughter, but disagreements about how caregiving needs should be met and an unequal sharing of caregiving responsibilities spilled over into other roles, especially those of parent and sibling. More time and effort were invested in activities in the self-care/home maintenance category because caregivers had to perform obligatory tasks previously done by care recipients. In the health and wellness category, strategies such as attendance at support groups, self-education, prayer, and routinization of daily living were added to the therapy/wellness participant role. The utility of the RCA for intervention planning is illustrated in a companion article in which the identified changes in caregiver role participation were translated into health and wellness strategies that could be implemented by practitioners.[24]

Jackoway[20] administered the RCA (Version 1.0) to healthy, community-dwelling older adults (15 women), with a mean age of 77 (range 70 to 85). Eight of the men and six of the women were married. When participants were interviewed, the mean number of roles held was 24.5 (range 15 to 33), whereas 1 year prior to the interview the mean number of roles recalled was 25.3 (range 18 to 32). Eleven roles were most common (ie, held by > 80%): parent, grandparent, friend, member of a religious organization, personal-carer, cook, shopper, house cleaner, traveler, observer, walker. No one participated as a consultant, was self-employed full-time, or belonged to a support or self-help group. Participation in the social and family (renamed relationship in Version 2.0), organization, and leisure role categories tended to be concentrated in one or two of these categories rather than being evenly distributed. The primary deterrent to role participation was health, particularly visual impairment and loss of energy. Five subjects mentioned lack of time as a limiting factor and six subjects stated that they were already as active as they could or desired to be. Slightly more than half (56%) of the subjects experienced role loss, while about one-third (36%) experienced role gain. The majority of subjects perceived decreases (96%) and increases (88%) in the intensity of role participation. The most change was perceived in the organizational category, followed by health care, leisure, self-care (renamed self-care/home maintenance), family (renamed relationship), and vocational (renamed productive), with the specific roles lost most frequently being: acutely ill, neighbor, visitor, part-time worker, student, hobbyist, and episodically ill.

Bonder and Fisher[25] used the RCA (Version 1.0) to examine the activity balance of community-dwelling older adults (> 64 years), with and without disabling conditions. Of the 88 subjects, 33% were women and 80% were Caucasian. Most subjects (70 of 88) listed roles in at least four categories. The mean number of roles was 6.4 (range 3 to 11). Of the 45 roles surveyed, 35 were mentioned at least once, suggesting that older adults fill a wide range of roles. Roles in the organizational and vocational (renamed productive) categories were mentioned least.

Mitcham and colleagues[26] studied community-dwelling elderly (n = 10; 9 women) of advanced age (mean age = 85). Over 5 years, in the family and social (renamed relationship) category, participants were no longer in the spousal or son/daughter roles (not surprising given the advanced age of the sample) and declines were evidenced in the roles of friend, sibling, visitor, and pet owner. All participants were active in religious and senior citizen organizations; however, this was likely attributable to sample selection from these sites. Decreased participation was observed in all roles, except senior citizen, political, and support/self-help groups; participation in the latter two organizations was low. The vocational (renamed productive) category was fulfilled through volunteering and losses occurred in spousal caregiving. In leisure, declines occurred in the roles of hobbyist, collector, traveler, event attender, game player, and walker, but not in observer, and there was no participation in sports. Subjects were active in self-care roles, except for that of repair person. In home maintenance, declines were perceived in cooking, shopping, doing the laundry, driving, and gardening, while house cleaning and personal care were stable. In the organizational category, subjects were active in six roles, with no activity detected in professional or special-interest groups. In health care, an increase was seen for chronic care, a slight decrease in acute care, and stability in episodic conditions. In general, role changes were perceived as positive or neutral, perhaps due to the loss of roles that were not highly valued or were not perceived as appropriate in late life (eg, worker).

Summary

The RCA is a client-centered instrument that facilitates discussion about role participation between patients and occupational therapy practitioners. It helps practitioners to understand the social context of patients' life situations and the meaning of various roles and role changes for patients' overall quality of life. Knowledge of role values and performance provides a powerful tool for establishing intervention priorities and motivating patients to work toward achieving their priorities. Further research is needed on the RCA to determine its sensitivity for detecting change following occupational therapy and other rehabilitative interventions.

References

1. Jackoway IS, Rogers JC, Snow T. The Role Change Assessment: an interview tool for evaluating older adults. *Occupational Therapy in Mental Health*. 1987;7:17-37.
2. Rogers JC, Holm MB. The Role Change Assessment (Version 2.0): An Interview Tool for Evaluating Older Adults. Pittsburgh, PA: Unpublished role assessment tool; 1995.
3. Reed KL, Sanderson SN. *Concepts of Occupational Therapy*. 4th ed. Philadelphia, PA: Lippincott Williams & Wilkins; 1999.
4. Bonder BR, Wagner MB. *Functional Performance of Older Adults*. 2nd ed. Philadelphia, PA: F.A. Davis Co; 2001.
5. Ebersole P, Hess P, Luggen AS. *Toward Healthy Aging: Human Needs and Nursing Response*. 6th ed. St. Louis, MO: Mosby; 2004.
6. Blau ZS. *Aging in a Changing Society*. New York, NY: Franklin Watts; 1981.
7. American Occupational Therapy Association. *Occupational Therapy Practice Framework: Domain & Process*. Bethesda, MD: AOTA Press; 2002.
8. Rogers JC, Holm MB. Role Change Assessment: an interview tool for older adults. In: Hemphill-Pearson BJ, ed. *Assessments in Occupational Therapy Mental Health: An Integrative Approach*. Thorofare, NJ: SLACK Incorporated; 1999:73-82.
9. Bailey D. *Research for the Health Professional: A Practical Guide*. 2nd ed. Philadelphia, PA: F.A. Davis; 1991.
10. Kuzel AJ, Like RC. Standards of trustworthiness for qualitative studies in primary care. In: Norton PG, Stewart F, Tudiver MJ, Bass MJ, Dunn EV, eds. *Primary Care Research: Traditional and Innovative Approaches*. Newbury Park, Calif: Sage; 1991:138-158.
11. Albrecht R. The social roles of old people. *J Gerontol*. 1951;6:138-145.
12. Cavan RS, Burgess EW, Havighurst RJ, Holdhammer H. *Personal Adjustment in Old Age*. Chicago, IL: Science Research Associates; 1949.
13. Clark M, Anderson B. *Culture and Aging: An Anthropological Study of Older Americans*. New York, NY: Arno Press; 1980.
14. Cumming E, Henry W. *Growing Old: The Process of Disengagement*. New York, NY: Basic Books; 1961.
15. Havighurst RJ, Albrecht R. *Older People*. New York, NY: Longmans, Green and Co; 1953.
16. Havighurst RJ, Neugarten BL, Bengtson VL. A cross-national study of adjustment to retirement. *Gerontologist*. 1966;6:137-138.
17. Morgan LA. Social roles in later life: some recent research trends. In: Eisdorfer C, ed. *Annu Rev Gerontol Geriatr*. 1982;3:55-79.
18. Oakley F. The Model of Human Occupation in Psychiatry. Unpublished master's project. Richmond, Va: Department of Occupational Therapy, Virginia Commonwealth University; 1982.
19. Williams RH, Wirths CG. *Lives Through the Years*. New York, NY: Atherton; 1965.
20. Jackoway IS. Role Change in Older Adults. Unpublished master's thesis. Chapel Hill, NC: Division of Occupational Therapy, University of North Carolina, 1985.
21. Cantril H. *The Pattern of Human Concerns*. New Brunswick, NJ: Rutgers University Press; 1965.
22. Baltes PB, Baltes MM. Psychological perspectives on successful aging: the model of selective optimization with compensation. In: Baltes PB, Baltes MM. *Successful Aging: Perspectives From the Behavioral Sciences*. Cambridge, England: Cambridge University Press; 1990:1-34.
23. Hogan VM, Lisy ED, Savannah RL, Henry L, Kuo F, Fisher GS. Role change experienced by family caregivers of adults with Alzheimer's Disease: implications for occupational therapy. *Phys Occup Ther Geriatr*. 2003;22:21-44.
24. Kuo F, Fisher GS. Meeting the needs of caregivers of individuals with Alzheimer's Disease: recommendations for health care providers. *California Journal of Health Promotion*. 2004;2:82-91.
25. Bonder BR, Fisher AG. Roles and activities of the elderly. *Gerontologist*. 1990;30:139A.
26. Mitcham MD, Cartin AE, Krause CA, Mannix CV, Mayhugh ME, Melton PS. The Effects of Role Changes on the Life Satisfaction of Independent Elderly Adults. Paper presented at the Great Southern Occupational Therapy Conference, Lexington, KY: October 27, 1994.

PART III:
PSYCHOLOGICAL ASSESSMENTS

5

JOURNALING AS AN ASSESSMENT TOOL IN MENTAL HEALTH

Kristine Haertl, PhD, OTR/L

"Be patient and compassionate towards yourself and each other. Help each other learn to think and write and solve problems, and the journal will become a tool that your friends and partners honor for the benefits they see it bringing to them as you become more fully yourself, and more fully their companion." Baldwin C. One to One: A New and Updated Edition of the Classic Self-Understanding Through Journal Writing. *New York, NY: M. Evans and Company; 1991.*

Introduction

The power of the written word transcends time and space. Historically, cultures have developed written forms and symbols as means of communication, personal expression, and thought. Writing is powerful; it influences our perceptions, constructs, and worldview. Such forms of written communication may be expressed in the private, public, or personal realm. Personal writing is a unique occupational tool that may be used to enhance personal growth. The following chapter presents an innovative approach related to the use of journal writing in dynamic assessment and intervention within occupational therapy.

The term *journal* refers to a form of personal writing that expresses perceptions, experiences, dreams, and creativity from the perspective of the self. The word comes from the French root word "jour," meaning day,[1] and is often used to depict a form of daily writing and reflection. The literature reveals a variety of definitions of journal. Rainer[2] often used the terms "diary" and "journal" interchangeably, whereas other authors have distinguished a journal from diary writing, identifying the diary as a more formal type of daily writing focused on external events and a journal as writing focused within.[3,4] Murray asserted, "journaling is primarily a body/mind/spirit (metaphysical) activity where the journal keeper makes sense of living."[5(p69)] The use of journal writing is often instrumental in developing insight and working on personal goals, and may be used as a therapeutic tool in rehabilitation.

In personal and rehabilitative writing, the journal may take on a variety of formats including bound journals, computer-based private journals, and Internet-based journals. Decisions on the types and formats of journals used are highly personal and based on individual preference, the goals of journaling, and utility of the journal. Similar to personal journals, the format of the journal within a therapeutic setting will depend on the goals of therapy and a collaborative effort among the patient, therapist, and any other identified key persons (eg, other individuals in a journal-writing group). Journal writing has often been used in mental health as a form of intervention, yet within therapy the journal provides a unique tool for ongoing assessment amidst the intervention process.

Journal Writing and Mental Health

HISTORICAL ROOTS

Writing has been long recognized for its therapeutic properties, yet the use of journal writing for personal growth largely came about in the 20th century.[2] Historically, therapeutic writing was mainly used within the context of self-help approaches implementing cognitive and behavioral techniques.[6] Additional applications have focused on psychoanalytic Freudian and cognitive Adlerian approaches emphasizing the relationship between writing and psychological adjustment.[7]

Perhaps one of the most well-known applications of journal writing to self-development in the past century is the intensive journal process developed by Ira Progoff, a psychologist who specialized in the development of therapeutic writing applications.[8,9] Progoff spent decades developing his techniques utilizing theoretical principles from depth psychology. Progoff's Intensive Journal process involves the use of multiple sections within the journal designed to look at the self from different perspectives. Progoff emphasized the importance of daily logs, meditations, life dimensions, spirituality, dreams, and reflections in working toward personal growth through both the process and product of journal writing. His journal writing techniques continue to be used in various forms throughout the world.

Current Applications and Research

Current literature and research on therapeutic applications of writing are largely focused within psychology and counseling and are based on the use of various writing techniques in both individual and group therapy.[10-15] Applications of reflective and journal writing strategies have also been extensively used in the academic realm in order to facilitate critical-thinking skills in students within the classroom and fieldwork settings.[16-19] Writing strategies used within clinical and academic settings often focus on developing personal insight on the part of the patient or student. Insight may be gained by personal reflection and analysis, cooperative dialogue and feedback with the therapist or teacher, or through use of peer feedback from other patients or students. Within these settings, individual, environmental, and therapeutic factors lead to development of the purpose of the assigned writing, and ultimately to the selection of the format of writing, reflection, and feedback.

Wright and Chung defined writing therapy as "client expressive and reflective writing, whether self-generated or suggested by a therapist/researcher."[6(p279)] Research on the use of therapeutic writing suggests promising results in a variety of areas, yet continued research is needed, particularly in the rehabilitative fields. One of the most well-known studies on the use of writing within psychotherapeutic approaches is that of Pennbaker (as cited by L'Abate[13]) in his studies of undergraduate students who participated in a regimented program of writing on stressful/traumatic events.[13] His studies demonstrated statistically significant improvement in physiological measures (eg, blood pressure and skin conductance) in students who wrote about personal traumatic events. A subsequent meta-analysis by Smyth suggested that the effect sizes of studies on personal writing about stressful events seem to imply that expressive writing may lead to improved psychological health and well-being.[20]

Additional research on therapeutic writing techniques has demonstrated a variety of benefits. Brady and Sky found in a qualitative study of 15 older learners (average age = 69.2) that journal writing facilitated improved personal coping skills with daily life and contributed to self-expression and the ability to reflect on and integrate meaning in life.[21] Hall and Hawley conducted a study on the use of interactive process notes (IPN), which involved peer sharing of personal writing within a group setting.[11] The study suggested that the use of interactive process notes might facilitate increased patient insight, yet drawbacks include questions of confidentiality among the patient, peers, and the group facilitator. Wright reviewed research on therapeutic outcomes of writing and cited a number of research studies suggesting benefits of therapeutic writing to include: (1) greater patient control within the therapeutic relationship, (2) the provision for an outlet of emotional expression, and (3) increased patient participation in the healing process.[22] Additional applications of therapeutic writing include use of poetry therapy, bibliotherapy, expressive forms of writing, and structured workbooks.[23] As the use of writing continues to increase in psychological and mental health settings, increased research is needed, particularly within the rehabilitation fields.

Application to Occupational Therapy

The intrinsically personal nature of writing is well-suited to reflective client-centered practice and may be used in academic and clinical realms. Although expressive writing techniques and journaling may be included in the use of meaningful occupations within the context of the therapeutic relationship, little is written on the use of writing in occupational therapy settings. Denshire wrote of the power of personal reflective writing and its influence on the role of a therapist.[24] The author asserted the importance of personal reflection in developing subjective ways of knowing and valuing the personal within the therapy context. Similarly, client-centered occupation-based frames of reference such as the Person-Environment-Occupational Performance (PEOP) Model,[25] the Ecology of Human Performance Process Model,[26] and the Model of Human Occupation (MOHO),[27] all stress the importance of meaningful occupational engagement within the therapeutic context involving patient choice, perspective, and meaning. Through use of a journal, the patient is afforded opportunities to express personal thoughts, feelings, and ideas in a context that may feel safer than direct self-report. The patient has a unique opportunity to develop a relationship with the journal itself, a relationship that is sustainable over time.[28]

Haiman, Lambert, and Rodrigues wrote of the benefits of using various expressive techniques such as poetry and journal writing in adolescent mental health occupational therapy and suggested that writing techniques encourage emotional expression and personal exploration.[29] Such techniques may be applied in the rehabilitation setting to a variety of populations across the lifespan.[5,21,30-32]

JOURNAL WRITING ON THE OCCUPATIONAL THERAPY EVALUATION–INTERVENTION CONTINUUM

The evaluation process refers to the entire spectrum of information gathering, through use of historical information, interviews, observations, and formal assessments, whereas assessments denote use of a particular tool or technique. Assessments are often thought of as a reflection of patient function in a particular context and time. Assessment results may be fairly static when the patient is at baseline and function remains stable over time, yet often mental health patients are in a perpetual state of fluctuation in daily function; such variability lends itself well to means of assessment that measure change over time. Cohn, Schell, and Neistadt wrote of the dynamic interactive state of evaluation when used repeatedly throughout the therapy process.[33] The use of repeated evaluations assists the therapist and patient in measuring change as related to personal therapeutic goals. Given the fact that the nature of journal writing implies an ongoing practice, literature most often presents it in the context of intervention, yet the fluidity of journal writing provides opportunities for use throughout the evaluation-intervention continuum.

Within occupation-based practice, therapists seek to engage patients in meaningful activities throughout the therapeutic process. Patient interest and follow-through with journal assignments will vary based on personal preference, previous experience with writing, and the context in which it is presented. Given the highly personalized ongoing nature of journal writing, it is well-suited for use both as a dynamic means of assessment within the evaluative process, and as a unique intervention tool applicable to a variety of theoretical perspectives.

L'Abate presented four types of writing assignments often used in therapy: (1) open-ended writing, (2) focused writing, (3) guided writing, and (4) programmed writing.[13] *Open-ended* writing techniques are more free-flowing and patient-generated, such as the techniques used from psychodynamic perspectives. *Focused* and *guided* techniques provide the patient with some direction with relation to the writing content (eg, write about how you feel when you are depressed; answer the following questions, etc), yet allow the patient freedom within the guided writing. *Programmed* writing techniques often include prescriptive worksheets or a series of homework assignments designed for a specific purpose. The therapist must consider patient factors along with theoretical perspectives in determining the type, format, and duration of journal writing that will take place.

Frame of Reference and Theoretical Perspectives

In order to use journal writing within the evaluation and intervention continuum, therapists should have an understanding of journal writing, its techniques and applications, ethical and patient considerations, and should have a theoretical basis for which the journal will be used (Table 5-1). Information and resources related to journal writing are presented in Appendix A.

Table 5-1
Key Questions the Therapist Should Ask Prior to the Use of Journal Writing

1. What is my knowledge and use of journal writing as an assessment and intervention tool?

2. What are the therapeutic needs of the patient, and how will use of the journal meet these needs?

3. What form of journal will be used and how often? (eg, computer-based/Internet, hardbound, homework-based, structured assignments, etc)

4. Who will the journal be shared with? (eg, patient, therapist, peers, others)

5. What level of confidentiality will be maintained in use of the journal?

6. Do the patient's occupational profile and other factors lend themselves to use of the journal? (eg, consider the patient's writing skills, capacity for insight, motivation)

7. Is the patient interested in the use of the journal, and is follow-through likely?

8. What is the underlying theoretical background/frame of reference used?

The following is a brief summary of possible applications for use of a journal within the evaluation-intervention continuum. The techniques are only a sample of those available within the journal, and although they are presented within a specific frame of reference, many techniques are applicable across several therapeutic approaches.

OBJECT RELATIONS/PSYCHODYNAMIC TECHNIQUES

The application of psychodynamic principles to occupational therapy practice assumes that psychological constructs contribute to an individual's occupational and social behaviors.[34] The use of expressive and projective journal techniques within this approach may bring up thoughts and emotions that are within the unconscious or subconscious.[9,34,35] The therapist serves as a guide within this approach, and not an analyst. Through the use of therapeutic writing within this frame of reference, the therapist seeks to achieve a collaborative relationship with the patient in order to "mutually assume responsibility for assessment, identification of intervention goals, and development of an intervention plan, and to work together cooperatively during the intervention process."[34(p91)]

Stream of Consciousness

Stream of consciousness writing comes out of psychodynamic principles of Freud and includes techniques such as flow writing, expressive writing, and dream exploration.[35,36] A related form of expression in the journal, *map of consciousness*, includes not only the use of words, but also encourages creative spontaneous expression including use of drawings, diagrams, and symbols in conjunction with the use of words.[3] In both stream of consciousness and map of consciousness, patients are encouraged to explore areas of the unconscious through free-form writing, often initiated with a particular word or topic. Once the idea is introduced, the patient is encouraged to write or draw whatever comes to mind. One of the most common types of stream of consciousness writing is free writing, or flow writing.

Flow Writing and Free Writing

Flow writing and *free writing* are terms used to denote writing techniques within the journal that encourage the free expression of thought over a period of time. The patient is encouraged to write whatever comes to mind. The patient may be given a specific topic to write about, but generally there is a fair amount of freedom allowed within this type of journal entry. Patients may be given a set amount of time to write[37] or may be encouraged to write as long as they would like to do so. Benefits of flow writing include the opportunity for free expression of thoughts and feelings and the ability to access the unconscious.[2,35] This technique may also be helpful when the patient/writer experiences writer's block within the journal.[2] When used in the mental health setting, the patient and therapist may wish to revisit the entry immediately after it is written, or may choose to wait for a period of time, as it allows the patient time between the writing and review in order to explore the entry for potential themes, meanings, and insights.

Expressive Writing

Forms of expressive and creative writing may be used within the journal through a variety of techniques including the writing of stories, poetry, and narratives. Art therapist Dr. Lucia Cappachoine has written several books on creativity and journal writing, and introduced a creative journal approach designed for feelings exploration through use of writing and drawing exercises.[38] Of most notable interest in her technique is the encouragement of use of the nondominant hand, forcing expanded use of the creative means within the brain. According to Campbell,[39] the use of the nondominant hand encourages recruitment of the nondominant side of the brain. Such expression may be more difficult for the journal writer, but may tap into some unconscious creative areas that are not often used. Additional techniques within the journal should explore personal expression regarding topics of meaning, areas of difficulty, and plans for future goals.

Dream Exploration

Journals may be used as an access to the unconscious, bridging the dream life to our waking hours.[2,8,35] The use of dream exploration and dream analysis comes out of the psychoanalytic applications of psychology and is best used by trained therapists. Occupational therapists generally are not trained in dream analysis; however, the patient may wish to explore dreams within the journal. Through the recording of dreams, patients may gain insights into themes of importance in their lives. Adams suggested techniques for improving dream recall including:

1. Keeping a notebook and pen by the bed
2. Recording the dream immediately upon awakening, even if in the middle of the night
3. Going to sleep with the intention of remembering your dreams
4. Visualizing writing down the dreams upon awaking
5. Writing whatever comes to you upon wakening (do not censor)
6. Being good-natured in the process of dream recall.[35]

Often dreams may be frightening or confusing. Progoff emphasized the importance of recording the dreams without initial judgment or analysis and asserted, "…to do that would, in the first place, have the effect of rationalizing the symbolic material and thus violating the fact that its nature is inherently non-rational."[9(p203)] The author stressed the importance of recording dream materials in a nonbiased manner and revisiting the mate-

Table 5-2
Questions to Consider When Using Creative Expressive Entries

1. What was the experience of the patient during the writing process? Was it therapeutic?
2. What are the patient's thoughts, feelings, and experiences in relation to the process and product of the writing?
3. What does this entry say about patient events, experiences, thoughts, feelings, and ego functions?
4. Are there themes that relate to other journal entries and/or past or current experience?
5. What does this entry say about patient meaning, and how does this apply to identified strengths, needs, and goals?
6. What insights can be gained from this entry? How can these insights be utilized in the therapeutic process and in pursuit of improved occupational performance?
7. Where will the therapeutic writing process go from here?

rial later, recording any insights without overanalysis. In addition to dream logs, the use of meditation or twilight imagery may be used to invite thoughts, images, and dreams in a state between the sleep and wake cycle.[2,8,9] *Twilight imagery* is a term used to denote a state between levels of consciousness.[9] The journal writer enters the state through a process of meditation and imagery that may bring about images that later are reviewed for correlation with life events and themes of meaning.

Special Considerations in Applying Psychodynamic Applications to Assessment

Within the psychodynamic framework, therapists uphold the importance of developing patient insight, and therefore patient capacity for realistic thinking and development of insight should be considered.[34] Expressive journal entries must be considered in the context of the environment, patient factors, and personal meaning. The therapist and patient work together in a collaborative relationship, identifying themes that may be of importance with relationship to life history, current experience, and therapeutic goals. When using creative expressive entries within the journal, questions for consideration are included in Table 5-2.

If expressive writing techniques are used in the assessment process, the patient and therapist must maintain the collaborative relationship throughout the planning, writing, and discussing of the journal. Therapists should assure that the writing does not bring up issues or questions that compromise the patient's ability to cope, and therefore ethical considerations (presented later in the chapter) must be adhered to. Journal entries and follow-up dialogue are often rich sources of information regarding patient perception and sources of meaning, cognitive status, dynamic changes within the patient's psyche, and potential areas for goal and intervention planning. In using the journal as an assessment tool, dialogue and teamwork must be maintained at all times among the patient, therapist, and intervention team.

COGNITIVE BEHAVIORAL TECHNIQUES

The cognitive behavioral frame of reference assumes that: (1) thinking influences behavior, (2) that thinking can be self-regulated, and (3) desired behavioral change may occur through structured learning and acquired skills.[40] This frame of reference often involves skill building through the use of structured homework assignments, the use of daily personal tracking sheets, and the teaching of coping skills such as relaxation training and exercise. Use of therapeutic writing and journal techniques may involve structured assignments followed by self-reflection, group interaction, or feedback and dialogue between the patient and therapist. A key focus within this frame of reference is the development of personal insight and skills in order to maximize function and quality of life through the development of coping skills and meaningful healthy occupational patterns.

Homework/Structured Journal Writing

According to L'Abate, the use of writing assignments is advantageous in the provision for structure in therapy, yet it is important that such assignments do not over-control the assessment and intervention process.[13] In order to remain dynamic and client-centered, occupational therapists must select and adapt journal assignments based on the context and the patient's needs and desires.

There are several resources available to guide structured journal writing.[1,41,42] Therapists may choose to utilize prescriptive journal assignments, or may wish to adapt homework assignments based on the goals of the assessment and intervention process. Typically, patients engage in journal homework as part of an ongoing assessment and intervention process within individual or group therapy. If used as a part of a group, decisions should be made as to how confidentiality will be maintained and how much of the journal will be shared with the therapist and peers. Through the use of homework, patients are often asked to complete a structured writing assignment with the intention of later revisiting the assignment for personal analysis or feedback from peers or the therapist. Assignments may be used to gauge and track progress on personal goals, or may be used in order to further the assessment and intervention process through the development of new goals and practice of skill building. Appendix A provides suggested resources to help the facilitation of structured journal writing.

Lists

The use of lists within the journal provides a means to organize thoughts around a particular topic. Lists are powerful tools due to their simplistic, informative, and efficient properties.[39] Lists may be used for a variety of purposes, including self-expression, such as in the instance of exploring anxiety (eg, 10 things that I am stressed about right now); for problem solving (eg, five things I can do to cope with my stress); or for the development of insight (eg, five key events in my life). The structuring of lists within the journal may include lists of short words, phrases, or sentences (eg, list of friends) or more detailed lists (eg, 10 favorite memories from college). Progoff introduced a type of list he termed *steppingstones*.[8,9] Journal writers are encouraged to list significant events that have occurred in their lives. The list of steppingstones is akin to looking at personal marker events in one's life, a practice that fits well not only into the cognitive behavioral frame of reference, but also into developmental theories and frames of reference. Following the list of steppingstones, the journal writer and therapist review the journal entry for themes of importance throughout the lifespan, and identify areas for further exploration in the assessment-intervention continuum.

Adams[35] asserted the utility of using longer lists within journal writing and introduced an additional listing technique titled "Lists of 100." Examples of lists she identified include lists of fears, lists of stressors, and lists of things never grieved. Adams suggested that use of extensive lists often provides greater depth and unfolds into three parts: (1) things held in the conscious mind (generally the first third of the list), (2) repetition and themes that arise in the list, and (3) things that arise from the subconscious. Extensive lists may be used within the journal in order to assess for themes, information, insights, and consideration for future goal planning.

Clustering

Similar to lists, *clustering* is a writing technique that may be used to organize thoughts and feelings around a particular topic. Clustering is the use of cognitive mapping strategies and involves the connection of words and topics to similar words and topics.[35,39] The use of clustering is not isolated to journal writing, as it is often used in academic settings to facilitate student learning of a topic. Campbell suggested the use of clustering as a means of undercutting tension or anxiety often caused by writing.[39] Perhaps one of the most basic techniques is the mapping of words, where one word is placed in a box and lines are drawn to additional boxes with associated words. Although clustering is a useful tool, it should not be overused in the journal, as it is highly structured and limits free expression of thought. It is, however, a useful tool for organizing thoughts and beginning exploration of a particular topic.

Dialogue

Progoff introduced the technique of using dialogue within the journal in order to explore relationships with other persons, with the self, or with inanimate objects.[8,9] Generally, when selecting a source for dialogue, a person or object is chosen with which there is unfinished business, a significant event, or some area that needs more insight. Progoff discussed the use of dialogue with persons (relationships), works (significant activities in life), the body, society, and events. Adams suggested additional areas for dialogue, including emotions, objects, subpersonalities/symbols, and areas of resistance.[35] In order to engage in the dialogue, Adams suggested the importance of taking time to enter into a state in which the journal writer is prepared to write the dialogue. The use of imagery and meditation may be helpful, and it is important for the writer to be gentle on the self when engaged in the process. Following the writing of the dialogue, the writer (and possibly therapist) should revisit the dialogue and consider the questions in Table 5-3.

The following presents an example of a short journal dialogue between a 36-year-old depressed mother (Jane), and her deceased 18-year-old son (Mark), who died in an accident while under the influence of alcohol:

Me: Daily my stomach curls, I sob, and I don't think there is a reason to go on. I can't deny that I am angry you are dead, I question why you always drank, and some days I want to scream "I told you so!!" but it cuts me apart to know you will never hear my voice again.

Mark: You're one to talk you hypocrite!! I never drank that much, and you were always so hard on me, I know you never cared as much for me as you did for your job!! It seemed that you were always working, never home, and you know that you GUZZLED TOO!!!

Table 5-3
Questions Following Dialogue

1. Is there anything more to be written?
2. What thoughts and emotions were experienced during the writing, following the writing, and now?
3. What perceptions and insights does the dialogue present?
4. Is there unfinished business to attend to?
5. What do you hope to gain from the dialogue?
6. What strategies can be used for personal growth following the dialogue process?

Me: (crying) I'm sorry! I did my best! Why will no one forgive me? Why can't I cope? Why is my life full of eating, sleeping, and drinking? I can't go on!!!

Following an extended version of this excerpt, Jane and the therapist identified key areas for intervention planning and goal setting, including: (1) her chemical dependency issues, (2) stress management, and (3) finding meaningful occupational activities within a daily schedule in order to improve her quality of life. In addition to the occupational therapy approach, the entire team made a collective plan as to how to address her issues of grief/loss, self-esteem, depression, and chemical dependency. The use of a small journal excerpt provided a wealth of information within the assessment process.

Unsent Letters

A technique similar to dialogue is the use of unsent letters within the journal. The patient is encouraged to write a letter designed for one-way communication to someone/ something of significance. The letter may be written about a past hurt, about a time of meaning, or about continued questions in life. According to Adams, "unsent letters are marvelous tools for the 'three C's'—catharsis, completion, and clarity."[35(p172)] Such letters can help bring closure to difficult issues, or may be used to bring new insights to something or some relationship that has caused hurt, anxiety, stress, or some other psychological need that should be expressed. Unsent letters are meant for the individual writer and are generally not intended to actually be sent to the person of correspondence; however, the journal may also be used to write a practice letter to someone with whom correspondence, confrontation, or communication is anticipated to be difficult. The use of the journal through this means can provide a venue for patients to self-evaluate with the therapist the patterns of communication and to consider healthy means of expression. Rainer stressed that therapists and patients should caution against overuse of unsent letters because they may encourage a preoccupation with the journal and avoidance of actual expression of feelings to the individuals with whom communication is intended.[3] Therapists using the unsent letters technique should explore with the patient the significance of the letter as related to occupational themes, social relationships, life satisfaction, and areas for future work.

Reflective Writing

There are many types of reflection that may occur within the journal. Progoff spoke of the importance of revisiting the journal in order to develop new insights and add new entries based on reflections of previous writing.[8,9] Therapists may work with patients to structure the journal entries in order to have space for writing future insights upon the revisiting of the journal entries. One such technique, the double entry, utilizes half a page for the actual writing and leaves half the page blank for future reflections and insights. Reflections may be retroactive based on a particular journal entry, or may be single entries designed to reflect on any area of life, therapy, or personal significance. Following the reflections, the patient and therapist work together to assess progress toward goals, personal growth, and areas for future development.

Use of Writing in Dialectical Behavioral Therapy

Dialectical behavioral therapy (DBT) is a broad cognitive behavioral strategy originally designed to treat patients with borderline personality disorder, but it since has been applied to a number of populations, including those with depression, substance abuse, and eating disorders. Marsha Linehan developed the method based on the premise that individuals who have lived in invalidating environments often develop maladaptive skills for coping and emotional regulation.[43] Use of the DBT program generally involves a structured, weekly psychotherapy session as well as an intensive group session designed to teach adaptive coping skills such as emotional regulation, interpersonal effectiveness, and assertiveness training. Occupational therapists are often involved as facilitators of the skill-training component of DBT. Within the group, patients use a diary card to track incidents, events, and reactions, and in retrospect often evaluate their performance in the situation. The group also involves a series of homework sheets and may incorporate the use of therapeutic writing or a journal in order to facilitate insight related to the skills taught. A key consideration when facilitating DBT groups is the impact of skills training on occupational performance and the maintenance of open communication with the patient's psychologist and other team members. Consistency of approach is of importance when facilitating skills training and therapeutic writing applications.

Additional Considerations Within the Cognitive Behavioral Frame of Reference

Within the cognitive behavioral frame of reference, a key focus is the development of insight in order to influence growth and change. The journal and homework assignments are often incorporated in stages designed to: (1) bring about awareness, (2) practice adaptive skills, and (3) develop an internal locus of control designed to follow through with the skills throughout life. In order for the achievement of such goals to be met, the therapist continually works with the patient to assess progress through review and discussion of the homework and journal assignments. Progress will depend on patient motivation, capacity for insight, the therapeutic relationship, and contextual factors. Academic literature identifies various factors necessary for individual capacity and willingness to reflect including: (1) developmental level, (2) perceived trustworthiness of the teacher (therapist), (3) the clarity of expectations, and (4) the quality of the feedback process.[44] When utilizing reflective practice within occupational therapy, therapists should consider the patient's capacity for insight, willingness to journal, and amount of structure needed to meet the needs of the patient, context, and therapeutic process.

SPIRITUALITY

Often, mental health patients have to deal with grief, loss, and bereavement related to their illness, personal trauma, and/or a chasm between their goals for the self, conceptualizations of the perceived self, and current life events contributing to the actual self. The journal is a powerful place to work through bereavement and loss, find a place of meaning, and explore personal spirituality and belief systems.

The American Occupational Therapy Association's *Occupational Therapy Practice Framework* acknowledges the spiritual dimensions of our lives in the contexts section within the *Framework*.[45] Personal spirituality affects the development of the self and influences occupational patterns within our lives. The journal is a powerful tool for exploration of spirituality and matters of personal meaning. Baldwin wrote of the power of the journal to facilitate our exploration of personal meaning within and beyond ourselves.[37] The author asserted, "spiritual writing expands the interior conversation of consciousness to include your relationship with the sacred...You are in conversation with something you perceive as beyond, or deep within, yourself. It is this inclusion of the sacred that spiritualizes the writing."[37(p23)] Through the use of spiritual questions, reflections, and expressive writing, patients may work with the therapist to gain insight into areas of meaning relating to personal existence. Occupational therapists are not formal spiritual leaders, yet issues of spirituality, value, and meaning should be addressed, as they are intrinsic to occupational performance and quality of life. As themes of meaning unfold within the journal, the therapist and patient work together to develop goals and interventions surrounding lifestyle, meaningful activities, and occupations that contribute to personal quality of life, wellness, and ability to cope with loss, work through grief, and explore spiritual matters as they relate to individual occupational performance.

Applying Journal Writing to Occupational Therapy Assessment

The use of the journal in mental health assessment is a dynamic process and should flow from assessment to intervention. Prior to utilizing the journal for assessment, therapists must determine how the journal will fit into the evaluation-intervention continuum. Decisions must be made on the journal format, theoretical approach, patient readiness, and utility to achieve desired outcomes. By definition, the journal is a fluid, ongoing process, and therefore structure must be built into therapy in order to assure regular journal entries and opportunities for assessment, goal planning, and intervention. Assessment of the journal should be a collaborative process between the therapist and patient, and if applicable, peers. Some individuals choose to use therapeutic writing within a group format, and therefore decisions must be made as to how much of the journal is shared with peers and who partakes in the feedback process. Generally the assessment process is ongoing and involves looking at original entries, collaborating with the patient to develop a goal plan, and periodically revisiting future entries to track progress. Patients may also be asked to engage in formal self-assessments within the journal, and therefore structured questions or goals may be written into the journal (eg, tracking sheets) and set up for patient self-evaluation.

Schneider and Stone suggested that various journal techniques work best within three separate stages of therapeutic change: (1) the reflection stage, (2) the cognitive reconstruction stage, and (3) the creative construction stage.[7] Within the first stage, patients engage in expressive techniques designed to look at perceptions, views, and experiences. This first stage may be used as a means of assessment by which the patient's current view of the self, key life issues, strengths, and needs are addressed. Through the writing process and the revisiting of entries, the patient and therapist develop new insights and are challenged to recognize, interpret, and assimilate the insights into their view on life. During the reconstruction stage, patients use the insights gained and develop new insights, outlooks, and goals for themselves. During the last stage, the therapist and patient work together to help the patient develop an internal locus of control (empowerment of the patient from within) in order to utilize personal skills in meaningful occupational patterns. Throughout this process, the patient is encouraged to practice skills including positive coping, healthy decision making, and meaningful occupational engagement. The journal provides a unique means for ongoing opportunities for expression, insight, and personal growth.

FORMAT

Journals may take a variety of forms, including: (1) computer-based journals, (2) Internet-based journals, (3) hard copy journals, and (4) structured workbooks. In addition to the format of the journal, therapists must consider the structure for assessment and intervention including the therapeutic approach, theoretical application, and whether the journal process will be done individually or within a group. If journal writing is introduced in a group, it is often easiest to have all patients use the same journal techniques, yet Stone asserted the importance of individualizing the journaling approach in order to maximize follow-through during and post-therapy.[32] As a result, the use of groups should have some consistency in approach, yet enough freedom for patient expression and individuality. Decisions must also be made as to whether groups will involve face-to-face interactions or the use of a computer-based journal. The use of Internet journal sites or specialized software often allows patients to determine which entries are public and which are private. Such flexibility may be useful in both individual and group journal approaches, and offers the patient freedom for personal expression and privacy, an area integral to personal journal writing.[1] The danger of using an Internet-based journal in a group format is that the group facilitator has less control over the group exchange, particularly in asynchronous formats, and therefore the therapist must use caution when setting up Internet-based journal groups in order to adequately facilitate and structure the process for entry submissions, as well as facilitate ongoing interchange. If journal groups are used, particularly Internet-based groups, careful selection must take place regarding the patients' ability for insight, capacity for empathy in social interaction, and patient skill related to conflict management and assertiveness. With careful set-up, structure, and patient selection, groups can be an excellent way to develop patient insight and promote empowerment within a peer-support model.

SELF-ASSESSMENT

Throughout the journal process, patients should be encouraged to partake in self-assessment. The addition of reflective questions is often used in academia and has utility in therapeutic writing as well. An example of self-reflection may include the use of a prescribed journal entry in order to reflect on insights gained from a series of prior journal entries and personal experiences within a coping skills group. Sample reflective questions are included in Table 5-4.

The use of self-assessment techniques may later be shared with the group and/or therapist so that the patient can be held accountable for personal goals. The group may also be structured for open discussion and feedback regarding the patients' self-assessment and may be used to consider current progress and future goals. The use of didactic

---

Table 5-4

Sample Reflective Questions

1. What did I learn from my journal entries and this group regarding my current coping patterns and how they influence my daily life?
2. What coping skills have been most successful for me to avoid maladaptive behaviors?
3. What progress have I made on my goal to (list goal)?
4. Have I completed or do I need to revise or change my goals?
5. What is my plan in order to address these goals for the next week?

---

processes and periodic feedback may facilitate self-understanding as well as opportunities to practice healthy social interactions.

Additional means of self-assessment within the journal include the use of reflective entries, tracking sheets, checklists, and ongoing discussions with the therapist. When utilizing the journal for insight and self-assessment, it is important for the therapist to provide clear expectations and feedback regarding the purpose of the journal, the means by which it will be used, the expectations, and the depth of reflection expected.[46] Providing clear expectations and use of a collaborative approach is imperative in order to maximize meaningful use of the journal.

Additional Considerations

In today's psychosocial practice, there is often a blending of roles and intervention approaches in the mental health service team. The use of journal writing is not unique to occupational therapy, and much of the writing on its therapeutic applications is within the fields of clinical and counseling psychology. Journaling is, however, well-suited to occupational therapy, particularly when considered as a means of meaningful occupational engagement as well as a conduit toward the provision of improved occupational performance. The use of journal writing within the assessment-intervention continuum should: (1) have meaning to the patient, (2) consider the process and product of the journal within the *Framework*,[45] and (3) be linked to evaluation and intervention goals aimed at improving occupational performance, life satisfaction, and quality of life. As the patient engages in the journal process throughout therapy, a plan should be in place to consider the future utility of journaling as an ongoing part of the individual's daily life postdischarge.

ETHICAL IMPLICATIONS

In deciding whether to use journal writing, a therapist must take into account ethical considerations such as: (1) the expertise of the therapist, (2) the appropriateness of journal writing for the context and the patient, and (3) consideration of means by which it will be used. L'Abate identified a potential barrier in use of journal writing regarding the patient's willingness or unwillingness to engage in the writing process.[13] In utilizing a patient-centered approach, the decision to use journal writing and the format that will be used should involve patient input. Discussions should be centered on expectations, the journal format, and the degree of confidentiality that will be maintained. Therapists must caution against promising confidentiality if the patient's safety or the safety of others is put at risk, and therefore clear guidelines, expectations, confidentiality, and boundaries must be established prior to the onset of therapy. If the journal is used within a group, additional considerations include: (1) the establishment of trust and confidentiality codes within the group, (2) the freedom for patients to determine how much will be personally shared, and (3) the provision for a structured group process, conversation, and conflict management should an uncomfortable topic emerge within the group. In order for trust to be developed, the therapist must also facilitate and educate patients within a group on the importance of nonjudgmental attitudes within the group process. Patients should have some capacity for insight and empathy when assigned to groups utilizing shared writing strategies.

Additional confidentiality concerns include patient privacy regarding the accessibility of the journal to others. If patients are in a facility with shared bedrooms, concerns may arise as to whether others would have access to the journal. The therapist and patient should establish a plan for how the journal will be kept safe from others, what sections of the journal may be completely private (patient access only), and what sections will be accessible to the therapist or to others (if in a group setting). Often in a group, the actual journal is not shared, but patients have freedom to openly discuss particular insights or journal entries that are meaningful to the group.

THERAPIST EXPERTISE

Within the therapeutic process, the occupational therapist must utilize clinical reasoning and a therapeutic approach to determine means to facilitate desired change.[34] Although there is evidence to support the benefits of journal writing,[20,21] little is written on conceptualizations of the use of a journal and therapeutic writing in occupational therapy. Occupational therapists are uniquely trained in the study of occupation in conjunction with the person, environment, and context, and therefore have a unique set of skills in order to determine meaning, useful engagement, and the utility of writing within the therapeutic process. However, when utilizing any means of assessment and intervention, therapists must consider their own expertise. Key questions within the use of journal writing include:

1. What is the therapist's expertise?
2. Is the use of journal writing suited to this population and setting?
3. How will the therapeutic approach be unique to occupational therapy?
4. How will this approach be assimilated into the team approach and modalities used by other professionals working with the patient?

It is imperative that the therapist has a rationale and theoretical basis for the use of journal writing within therapy and has the capacity and skills to educate the patient, other team members, and the public regarding its use. Several workshops, organizations, books, and resources exist in order to provide support and education in the use of journal writing (see Appendix A).

Case Study

Marcy is a 19-year-old female recently admitted to New Start Day Program for depression, suicidal ideation, and anorexia nervosa. Marcy recently graduated from high school with high honors and numerous athletic awards in gymnastics. In addition to athletics, she was the editor of the school newsletter and a participant in the poetry club. She originally planned to attend a large local university, but due to increasing depression and medical concerns secondary to her drop in weight (5′ 6″, 95 pounds), her primary physician convinced her to take a semester off.

Marcy grew up in a single-parent household with one younger sister. Her father left when she was 5, and she hasn't seen him since. Marcy has been on antidepressants for about a year but has never had a psychiatric hospitalization, nor has she ever attended day treatment. She did briefly see a counselor at school, and the question of her eating patterns came up, but at the time she was not referred for medical intervention. During the summer following graduation, she reported increased feelings of stress and depression related to a fear of failure and recent separation from her best friend, who has moved away to college. Her general practitioner referred her to the New Start program, given its multidisciplinary approach and comprehensive services including psychiatric, residential, vocational, and recreational programs. As part of the regular day program, Marcy was referred for occupational therapy assessment and intervention.

In the initial occupational therapy interview, Marcy admitted being depressed but had difficulty verbalizing her feelings and the events surrounding the depression and eating disorder. She indicated interests in writing, poetry, literature, and exercise, yet admitted that she didn't feel much like participating in any leisure activities. Given her writing interests, she agreed to participate in journal activities as part of her ongoing assessment and intervention. As part of an assessment battery during the second week of therapy, Marcy completed an unsent letter journal entry to her father. The following is a short excerpt:

Dear Dad,

They say I'm sick but I feel fine, just a little depressed, that's all. I shouldn't be here anyways; I should be in class working on a degree in education. Why is it that no matter how much I try, I always screw things up? Anyways, you wouldn't care, you never call and mom never mentions your name. I wanted to go to college, and now I've screwed that up too; it seems the world hates me, that's all. My life is crap. I sleep, get up, watch TV, and listen to tunes. Jonna [Marcy's friend] is gone and there's nothing to do. I never write anymore and have no energy. So what's the big deal? They say I don't eat, I eat fine, they say I'm not ready for school, they say, they say, they say!!! Why doesn't anybody ever listen to me?!!

Following her writing, Marcy was asked to complete a reflection indicating any insights she had from her letter. Due to her depression, the occupational therapist decided she would need a structured format for reflection, and therefore she was asked to consider the following questions:

1. What feelings and memories came to you as you were writing?
2. What feelings do you have now?
3. What does this entry say about what is important to you?

4. Is your lifestyle how you would like it to be?

5. What could you change?

6. What are your goals?

7. How can we work toward the goals in occupational therapy?

8. Was the process of writing helpful? If so, how?

Marcy identified that she was angry, frustrated, and depressed as she wrote her entry. Although she initially identified magnified feelings of depression during the writing process, she stated that writing helped her sort through some things that were bothering her, including the lack of communication with her father, the feeling of helplessness and failure to achieve her goals, the loss of control, and the lack of pleasure in her life. From the initial assessment entry, the occupational therapist developed an occupational profile[45] that identified occupational barriers, including her depression, eating disorders, self-concept, and family issues, all of which posed difficulties in successfully achieving her goals to attend school and create a meaningful life. Strengths and interests identified included Marcy's athleticism, intelligence, interest in writing and poetry, and willingness to engage in therapy. It was determined that the role of the family would need to be further explored. The therapist collaborated with Marcy and identified initial goal areas, including the development of coping skills, increased meaningful engagement in activities of interest, and development of a plan for return to school. In addition, Marcy was to work on her eating disorder concerns in therapy and in collaboration with the entire treatment team. A plan was developed for Marcy to attend DBT treatment, to engage in ongoing journal writing, and to work individually with the therapist in order to examine lifestyle patterns and means to enhance her quality of life through meaningful activities.

Questions for the Reader

1. Do you agree with the use of the journal in this case? Why or why not?

2. What other information would you need to know in approaching Marcy for assessment?

3. What additional journal writing techniques might you use in this instance?

4. Do you believe Marcy would have been a candidate for a journal group? Why or why not? What ethical concerns may arise?

5. How would you collaborate with the intervention team in your occupational therapy approach with this patient?

Summary

The journal provides a unique tool within the occupational therapy evaluation-intervention continuum. As therapists' use of writing within occupational therapy continues, research is needed regarding the unique role, efficacy, and utility of the journal in practice. Journal writing is highly individualized and fits well into patient-centered practice, yet should be used in conjunction with other, more formal means of assessment. Through the use of the journal, patients can gain insight, work on personal goals, and have an ongoing venue for reflection and personal growth that can be carried throughout life.

References

1. Bender S. *A Year in the Life: Journaling for Self-Discovery.* Cincinnati, OH: Walking Stick Press; 2000.
2. Rainer T. *The New Diary: How to use a Journal for Self-Guidance and Expanded Creativity.* Los Angeles, CA: Penguin Putnam; 1978.
3. Baldwin C. *One to One: A New and Updated Edition of the Classic Self-understanding Through Journal Writing.* New York, NY: M. Evans and Company; 1991.
4. Miller JE. *The Rewarding Practice of Journal Writing: A Guide for Starting and Keeping Your Personal Journal.* Fort Wayne, IN: Willowgreen Publishing; 1998.
5. Murray S. The benefits of journaling: "stories are medicine" "art is medicine." *Parks Recreation.* 1997;32:68-75.
6. Wright J, Chung MC. Master or mystery? therapeutic writing: a review of the literature. *Br J Guidance Counsel.* 2001;29:277-291.
7. Schneider MF, Stone M. Processes and techniques of journal writing in Adlerian therapy. *J Indiv Psychol.* 1998;54:511-531.
8. Progoff I. *At a Journal Workshop: The Basic Text and Guide for Using the Intensive Journal.* New York, NY: Dialogue House; 1975.
9. Progoff I. *At a Journal Workshop: Writing to Access the Power of the Unconscious and Evoke Creative Ability.* New York, NY: Penguin Putnam Books; 1992.
10. Bacigalupe G. Writing in therapy: a participatory approach. *J Family Ther.* 1996;18:361-373.
11. Hall J, Hawley L. Interactive process notes: an innovative tool in counseling groups. *J Spec Group Work.* 2004;29:193-205.
12. Jordan KB, L'Abate L. Programmed writing and therapy with symbiotically enmeshed patients. *Am J Psychother.* 1995;49:225-236.
13. L'Abate L. The use of writing in psychotherapy. *Am J Psychother.* 1991;45:87-98.
14. L'Abate L. Taking the bull by the horns: beyond talk in psychological interventions. *Fam J Counseling Ther Couples Families.* 1999;7:206-220.
15. Ullrich PM, Lutgendorf S K. Journaling about stressful events: effects of cognitive processing and emotional expression. *Ann Behav Med.* 2002;24:244-250.
16. Griffith BA, Frieden G. Facilitating reflective thinking in counselor education. *Counselor Educ Supervision.* 2000;40:82-93.
17. Ritchie MA. Faculty and student dialogue through journal writing. *J Spec Ped Nurs.* 2003;8:5-12.
18. Ruthman J, Jackson J, Cluskey M, Flannigan P, Folse VN, Bunten J. Using clinical journaling to capture critical thinking across the curriculum. *Nurs Educ Perspect.* 2004;25:120-123.
19. Spalding E, Wilson A. Demystifying reflection: a study of pedagogical strategies that encourage reflective journal writing. *Teachers College Record.* 2002;104:1393-1421.
20. Smyth JM. Written emotional expression: effect sizes, outcome types, and moderating variables. *J Consult Clin Psychol.* 1998;66:174-184.
21. Brady EM, Sky HZ. Journal writing among older learners. *Educ Gerontol.* 2003;29:151-163.
22. Wright J. Online counseling: learning from writing therapy. *Br J Guidance Counsel.* 2002;30:285-298.
23. McArdle S, Byrt R. Fiction, poetry, and mental health: expressive and therapeutic uses of literature. *J Psychiatr Ment Health Nurs.* 2001;8:517-524.
24. Denshire S. Reflections on the confluence of personal and professional. *Australian Occup Ther J.* 2002;49:212-216.
25. Christiansen C, Baum C. Person-Environment Occupational Performance: A conceptual model for practice. In: Christiansen C, Baum C, eds. *Occupational Therapy: Enabling Function and Well Being.* 2nd ed. Thorofare, NJ: SLACK Incorporated; 1997:47-70.
26. Fearing VG, Law M, Clark J. An occupational performance process model: fostering client and therapist alliances. *Can J Occup Ther.* 1997;64: 7-15.
27. Kielhofner G. *A Model of Human Occupation: Theory and Application.* 3rd ed. Baltimore, MD: Lippincott Williams & Wilkins; 2002.
28. Thompson K. Journal writing as a therapeutic tool. In: Bolton G, Howlett S, Lago C, Wright J, eds. *Writing Cures: An Introductory Handbook of Writing in Counseling and Therapy.* New York, NY: Brunner-Routledge; 2004:72-84.
29. Haiman S, Lambert WL, Rodrigues BJ. Mental health of adolescents. In: Cara E, McCrae A, eds. *Psychosocial Occupational Therapy: A Clinical Practice.* 2nd ed. Clifton Park, NY: Thomson Delmar Learning; 2005;298-333.

30. Cara E. Mood disorders. In: Cara E, McCrae A, eds. *Psychosocial Occupational Therapy: A Clinical Practice.* 2nd ed. Clifton Park, NY: Thomson Delmar Learning; 2005:162-192.

31. Levitt VB. Anxiety disorders. In: Cara E, McCrae A, eds. *Psychosocial Occupational Therapy: A Clinical Practice.* 2nd ed. Clifton Park, NY: Thomson Delmar Learning; 2005:1193-234.

32. Stone M. Journaling with clients. *J Indiv Psychol.* 1998;54:535-545.

33. Cohn ES, Schell BA, Neistadt M. Introduction to evaluation and interviewing. In: Crepeau E, Cohn E, Schell B, eds. *Willard & Spackman's Occupational Therapy.* 10th ed. Philadelphia PA: Lippincott Williams & Wilkins; 2003: 279-297.

34. Bruce MA, Borg B. *Psychosocial Frames of Reference: Core for Occupation Based Practice.* Thorofare, NJ: SLACK Incorporated; 2002.

35. Adams K. *Journal to the Self: Twenty-Two Paths to Personal Growth.* New York, NY: Warner Books; 1990.

36. Senn LC. *The Many Faces of Journaling: Topics and Techniques for Personal Journal Writing.* St. Louis, MO: Pen Central Press; 2001.

37. Baldwin C. *Life's Companion: Journal Writing as a Spiritual Quest.* New York, NY: Bantam Books; 1991.

38. Cappacchione L. *The Creative Journal: The Art of Finding Yourself.* 2nd ed. Hollywood, CA: Newcastle Publications; 1989.

39. Campbell A. *Your Corner of the Universe: A Guide to Self-Therapy Through Journal Writing.* Lincoln, NE: ASJA Press; 2000.

40. Stein F, Cutler SK. *Psychosocial Occupational Therapy: A Holistic Approach.* 2nd ed. Albany, NY: Delmar; 2002.

41. Adams K. *The Way of the Journal: A Journal Therapy Workbook for Healing.* 2nd ed. Baltimore, MD: Sidran Institute Press; 1998.

42. Jacobs B. *Writing for Emotional Balance.* Oakland, CA: New Harbinger Publications; 2004.

43. Linehan MM. *Skills Training Manual for Treating Borderline Personality Disorder.* New York, NY: The Guilford Press; 1993.

44. Paterson BL. Developing and maintaining reflection in clinical journals. *Nurse Educ Today.* 1995;15:211-220.

45. American Occupational Therapy Association. Occupational therapy practice framework: domain and process. *Am J Occup Ther.* 2002;56:609-639.

46. Srimavin W, Darasawang P. Developing self-assessment through journal writing. Published Proceedings of the 2003 Independent Learning Conference. 2004. Retrieved August 24, 2005. Available at: http://www.independentlearning.org/ila03/ila03_srimavin_and_pornapit.pdf.

6

EXPRESSIVE MEDIA USED AS ASSESSMENT IN MENTAL HEALTH

Frances Reynolds, PhD

"The creative act can be an affirmation of purpose and meaning in the face of risk, loss, and disaster...The creative act is a gift for those who are capable of recognizing and receiving it." Kastenbaum R. Riding the tiger: the challenge of creative renewal in the later years. In: Bloom M, Gullotta T, eds. Promoting Creativity Across the Lifespan. *Washington: CWLA Press; 2001:277-309.*

Introduction

Expressive media typically include visual art-making (drawing, painting, or clay), photography, creative writing, music, drama, movement, sand-tray, computer graphics, and dance, although nearly any freely chosen activity can be self-expressive.[1,2] Occupational therapists that I interviewed when preparing this chapter also mentioned card making, beadwork, mosaics, glass painting, embossing, enameling, and many other activities as forms of expressive media. This chapter will mostly focus on visual arts-based assessments because there is more published information about their use, reliability, and validity. The terms *expressive* and *creative* therapies are often used interchangeably, and this practice will be continued in this chapter. However, a distinction is made by Feder and Feder,[3] who suggest that the term expressive emphasizes communication (of self, ideas, or feelings), whereas creativity may be thought to connote problem solving, inventiveness, and imagination (see discussion by Creek[4]). Yet perhaps personal expression through art, drama, and other media is inherently creative to the extent that the person puts together words and images in active, novel, and personally meaningful ways.

Historically, occupational therapists emphasized the therapeutic benefits of self-expression through arts and crafts, yet such activities seem to have declined in recent years.[5,6] There is very little published work on occupational therapists' current use of expressive media in assessment. Hence, this chapter will not only draw upon published research and clinical opinion pieces, but also interviews with practicing occupational therapists who are using expressive media to assess adult patients in mental health settings.

Certain standardized assessments can be carried out to evaluate patients' occupational performance when they are engaged with expressive media either individually or in groups. For example, the Canadian Occupational Performance Measure (COPM), Occupational Therapy Task Observation Scale (OTTOS), and Comprehensive Occupational Therapy Evaluation (COTE) have been found useful.[2] This chapter will explore formal and informal assessments that are grounded more directly in patients' use of creative or expressive media.

Many debates exist among therapists about the appropriate use of expressive media in assessment. For example, there is controversy about the relative merits of formal or informal assessments, and whether assessments should be based on single or multiple media. Therapists also differ in their preparedness to offer interpretive or descriptive responses to patients' creative or expressive work. Some assess content, while others focus more on process issues. Creative or expressive arts assessments have been used in various ways in mental health settings, eg, as an aid to formal psychiatric diagnosis, to guide treatment decisions, or—in a more idiographic way—to enable therapists to enter the patient's subjective world more successfully and, above all, to communicate in greater depth with the patient and thereby build an empathic alliance.[3]

To some extent, therapists' varied uses of expressive media in assessment reflect their diverse theoretical positions. These include occupational science, existentialism, behavioral perspectives, and various psychodynamic theories, including the Freudian perspective, Jung's analytic approach, and object relations theory.[3,7] The functions of expressive media within assessment are viewed rather differently from these various vantage points. While occupational therapists mostly subscribe to the humanistic, patient-centered perspective, other psychological theories explicitly inform practice in some settings, especially where multiprofessional practice occurs (such as shared sessions with psychodynamically trained art therapists). It is particularly important to have some understanding of the concepts derived from psychodynamic perspectives, as these can be used quite intuitively, and not necessarily correctly. For example, a therapist who observes a patient smothering a picture in black paint might infer that depression or grief is being expressed. Such an interpretation has been guided by the therapist's implicit or explicit understanding of psychodynamic theory and its focus on the symbolic workings of the unconscious mind.

The Therapeutic Use of Expressive Media Within Occupational Therapy

Why are expressive or creative media used in occupational therapy in mental health settings? Therapists have many specific goals, but these can perhaps be grouped into two broad categories: (1) helping patients gain greater competence (and satisfaction) in skills and activities that can be used in everyday life, and (2) promoting psychotherapeutic change.[8]

In relation to promoting life roles and meaningful activities, expressive media such as art can help patients to acquire (or rediscover) creative and social skills that will reduce occupational deprivation and thereby enhance quality of life.[9] Patients gain self-esteem through making choices and seeing the visible results of expressive or creative work; they also experience control, mastery, achievement, and autonomy, all of which strengthen identity and build well-being.[10] The deep concentration required by many expressive or creative activities can be calming, reducing self-consciousness and unproductive cognitive rumination on personal problems and promoting positive experiences of flow.[2,11,12] On a deeper psychotherapeutic level, patients have been observed to express troubling feelings more openly through nonverbal arts media than through words.[6,13] Yet, patients also have considerable control over their level of engagement and disclosure during expressive activities, and this control helps to reduce feelings of passivity that are prevalent among those in mental health settings. Patients who find it difficult to interact with others may be able to relate with more confidence to inanimate artwork and thereby find an expressive outlet within creative activity.[10] Occupational therapists who are guided by a psychodynamic perspective argue that patients use art and other media to project and work through unconscious feelings about themselves and the outer world.[13]

PERSPECTIVES THAT INFORM THE USE OF EXPRESSIVE MEDIA TO ASSESS PATIENTS IN MENTAL HEALTH SETTINGS

In order to support patients' participation in meaningful roles and occupations within everyday life, occupational therapists need to develop a profound understanding of their "concerns, problems and risks."[14(p614)] Patient-centered assessments are valued for focusing on patients' strengths and priorities as well as vulnerabilities. However, in mental health settings where patients may have limited awareness of their problems or choices, additional frameworks are sometimes used to guide practice.

Therapists whose practices are informed by psychodynamic concepts may consider it appropriate to interpret both the content and process of patients' art and other expressive work, looking for symbolic communications in order to develop a more in-depth understanding of patients' concerns.[15] The psychodynamic perspective embraces a number of distinct theories, including those of Freud, Jung, and the object relations school.

Freud proposed that psychological distress and behavioral disturbance have roots in unconscious conflicts that exist beneath the reach of conscious awareness. A number of unconscious defense mechanisms, such as repression and projection, keep such conflicts hidden from the person. From this perspective, expressive media (eg, drawing, sand-tray, and clay-work) enable the patient to express fantasies and troubling feelings symbolically. Because patients have little awareness, by definition, of such psychodynamic processes, their self-expressive work is less edited and therefore more revealing of their inner states. Freud also proposed that repressed or conflictual experiences could be expressed in disguised ways through condensed or indirect (displaced) images. The surface (or *manifest*) content of visual imagery tends to disguise the underlying (or *latent*) message. Many formal assessments (such as the Draw-a-Person test) rest on the assumption that the patient is engaged in a symbolic representation of the self. Occupational therapists' informal observations may also be informed by such psychodynamic concepts. For example, Harries offered a sensitive analysis of drawings made by an anorexic patient during occupational therapy.[13] Harries suggested that certain images revealed the young woman's dependency upon her parents and her ambivalence about leaving home. The patient did not (or could not) directly verbalize such issues in early therapy sessions. She drew friends initially as stick figures. Why these figures lacked substance could be interpreted in many ways.

Freud also proposed that both patient and therapist project their own unresolved feelings onto each other in a process known as *transference* and *countertransference*. Robbins defines transference as the "emotions, attitudes, or perceptions from the past that the patient brings to the relationship."[16(p147)] For example, a patient may feel negatively judged by the therapist when he or she has had a long family history of criticism or abuse. Robbins describes countertransference as the "total emotional response of the therapist to the patient."[16(p147)] Some therapists argue that it is important to be sensitive to the feelings that the patient's expressive work arouse in him- or herself, as these feelings offer insights regarding the patient's unspoken experiences, such as being bullied or frightened. Case described working with a 14-year-old adolescent in art therapy.[17] She said, "Much of my understanding of him comes from my feelings in the session and sense of how he experiences me."[17(p31)] However, countertransference also carries a risk of over-interpreting patients' expressive artwork. Therapists need to guard against projecting their own preoccupations and fantasies rather than accurately assessing the patient's own issues.

Some therapists working with expressive media draw upon the concepts of Jung.[18] Jung argued that people expressed their deepest concerns obliquely through art and other forms of expressive media. In contrast to Freud, Jung was more positive about the processes occurring within the unconscious mind, believing that creative, healing forces were present. He also proposed that people make use of collective as well as personal symbolism in their expressive work, such as drawing on archetypes to communicate human experiences like death and fear.

The object relations school has focused more upon the role of the therapeutic relationship in helping patients to understand how relationships have functioned in their lives outside of therapy and to find ways of managing appropriate levels of intimacy. From this perspective, the therapist provides a *holding environment*, increasing the patient's sense of emotional safety and facilitating exploration of feelings. Object relations theory also proposes that the expressive medium (eg, painting) can act as a container for difficult feelings.[19] Winnicott conceptualized artwork as a *transitional* object, enabling inner feelings to be externalized, distanced, and thereby rendered less powerful. Interested readers may refer to Malchiodi for further details.[7]

The *behaviorist* perspective eschews both biomedical diagnosis and also the notion of unconscious personality structures or conflicts. Instead, therapists focus on describing observable problematic or adaptive behavior, noting its context, frequency, triggers, and consequences. Few occupational therapists appear to rely totally on behaviorist theory. Nevertheless, the perspective is useful in emphasizing that self-expression (via any medium, verbal or nonverbal) is a form of behavior. Much can be learned about the patient from careful observation. For example, a patient who usually has problems concentrating might be observed to attend to an art making task for a long period. A socially withdrawn patient might make brief eye contact or ask others for equipment during an art session. This information would not be interpreted for any deeper meaning, but it potentially demonstrates therapeutic change and could therefore be used to guide further therapeutic interventions and choice of meaningful occupation. Case describes working with an adolescent whose challenging behavior subsided during an art session.[17] The patient started out almost monosyllabic and perceptibly shaking. As the painting progressed, his hand steadied and the wariness subsided. The young man became willing to talk about the painting he had created, and an embryonic therapeutic relationship began. While the therapist was attentive to possible meanings in the artwork, she was also carefully observing behavioral changes in the adolescent patient.

The *humanistic* or *existential* perspective regards patients as the authors of their own life and the "experts" on their own concerns. From this perspective, the therapist's own interpretation of the meaning of the patient's artwork or other expressive product is largely seen as inappropriate. Instead, the therapist encourages the patient to find his or her own meanings in the activity, to enhance self-insight, choice, and control. The humanistic perspective also encourages therapists to focus on patients' strengths as well as vulnerabilities. Patients communicate self-insights, aesthetic judgments, and other strengths and skills when working with expressive media, as well as their preoccupations and anxieties. Some occupational therapists ask patients to review the meanings of their expressive work even when they accept that the significance of some communications are symbolic and difficult for patients to decode.[13] The nonjudgmental acceptance of a patient's artwork helps the patient also to feel unconditionally accepted as a person with worth.[11]

Why Assess Mental Health Using Expressive Media?

Expressive media can be used to assess patients' cognitive abilities, emotional concerns, occupational preferences, skills, and interests, as well as life experiences, and may complement traditional interview techniques.[3]

However, expressive media may also have a more distinctive role to play, specifically in giving voice to less consciously available material. For example, expressive media offer a means of:

- Communicating the inexpressible: some traumatic experiences such as abuse and loss cannot be verbalized successfully, either because the patient is too fearful to confront the experience directly or because words are not sufficient to capture the feelings involved.[11]

- Containing potentially overwhelming emotions within the art materials or creative encounter, thereby enhancing psychological security and enabling self-expression.[19]

- Enabling oblique or indirect self-expression (eg, the use of metaphors, symbols, and archetypes that externalize inner turmoil and hurt, bypassing internal censorship or psychological defenses).[20,21]

- Giving disenfranchised and stigmatized people "a voice in the world."[22]

- Revealing patients' strengths as well as vulnerabilities (eg, responsiveness, self-confidence, cognitive problem-solving strategies, and collaborative skills, as well as fears or self-defeating fantasies).[1]

- Working "at the patient's level of comfort."[3(p246)]

However, creative or expressive products do not simply reflect the maker.[20] The social and physical environment, the patient's relationship with the therapist (and other group members), perceived audience, and other factors all play a part in the process.[23] This makes interpretation of the patient's response to expressive media uncertain and raises the debate about the reliability and validity of arts-based assessments.

Oster and Gould emphasize that "a thorough assessment involves sampling a wide range of an individual's cognitive and emotional resources and attempting to integrate these discrete bits of information."[24(p15)] Different expressive media may play distinctive roles in the assessment process because they present different challenges for patients.[1] For example, watercolor painting demands a tolerance for spontaneity, and so this medium may be too anxiety-provoking for patients with shaky boundaries, a need for containment, or obsessional neatness.[19] Patients face social challenges when working collaboratively in drama and music. Some creative media may be considered demeaning or age-inappropriate by patients. These factors should all affect the choice of assessment medium for the individual patient and suggest that very cautious inferences are made about patients' functioning when a single medium is used.

Formal and Informal Assessments Using Expressive Media

Formal assessments comprise both projective and standardized psychometric tools. Many such test designers propose that particular creative strategies and themes within the expressive work signify common psychological issues. Some formal tests have been used as an aid to the diagnosis of mental health problems, and going beyond biomedical diagnosis, to identify particular strengths and vulnerabilities within patients. While there has been little published evidence about their use among occupational therapists, creative arts therapists have conducted an increasing amount of research into the reliability and validity of such tests, with the intention of establishing predictive patterns and norms. Such information, if valid and reliable, may arguably enhance occupational therapy practice.

Expressive media have also been used in more informal ways to contribute to the assessment of mental health. It is widely accepted among practitioners using expressive media that they have a distinctive role to play in the holistic assessment process. For example, patients may feel emotionally safer when engaged in creative work rather than in face-to-face verbal interaction, and they may therefore be less guarded in their response. If less anxious and psychologically defended, the patient is more likely to reveal personal concerns and experiences and to demonstrate more optimal functioning. The occupational therapist thereby gains valuable information about the patient's strengths as well as vulnerabilities. Careful observation of the patient engaged in an expressive medium contributes to a detailed idiographic assessment.

As with the formal use of creative arts assessments, there is relatively little published research in the occupational therapy literature about using expressive media for informal assessment. Therapists using expressive media in nonstandardized ways are reliant on intuition, past experience, and clinical reasoning when making sense of the patient's expressive process or products. Assessment tends to be closely intertwined with the therapeutic process and relationship. There also appears to be a greater willingness among therapists working in this way to assume that patients are open to change and that, where possible, patients participate in the assessment process through reflecting on their own creative experience. Therapists making informal use of expressive media within assessment are more likely to integrate their own observations with patients' views and narratives, rather than relying on their own "expert" opinion alone. These issues will be further explored, drawing on interviews with occupational therapists.

FORMAL ASSESSMENTS

Several standardized creative arts assessments have been proposed, mostly using the visual arts such as drawing and painting. Some of these are considered to be projective techniques. Projective techniques are less structured activities in which patients are assumed to express unconscious issues. Therapists working with such tests attempt to gain insight into these deep-seated concerns through interpreting the meanings of the images or stories created. However, other creative arts therapists have queried the validity of projective tests and advocate descriptive assessments of the creative form rather than content of the work (such as the patient's use of color and space in a piece of artwork rather than themes or meanings).

Projective Tests

Projective arts tests include House-Tree-Person, Draw-A-Person, Kinetic Family Drawing, and Draw-A-Person-Picking-An-Apple-From-A-Tree (PPAT).[25] Projective tests developed specifically by occupational therapists include the Azima Battery[26] and the Goodman Battery,[27] both of which include figure drawing and free, or spontaneous, drawings. The Lerner and Ross Magazine Picture Collage and Ehrenberg Comprehensive Assessment Process (which involves collage as well as other expressive activities) were also developed by occupational therapists. Further details are provided by Drake.[28] Lloyd and Papas[5] point out that little has been published in recent years about these assessments and that their validity and reliability are uncertain. They are mostly time-consuming, which presents a further barrier to regular use.

All projective tasks are relatively ambiguous, thereby facilitating in the patient expressions of personal concerns and traits such as hostility. The House-Tree-Person test, for example, invites patients to draw each of the three images on separate sheets of paper and then to offer verbal associations.[25] Polatajko and Kaiserman report a validation of its use by occupational therapists.[29]

Projective tests are mostly influenced by Jungian and object relations theories. While many therapists may readily accept that patients' issues are likely to be expressed in these relatively unstructured tasks, concerns remain about the specific interpretations that some authors suggest. For example, the house drawing in the House-Tree-Person (HTP) test has been interpreted as a symbolic representation of the patient's psyche, with the lower level more indicative of unconscious processes, and the tree drawing is supposed to express life role and life satisfaction (Buck, 1987, see review by Brooke[25]). Buck also proposed that the tree drawing is representational of the self, with knotholes and broken branches interpreted as indicating emotional trauma. In the absence of strong evidence, the validity of such interpretations may be questionable. Other authors suggest that it is safer to regard such images as a source of tentative hypotheses about a person's mental state.[3,23]

Some projective tests, such as the Diagnostic Drawing Series,[30] have been used as diagnostic tools to detect signs of schizophrenia, dissociative disorders, and attention deficit hyperactivity disorder (ADHD). In addition to affirming the *Diagnostic and Statistical Manual of Mental Disorders* (DSM-IV) diagnostic categories, projective tests have been used to reveal more specific cognitive and emotional processes such as anxiety, hostility, and reality distortion.[31] Some tests have undergone reliability and validity testing (eg, by Mills and colleagues[30]), but as Brooke[25] discusses, many have not.

The Draw-a-Person Test was developed by Machover in 1949.[32] As a projective test, it assumes that the patient expresses, in metaphorical or symbolic terms, aspects of his or her self-image or conceptualization of relationships through the image created. Some therapists offer interpretations of patients' responses based on clinical experience. Oster and Gould outline a number of features that are said to have significance.[24] These features include sketchy outlines and heavy shading, which may be associated with anxiety; tiny figures, which may signify high levels of insecurity; and teeth, which may indicate aggressiveness.

Certain standardized scoring systems have been developed, attempting to determine whether patients with specific diagnoses include particular elements in their Person drawings. For example, Lev-Wiesel and Shvero[31] compared the self-figure drawings of patients diagnosed as schizophrenic and nonpatients matched for age, gender, and level of education. The authors inferred certain differences between the groups, with schizophrenic patients' figure drawings having distinctive head shapes and unusual sizes, as well as exaggerated (or omitted) eyes and ears. Patients with mental health problems also tended to present broken or double outlines. However, this study did not really address whether patients were simply incorporating cultural stereotypes of the "insane" in creating these figures. Other potential influences in the schizophrenic group, such as medication, did not appear to be considered. Above all, efforts to link expressive imagery with diagnosis rest on acceptance of the validity of the DSM-IV diagnostic categories and the questionable assumption that symptomatology is directly expressed in artistic activities. This is open to doubt. There is perhaps "no more an art of the insane than there's an art of dyspeptics or of people with sore knees" (Dubuffet, quoted by Thomson[33(p38)]). Occupational therapists who prefer to focus on a patient's unique constellation of occupational goals, vulnerabilities, and competencies seem unlikely to use projective techniques in such a classificatory way. Furthermore, therapists should bear in mind that some projective tests undermine patients' performances through being time-consuming and exhausting, thereby raising evaluation anxiety.[25]

The Silver Drawing Test (SDT) seems to have undergone a lengthier process of validation than many other tests.[34] The tests were originally developed to assess the cognitive skills of children with hearing impairments, but have been subsequently used to assess depression and other emotional problems. Silver argues that drawing assessments help patients to articulate their needs and skills in ways that they might not be able to manage verbally. The assessments are unusual in presenting patients with an array of ready-made stimulus drawings, such as a parachute, tree, or dinosaur. Silver argues that the presentation of ready-made stimulus drawings is especially useful for patients who would otherwise feel too anxious to engage with unstructured expressive or creative tasks. In one version of the test, the patient chooses two pictures from the series of images and then draws a picture combining both of these choices. Other elements can be added if the patient so wishes. The patient finally offers a narrative about the image created, as well as a title. This form of assessment, with its visual and narrative elements, has been found useful in identifying depressive and aggressive tendencies in patients. Silver's scoring system is complex, and interested readers are advised to read the original work.[34] In brief, the patient's image can be scored on 5-point scales denoting conceptual level, successful coordination of the chosen images, creativity or playfulness, negative or positive emotional content, and types of fantasy about the self or identifications. Occupational therapists may find that its contained approach to encouraging self-expression is useful for providing patients in the early stages of therapy with an opportunity to create personal narratives within a relatively structured, emotionally safe activity.

Case Study

Holly, aged 38, was admitted to an inpatient mental health setting and diagnosed with depression and self-harming behavior. At the time of admission, she was very withdrawn, did not make eye contact, and lacked energy to carry out even basic self-care tasks. Clinical notes revealed that Holly had lost both parents to cancer during her adolescence. Her mother had died when she was 12. She then lost her father when she was 17. She was an only child and inherited a considerable amount of money on the death of her father. Within a few months, she married. She now recognizes that it was her urgent need for companionship that led her into early marriage. Unfortunately, her husband, a much older man, became very controlling and critical. He insisted that they invest her money in a small grocery store. They had two daughters early in the marriage. Holly experienced severe postnatal depression after each birth but did not receive inpatient care. From an occupational perspective, Holly suffered occupational alienation for all of her adult life, having never wanted to run a grocery store, with its long hours and lack of leisure time. A recent economic downturn resulted in the couple losing their business and their apartment above the store. At this point, Holly decided to leave her husband and find an alternative way of life. His response was to try to gain custody of the children. Exposed to this level of stress, Holly's tendency to self-harm became much worse and she was admitted as an inpatient.

The occupational therapist initially found it difficult to engage Holly in any meaningful task. She was very withdrawn and her concentration was poor. The therapist offered her the SDT cards and, with a little encouragement, Holly selected the dinosaur and parachute. With some wariness and little verbalization, she drew a large lumpy bag, and after a long hesitation, titled it, "The dinosaur finds a safe place." When asked to say a little about the picture, Holly paused and then said quietly, "The dinosaur has found the parachute and never wondered where it came from. He wraps himself up in it. [pause] He is enjoying the shady hiding place." From an assessment point of view, the picture and narrative suggested some playfulness and some positive emotional content, with the dinosaur both needing sanctuary and being able to find it. While any interpretation remains subjective, the content may have been revealing of the patient's need for a safe, containing hiding place. The task was effective in offering Holly an outward focus when she was so withdrawn and a means of expression. It helped Holly to show some initiative and created the beginnings of a working alliance between the patient and therapist.

Despite some limited research into the reliability and validity of projective test scoring, concerns remain. Therapists' interpretations of the hidden meanings within patients' expressive work seem vulnerable to subjectivity, theoretical position, and length of clinical experience. This is well-illustrated by Janie Rhyne's example of a social worker, qualified arts therapist, and student therapist each giving very different interpretations of a patient's artwork. She suggested that the differing interpretations occurred because the social worker "was looking at what was wrong...I was looking for what was right...[the student] was looking for approval."[3(p264)]

If the therapist searches for meaning within the patient's expressive work, it is important to be mindful that the content may be affected not only by mental health or psychopathology, but also by the patient's developmental stage, humor, conscious choice, noncompliance, level of art education, and many other influences. Interpretations of thematic content in artwork and creative writing also seem vulnerable to therapist projections and fantasies. Some authors have advocated scrapping the use of projective tests altogether.[35] Others argue that the wide range of available tests generally offers incompatible information.[36] On the other hand, projective tests may be useful as part of a sensitive, nonthreatening, idiographic approach to assessment.[5,23] If the therapist is comfortable with metaphor and uncertainty and brings hypotheses rather than certainties to the patient's expressive communications, then projective material can enhance the patient-centered assessment process.[37]

ASSESSING EXPRESSIVE FORM OR STRATEGY RATHER THAN CONTENT

Some authors of standardized tests using expressive media have advocated abandoning the interpretation of content, with its inherent ambiguities of meaning, and focusing instead on scoring the form or strategy of the art-making process. Gantt devised the

Formal Elements Art Therapy Scale (FEATS) with colleagues.[38,39] This is a detailed scoring system for analyzing a series, both of freely made pictures and also images created in response to instructions to draw a Person-Picking-an-Apple-from-a-Tree (PPAT). The test presents patients with a specified and limited range of art materials. Fourteen 5-point scales are used by therapists to assess aspects of expression such as prominence of color, amount of energy depicted, integration of elements, logic, and realism.

The research of Gantt suggests that there may be a graphic equivalent of symptoms.[38,39] For example, Gantt proposes that depressed or elevated mood may reveal itself in the absence or presence of prominent color; that decreased or excessive psychological energy may be inferred from ratings of use of space within a picture, level of detail, and amount of effort that would be required to reproduce the image; and that cognitive deficits may be reflected in perseveration, rotation of image, and poor line quality. These elements to artwork seem relatively easy for therapists to agree upon, enhancing reliability. Clusters of graphic features may suggest mental states such as depression (eg, drawings with limited details, use of monochrome, small images in relation to the size of the paper, low implied energy, and high logic). However, other authors put forward different interpretations of the meanings of creative strategies. For example, light touch (leading to faint drawing) has been held to be suggestive of dysthymia.[36] Other therapists argue that there is no one-to-one relationship between imagery used and clinical features (for example, that there is no specific imagery associated with suicidal thoughts or sexual abuse). Brooke[25] points out that the test does not appear to consider the influence of developmental stage or culture. Further research is needed to establish its value in an occupational therapy context.

Another example of a formal test that attends to dynamic processes of artistic self-expression rather than content is the Diagnostic Drawing Series developed by Cohen and colleagues.[37] The authors of this test intend that patients should have a high quality art experience to facilitate a greater range of artistic exploration. The assessment asks the patient to create a series of pictures consisting of a free choice image, a tree, and a representation of their current feelings. By asking about feelings directly, the patient is thought to have more opportunity to reflect and thereby to control the artwork. On completion of the series, the patient is invited to comment verbally. There is a comprehensive scoring system by which each of the three drawings is assessed on 36 dimensions. High inter-rater agreement has been found on many of these dimensions, such as the use of idiosyncratic color, blending, integration of elements, enclosure, use of written words in the picture, and unusual placement of objects. However, an occupational therapist might question what value these features have as an assessment tool regarding the patient's level of everyday functioning, vulnerabilities, therapeutic needs, or goals. In any case, there is some controversy about the diagnostic value of these expressive patterns. Whereas Gantt found that limited use of color was associated with depression, Cohen and colleagues suggested that schizophrenic patients tended to create "feeling" pictures in monochrome. Nevertheless, multiple rating scales can reveal changes over time (eg, as a result of therapy), and there may be additional value if patients offer comments on the changes that they perceive over time in their expressive work during a retrospective review process.[40]

Validity and reliability of scoring are also difficult to establish with formal assessments using expressive media other than art. For example, Read-Johnson[41] describes the Diagnostic Role-Playing Test, one element of which requires patients to act out five roles (such as "grandfather") using props. He proposed that this formal assessment is unstructured enough so that patients can project their concerns and problems into their role play. While the sequence of role-playing is fairly clear, it is far from obvious how a therapist can confidently infer states such as "fluid and rigid boundaries" or other clinically important information from their behavioral observations.

With increasing interest in the therapeutic uses of creative writing, occupational therapists may wish to explore how patients' poetry or other forms of writing could be used as an assessment tool. Hynes[42] describes a checklist approach to evaluating patients' strengths and problems from a poetry assignment. For example, the therapist may rate whether the poem conveys a complete, coherent idea or shows personal insight. However, as with certain approaches to rating visual artwork, there seems to be an unfounded assumption that poems are always coherent and expressive of personal concerns. Therapists need to be mindful that patients might choose not to focus on their own psychosocial problems. In creative tasks, they might derive relief from current anxieties by exploring positive experiences, external events, or an imaginary character. Patients might also choose to work on perplexing or surprising combinations of ideas in their poetry or other creative writing to demonstrate their intellectual capacities or to challenge what they might perceive as their "demoted status" as an adult with mental health problems. Nevertheless, the patient's level of motivation or engagement with the creative writing task, spontaneity or guardedness, degree of cooperation within a group, and other behaviors shown during a creative writing task provide valuable assessment data for the occupational therapist. However, doubts remain as to whether patients necessarily use creative writing projects as opportunities for working through deeper personal concerns or disturbing memories unless they explicitly agree to do so in therapy. The choice of assessment focus depends upon whether the patient is primarily engaging in art as a purposeful activity or as a form of psychotherapy.

The final example of a formal assessment process using expressive media is a *wagon-building* exercise.[43] This is a creative activity in which group members put together rods, wheels, and other construction materials to their own design. Rather than scoring the quality of the object produced, Clark-Schock and colleagues describe assessment by a multidisciplinary team, including an occupational therapist, which focuses more on the creative process. The scoring focuses on patients' demonstrated self-esteem and self-confidence during the task, level of cooperation with peers and therapist, reality orientation, concentration, frustration tolerance, attention to detail, planning, and motivation. This checklist approach illustrates how information can be obtained from an expressive activity that is of relevance to determining patients' strengths and needs and to formulating an individually tailored therapy plan.

USING EXPRESSIVE MEDIA IN NONSTANDARDIZED ASSESSMENT

As relatively few occupational therapists have written in recent years about formal or standardized assessments using expressive media, it might be inferred that nonstandardized assessment is more common in practice. However, this is difficult to ascertain, as few clinical accounts have been published about this approach. Nevertheless, arts therapists have written many articles illustrating their use of expressive media in the clinical assessment process, and their experiences may be relevant. Interviews with occupational therapists carried out in preparation for this chapter also inform this discussion. Some clinical accounts suggest the great potential of expressive activities for helping patients to disclose less edited, more personal material. The therapeutic context is vital, though. Patients must feel emotionally safe to explore, play, and perhaps even to have fun if they are to express themselves freely.[44] Patients are likely to explore expressive media more fully in a physically and socially supportive environment rather than in a sterile or stressful context.

Nonstandardized approaches vary considerably from almost entirely unstructured to relatively structured (where the patient is asked to focus on a specified creative task). However, unlike standardized assessment approaches where there are firm directives for administration and scoring, with nonstandardized approaches there is greater scope for taking an individualized, patient-centered approach, and for therapists to apply their clinical reasoning skills.

To give one example of a relatively structured approach to assessment, yet with non-standardized scoring, Arrington and Yorgin[45] asked orphaned and homeless children in Kiev to create a free choice picture and to paint their favorite kind of day. The authors reveal a sensitive awareness to the loss and abuse experienced by these children. They offer detailed psychodynamic interpretations of picture content based on their clinical experiences. For example, they propose that children's depictions of angular mountains suggest anger, that severe red "gashes" across the paintings communicate grief and loss, and that objects drawn as having tongues or smoke might betray sexual abuse. Clearly, the children have creative license when painting and may not intend these meanings. Although it can be argued that the therapists' interpretations have questionable validity from a strictly scientific viewpoint, they do seem to form part of a sensitive holistic assessment. However, therapists do need to be mindful that their interpretations are hypotheses rather than indisputable facts about patients' experiences. Other types of assessment information need to be collected and integrated with the information derived from the creative arts activity.

Occupational therapists who take an explicitly patient-centered approach are likely to resist making their own interpretations of the patient's self-expression. Instead, they may prefer to ask patients to reflect on their creative work. Natalie Rogers, a patient-centered therapist, argues that therapists need to have as much empathy when interacting with the patient's artwork as they do when interacting verbally with the patient.[46] The patient may be asked to "talk to the painting"[20] or write a poem about his or her art.[1] This reflective response may deepen the interaction between therapist and patient, offering opportunities for more sensitive assessment, developing insight on the part of the patient, as well as fostering the therapeutic relationship.

Case Study, Continued

Holly returned to the dinosaur theme in a subsequent expressive art session. She was given a free choice of theme to paint, and she decided to draw the dinosaur ripping up the parachute with huge, pointed teeth. She created a series of cartoon-like drawings depicting the dinosaur in various stages of tussling with the parachute. Two stick figures sometimes appeared in a shadowy background. The occupational therapist was tempted to interpret anger and hostility from the prominent representations of teeth and biting. The shadow figures seemed to the therapist as possible depictions of the patient's children, their insubstantial forms revealing an ambivalent relationship. Their sketchy outlines, according to the guidelines given for several projective tests, might indicate shaky boundaries, anxiety, or weak identifications.[24] Such interpretations, if made with great tentativeness rather than certainty, open up a rich array of possibilities for understanding the patient more fully. However, Holly offered a different commentary. She said that she had enjoyed thinking about the dinosaur in recent days. The dinosaur was enjoying making holes in the parachute to let daylight in. He could feel his power coming back. He didn't need his security blanket any more. The figures were people from space who had dropped the parachute and had come back for it. They were disappointed to see the mess it was in. As in the first session, Holly demonstrated a capacity for positive fantasy, and this time she injected some humor. Slowly, she was also discovering that drawing was a deeply satisfying occupation and that her self-confidence was re-building. The therapist found that they were able to communicate more openly through the artwork than when they directly referred to Holly's mental health problems and occupational goals. This helped to build trust in the therapeutic process, and promoted in Holly a more positive sense of self.

A relatively structured approach called Expressive Assessment has been described by Rosner Kelly.[44] This therapist argues that multiple media, such as art, music, drama, and movement, are needed for a holistic assessment. The patient's preferences for some media over others may reflect his or her comfort in using verbalization, action, or fantasy. This in itself can suggest treatment goals and meaningful activities. Rosner Kelly suggests that therapists use a series of creative processes (eg, six drawings, two dramatic role plays, three mimes) to enable the therapist to evaluate aspects of the patient's functioning, such as motivation, expressiveness, creativity, capacity to channel feelings productively, level of initiative, or need for support. However, this approach can be classified as relatively nonstandardized, as the therapist appears to have plenty of scope for individual interpretation about what behaviors to look for during the patient's engagement in this series of expressive activities.

Some phenomenological research, as well as autobiographical writing, has established that people can offer considerable insights into the surface and symbolic meanings of their artwork and can interpret, at least to some extent, the conflicts, losses, and anxieties they have expressed.[47,48] While so many assessments using the creative arts have been carried out solely by therapists, this research suggests that there is scope for asking patients to reflect on their experience of the creative process and the personal significance of their creative products.

In their interviews, several occupational therapists have emphasized the power of informal observation to assess change, especially when a consistent staff member works with patients over several sessions. In art and creative writing, the patient can approach the paper as a "playground," revealing (or even formulating) coping strategies and styles of functioning that are not necessarily demonstrated in more routine everyday tasks. Some patients are shocked at their disclosures; some are relieved; some are cautious and mistrustful. Such observations may suggest new goals in therapy to support further progress. When using expressive media, patients can choose to be a "different person," enhancing their repertoire of behavior and helping them to break free of confining labels and roles such as "mental health service user." These glimpses provide powerful clues regarding the patient's occupational potential. The patient's response to having choices (eg, among arts and crafts projects) can reveal his or her strengths and vulnerabilities, such as assertiveness or indecision. Many expressive media such as art and creative writing projects result in a visible product. How the patient reacts to this (for example, taking pride or anticipating criticism, disposing of the object, entrusting it to the therapist, or presenting it as a gift to a loved one) again offers the occupational therapist a wealth of patient-centered information.

Unfortunately, not all members of the multidisciplinary team value the observations derived from expressive activities. One occupational therapist ruefully commented that staff on the ward tended to "think drama, music, and art are associated with being happy clappy." However, in other settings, occupational therapists are aware that team members really appreciate knowing how differently patients can function in environments outside the ward, using expressive media.

Summary

This chapter has identified the value of expressive media (both process and product) for contributing to the nonthreatening, holistic assessment of the patient. Patients often find that expressive work offers a safe container into which to pour difficult feelings. Many find that they can at least temporarily escape the restricting labels that have been imposed by virtue of their mental health problems and explore other facets of identity.

Therapists working in this field ground their assessments in diverse theoretical frameworks. While the patient's occupational performance remains in central focus, many occupational therapists make use of psychodynamic, humanistic, and behavioral concepts to gain insights into the individual patient's strengths, vulnerabilities, hidden conflicts, and concerns, all of which have relevance to occupational performance. Yet, it is important to remain cautious rather than overconfident about interpreting the meanings of patients' expressive work. There are no "cookbook" answers to complex clinical issues.

Some formal or standardized assessments using expressive media have focused primarily on psychiatric diagnosis, making an awkward alignment between creative activity and the biomedical model. For patient-centered occupational therapists, the results of some standardized assessments (eg, patients' use of color, enclosure, and space) may provide limited information about therapeutic needs and goals. Despite some research, doubts remain about the reliability and validity of many assessment tools, particularly projective techniques. Nevertheless, some formal assessment tools (such as those developed by Silver[34]) have undergone validity checks, and they offer patients a relatively contained expressive opportunity, permitting creative self-expression through media other than words and offering therapists valuable insights into patients' concerns.

Many therapists observe that patients can reveal functional strengths and vulnerabilities through their engagement with expressive media. Aspects of cognitive performance including concentration, initiative, planning, and problem solving are demonstrated. Expressive media enable communications about emotions, autonomy, self-worth, and identity. Research also reveals that some patients are capable of deep reflection about the meanings of their creative work. Such reflections may offer sensitive insights into psychosocial issues, as well as create possible directions for therapeutic intervention. Patients tend to be less psychologically constricted when working with expressive media, and this enables the empathetic therapist to regard the person in a more multifaceted way, opening up therapeutic opportunities.

Some therapists work with expressive media toward psychotherapeutic goals and tend to use formal and informal assessments to understand the individual patient in-depth. Others use expressive media primarily as a therapeutic activity, enhancing the patient's occupational repertoire. Assessments in the latter case focus on patients' occupational deficits and performance strengths. Nevertheless, the two approaches to occupational therapy cannot be cleanly segregated. For example, a patient may choose to reveal very personal information in a creative writing group that aims to develop writing skills and self-esteem rather than offering psychotherapy. Similarly, patients may gain artistic skills and ultimately a new leisure occupation from working with paint in a more explicitly psychotherapeutic context.

Contextual factors are also important in the assessment process. Expressive work is highly affected by the perceived and intended audience, the patient's familiarity with the materials, the behavior of others in a group, the physical environment, and the quality of the therapeutic relationship with the therapist. Interpretations of content and process should be made cautiously, as the expressive performance that the therapist witnesses is not simply or solely a manifestation of the patient's level of functioning.

Despite the need for caution, many therapists are adamant that expressive media offer rich assessment opportunities in mental health contexts. One therapist interviewed by Schmid reflected on her use of expressive arts with patients: "I guarantee I [got to] know more about those people in that 1-hour session than any of us do in the other 2 weeks…it's all the stuff that they can't just talk out."[6(p86)]

This chapter ends with a plea for more published evidence in this field. There is a need for occupational therapists to devise and validate further formal assessment tools using expressive media and to research the tacit knowledge and informal assessments that they use in clinical practice. Publication of detailed case studies would also contribute to occupational therapists' sensitive use of expressive media in assessment.

Acknowledgments

The author would like to thank the following occupational therapists for generously sharing aspects of their practice: Polly Blaydes, Rebecca Brown, Wendy Bryant, Pauline Cooper, Tracy Holmes, Kate Leszkowski, Kee Hean Lim, and Christine Thomson. Your help has been invaluable.

References

1. Malchiodi C, ed. *Expressive Therapies*. New York, NY: Guilford Press; 2005.
2. Meiklejohn A. Creative therapies: is there a place for them in modern and evolving occupational therapy practice? *Mental Health Occupational Therapy*. 2004;9:4.
3. Feder B, Feder E. *The Art and Science of Evaluation in the Arts Therapies*. Springfield, IL: Charles C. Thomas; 1998.
4. Creek J. *Occupational Therapy and Mental Health*. New York, NY: Churchill Livingstone; 1997.
5. Lloyd C, Papas V. Art as therapy within occupational therapy in mental health settings: a review of the literature. *BJOT*. 1999;62:31-37.
6. Schmid T. Meanings of creativity within occupational therapy practice. *AOTJ*. 2004;51:80-88.
7. Malchiodi C. Psychoanalytic, analytic and object relations approaches. In: Malchiodi C, ed. *Handbook of Art Therapy*. New York, NY: Guilford Press; 2003:41-57.
8. MacDonald E. Focus on research: the use of art by occupational therapists working with adult patients in mental health. *British Journal of Occupational Therapy*. 2001;61:533.
9. Holder V. The use of creative activities within occupational therapy. *British Journal of Occupational Therapy*. 2001;64:103-105.
10. Mee J, Sumsion T, Craik C. Mental health patients confirm the value of occupation in building competence and self-identity. *British Journal of Occupational Therapy*. 2004;67:225-233.
11. Frye B. Art and multiple personality disorder: an expressive framework for occupational therapy. *Am J Occup Ther*. 1990; 44:1013-1022.
12. Thompson M, Blair S. Creative arts in occupational therapy: ancient history or contemporary practice? *Occup Ther Int*. 1998;5:49-65.
13. Harries P. Facilitating change in anorexia nervosa: the role of occupational therapy. *British Journal of Occupational Therapy*. 1992;55:334-339.
14. American Occupational Therapy Association. Occupational therapy practice framework: domain and process. *Am J Occup Ther*. 2002;56:609-639.
15. Atkinson K, Wells C. *Creative Therapies: A Psychodynamic Approach Within Occupational Therapy*. Cheltenham, England: Stanley Thornes; 2000.
16. Robbins A. Transference and countertransference within the schizoid phenomenon In: Robbins A, ed. *The Artist as Therapist*. London: Jessica Kingsley; 2000:145-186.
17. Case C. Brief encounters: thinking about images in assessment. *Inscape*. 1998;3:26-33.

18. Tuby M. Jung and the symbol: resolution of conflicting opposites. In: Pearson J, ed. *Discovering the Self Through Drama and Movement*. London: Jessica Kingsley; 1996:34-38.
19. Robbins A, Goffia-Girasek D. Materials as an extension of the holding environment. In: Robbins A, ed. *The Artist as Therapist*. London: Jessica Kingsley; 2000:104-115.
20. McNiff S. *Art and Medicine*. Boston, MA: Shambhala; 1992.
21. Bruscia K. Standards for clinical assessment in the arts therapies. *Art Psychother*. 1988;15:5-10.
22. Henare D, Hocking C, Smythe L. Chronic pain: understanding through the use of art. *British Journal of Occupational Therapy*. 2003;66:511-518.
23. Kaplan F. Art-based assessments. In: Malchiodi C, ed. *Handbook of Art Therapy*. New York, NY: Guilford Press; 2003:25-36.
24. Oster G, Gould P. *Using Drawings in Assessment and Therapy: A Guide For Mental Health Professionals*. New York, NY: Brunner/Mazel; 1987.
25. Brooke S. *Tools of the Trade: A Therapist's Guide to Art Therapy Assessments*. Springfield, IL: Charles C Thomas; 2004.
26. Cramer-Azima F. The Azima Battery: an overview. In: Hemphill BJ, ed. *The Evaluative Process In Psychiatric Occupational Therapy*. Thorofare, NJ: SLACK Incorporated; 1982: 57-61.
27. Evascus MG. The Goodman Battery. In: Hemphill BJ, ed. *The Evaluative Process In Psychiatric Occupational Therapy*. Thorofare, NJ: SLACK Incorporated; 1982:85-125.
28. Drake M. The use of expressive media as an assessment tool in mental health. In: Hemphill-Pearson BJ, ed. *Assessments in Occupational Therapy Mental Health: An Integrative Approach*. Thorofare, NJ: SLACK Incorporated; 1999:129-138.
29. Polatajko H, Kaiserman E. House-Tree-Person projective technique: a validation of its use in occupational therapy. *Can J Occup Ther*. 1986;53:197-207.
30. Mills A, Cohen B, Meneses J. Reliability and validity of the Diagnostic Drawing Series. *Art Psychother*. 1993;20:83-88.
31. Lev-Wiesel R, Shvero T. An exploratory study of self-figure drawings of individuals diagnosed with schizophrenia. *Art Psychother*. 2003;30:13-16.
32. Machover K. *Personality Projection in the Drawing of the Human Figure*. Springfield, IL: Charles C. Thomas; 1949.
33. Thomson M. *On Art and Therapy: An Exploration*. Chadlington, England: Free Association Books; 1997.
34. Silver R. *Three Art Assessments*. New York, NY: Brunner-Routledge; 2002.
35. Hunsley J, Lee C, Wood J. Controversial and questionable assessment techniques. In: Lilienfeld S, Lynn S, Lohr J, eds. *Science and Pseudoscience in Clinical Psychology*. New York, NY: Guilford Press; 2003:39-76.
36. Cohen B, Hammer J, Singer S. The Diagnostic Drawing Series: a systematic approach to art therapy evaluation and research. *Art Psychother*. 1988;15:11-21.
37. Groth-Marnatt G. *Handbook of Psychological Assessment*. 3rd ed. New York, NY: Wiley; 1997.
38. Gantt L. Brief report: The Formal Elements Art Therapy Scale: a measurement system for global variables in art. *Art Therapy: AATA Journal*. 2001;18:50-55.
39. Gantt L. The case for formal art therapy assessments. *Art Therapy: AATA Journal*. 2004;21:18-29.
40. Schaverien J. The retrospective review of pictures: data for research in art therapy. In: Payne H, ed. *Handbook of Inquiry in the Arts Therapies*. London: Jessica Kingsley; 1993:91-103.
41. Read-Johnson D. The diagnostic role-playing test. *Art Psychother*. 1988;15: 23-36.
42. Hynes A. Some considerations concerning assessment in poetry therapy and interactive bibliotherapy. *Art Psychother*. 1988;15:55-62.
43. Clark-Schock K, Turner Y, Bovee T. A multidisciplinary psychiatric assessment: the introductory group. *Art Psychother*. 1988;15:79-82.
44. Rosner Kelly C. Expressive therapy assessment. *Art Psychother*. 1988;15:63-70.
45. Arrington D, Yorgin P. Art therapy as a cross-cultural means to assess psychosocial health in homeless and orphaned children in Kiev. *Art Therapy: AATA Journal*. 2001;18:80-88.
46. Rogers N. *The Creative Connection: Expressive Arts as Healing*. Palo Alto, CA: Science and Behavior Books; 1999.
47. Reynolds F. Managing depression through needlecraft creative activities: a qualitative study. *Art Psychother*. 2000;27:107-114.
48. Reynolds F. Women's experiences of managing depression through textile artwork. *Mental Health Occupational Therapy*. 2002;7:7-9.

PART IV:
LEARNING ASSESSMENTS

THE PERFORMANCE ASSESSMENT OF SELF-CARE SKILLS (PASS)

Margo B. Holm, PhD, OTR/L, FAOTA, ABDA
Joan C. Rogers, PhD, OTR/L, FAOTA

"People may doubt what you say, but they will always believe what you do." ~ Anonymous

Introduction

The Performance Assessment of Self-Care Skills, Version 3.1 (PASS)[1] is a performance-based, criterion-referenced, observational tool designed to assist practitioners in documenting functional status and change. The PASS consists of 26 core tasks, categorized in 4 functional domains: 5 functional mobility (FM), 3 personal self-care (PSC), 14 instrumental activities of daily living (IADL) with a cognitive emphasis (CIADL), and 4 IADL with a physical emphasis (PIADL). Observed patient performance is rated for independence, safety, and adequacy. The PASS has two versions—the PASS-Clinic and the PASS-Home. Because the instrument was designed for practitioners to assess the types of assistance necessary for a patient to return to the community (PASS-Clinic) or remain in the community (PASS-Home), the instrument has a disproportionate emphasis on IADL. Both versions of the PASS include the same tasks, same subtask criteria, and the same directions. However, the task materials differ in each setting, with task materials being provided in the clinic and patients using many of their own task materials in their homes. The PASS is also designed to assist practitioners in treatment and discharge planning by identifying the type and amount of assistance required for successful task performance, as well as risks to safety and the specific point of task breakdown. Because the PASS is criterion-referenced (the patient is rated according to pre-established performance criteria versus a norm), it may be given in total, or selected tasks may be used alone or in combination. Tasks chosen for administration can thus be responsive to the need for the assessment, namely the reason for the referral, intervention planning, change in status, or discharge disposition. In addition to the 26 core tasks of the PASS, the developers have formulated a template for developing new PASS tasks.[2] In this chapter, we will describe the conceptual foundations of the PASS, its data collection and rating forms, its psychometric properties, and its utility in clinical practice.

Conceptual Foundations of the PASS

The PASS combines two conceptual foundations of assessment: interactive assessment and graduated prompting. *Interactive (dynamic) assessment*[3-5] is one conceptual basis for the design and structure of the PASS. The creator of the interactive assessment approach is considered by most to be Vygotsky (1896-1934), a Soviet psychologist.[6] Vygotsky described a zone of proximal (potential) development as the difference between a patient's independent performance on a test and the performance when the patient is assisted or guided on a test. Interactive assessment consists of establishing a patient's current level of performance without assistance, providing the type and amount of assistance required for improved performance, and documenting the outcome of the mediation on later task performance.[7] Most testing prohibits an assessor from assisting a patient during testing, but because the PASS uses interactive assessment, systematic assistance is encouraged when necessary. Moreover, the data collection and rating forms include space to document such assistance.

The second conceptual foundation used in the design and structure of the PASS is *graduated prompting*.[8,9] Graduated prompting incorporates a hierarchy of prompts that are used only when there is a breakdown in task performance and only in a specific sequence. Hierarchies can be based on the power of the assist,[10] the cost of the assist based on the interventionist's time, or the level of intrusiveness to the patient.[9] The layout and design of the PASS data collection and rating forms reflect both conceptual foundations.

Structure and Rating Scales of the PASS

STRUCTURE OF THE PASS

Conditions and Instructions

Each PASS task includes two types of directions for the assessment: Conditions and Instructions. *Conditions* includes the context for the task (eg, kitchen, bathroom, stairway), the materials (eg, utility bills, prescription bottle, wallet with real dollars and coins) and how they are to be arranged (eg, centered in front of the patient, on bed next to pillow, items available on the table), and the starting position of the patient (eg, seated at a table, positioned next to the foot of the bed, positioned at the bottom of the stairs). *Instructions* includes the standardized wording for the instructions to be given to the patient, as well as cues to the practitioner (eg, wait for response). The materials and equipment used in the PASS are common household items (eg, flashlight, mixing bowl, paring knife), and specifications, when relevant (eg, 1-quart sauce pan), are listed in the task Conditions. Items are purchased by the practitioner to develop the kit. The PASS-Clinic kit requires more items than the PASS-Home kit because in the home patients use many of their own items. Both kits include some adaptive equipment (eg, lighted magnifying glass, large button and display calculator), some of which may already be present in a clinic. It is recommended that the kit for the PASS-Home be transported in a small rolling suitcase.

Tasks, Subtasks, and Interactive Assessment

The 26 PASS core tasks (Table 7-1) consist of 163 criterion-referenced subtasks that the practitioner uses to rate performance.

Table 7-1

PASS Tasks Categorized by Functional Domain

Domain	Tasks
FM	Bed mobility
	Stair use
	Toilet transfers
	Bathtub and shower transfers
	Indoor walking
PSC	Oral hygiene
	Trimming toenails
	Dressing
CIADL	Shopping (money management)
	Bill paying by check (money management)
	Checkbook balancing (money management)
	Mailing (money management)
	Telephone use
	Medication management
	Obtaining critical information from the media (auditory current events)
	Obtaining critical information from the media (visual current events)
	Small repairs (home maintenance)
	Home safety (environmental awareness)
	Playing bingo (leisure)
	Oven use (meal preparation)
	Stovetop use (meal preparation)
	Use of sharp utensils (meal preparation)
PIADL	Cleanup after meal preparation (light housework)
	Changing bed linens (heavy housework)
	Sweeping (home maintenance)
	Bending, lifting, & carrying out the garbage (heavy housework)

Note: FM = Functional mobility; PSC = Personal self-care; CIADL = Instrumental activities of daily living (IADL) with a cognitive emphasis; PIADL = IADL with a physical emphasis.

Task subtasks vary between 2 and 12 subtasks, depending on the complexity of the task being observed. The patient is given standardized directions, and standardized task materials are presented in the clinic. In the home, however, patients use as many of their own task materials as possible. Independence in task performance is rated using an interactive assessment approach. When a patient is no longer able to proceed independently with a task (point of subtask breakdown), the practitioner begins the interactive assessment process using a nine-level system of graduated prompts to (1) facilitate initiation, continuation, or completion of task performance; (2) to alert the patient to safety concerns; and/or (3) to address concerns about task quality or inefficiency in task process. When prompts are necessary, the type and number of prompts needed to improve performance are recorded for each relevant subtask, which identifies the patient's potential for future task performance.[6] This blending of interactive assessment and graduated prompting yields a profile of patient performance that identifies the exact point of subtask breakdown, the type and number of prompts that the patient needed for successful task performance during the assessment, and the types of prompts that can support a patient's potential task performance. The profile of prompts recorded on the data-collection and rating forms identifies which prompts were beneficial to a patient, in other words, those that enabled, improved, or resulted in successful task performance. These data are critical for efficient intervention and discharge planning in today's health care environment.

DATA-COLLECTION AND RATING FORMS

PASS tasks are rated on three distinct concepts: Independence, Safety, and Adequacy of outcome. Each concept is scored on a predefined four-point ordinal scale (Table 7-2). For each PASS task, the data-collection and rating form includes a section for *Subtask Criteria, Independence Data, Safety Data,* and *Adequacy Data (Quality and Process)* as well as a section for the *Independence, Safety,* and *Adequacy Summary Scores.* Under *Subtask Criteria,* the observable criterion behaviors for each subtask are demarcated with a double underscore, and are the relevant behaviors for rating task Independence and Adequacy-Process. The criterion behaviors demarcated with a single underscore define the Adequacy-Quality with which the behaviors are to be carried out, with relevant examples for making that judgment in the parentheses that follow (Table 7-3).

Using the PASS Data Grids to Record Observations

On the data-collection and rating form, under Independence Data, for each subtask a grid of the hierarchical prompts is included for the practitioner to place a check mark each time a prompt is given for the patient to accomplish a subtask. The prompt hierarchy includes nine levels of graduated prompts. When a task cannot be performed independently, the practitioner provides the least powerful/intrusive type of assistance to facilitate task performance, safety, and/or adequacy. The types of prompts, beginning with the least assistive and progressing to the most assistive are: (1) verbal supportive, (2) verbal nondirective, (3) verbal directive, (4) gestures, (5) task object or environmental rearrangement, (6) demonstration, (7) physical guidance, (8) physical support, and (9) total assist (see Table 7-3). The grid is left blank if the patient needs no assistance.

Task safety is also anchored to each subtask. The practitioner again places a check mark in the *Safety Data* grid (not shown in Table 7-3) opposite the relevant subtask if any risks to safety are observed during task performance or if the practitioner is required to intervene because of a risk to patient safety or the environment. Therefore, the PASS helps to identify the specific aspect of task performance where safety concerns were evident. Likewise, task adequacy is also noted during task performance, and the *Adequacy Data* grid (not shown in Table 7-3) enables practitioners to place a check mark to identify task-adequacy problems related to the quality of subtask performance and/or the process of subtask performance. For each subtask criterion, sample quality standards are provided.

Table 7-2

Rating Scales for PASS Independence, Safety, and Adequacy

Score	Independence	Safety	Adequacy	
			Quality	Process
3	No assists given for task initiation, continuation, or completion	Safe practices were observed	Acceptable (standards met)	Subtasks performed with precision & economy of effort & action
2	No Level 7-9 assists given, but occasional Level 1-6 assists given	Minor risks were evident but no assistance provided	Acceptable (standards met, but improvement possible)	Subtasks generally performed w/precision & economy of effort & action; occasional lack of efficiency, redundant or extraneous action; no missing steps
1	No Level 9 assists given; occasional Level 7 or 8 assists given, or continuous Level 1-6 assists given	Risks to safety were observed and assistance given to prevent potential harm	Marginal (standards partially met)	Subtasks generally performed w/lack of precision and/or economy of effort & action; consistent extraneous or redundant actions; steps may be missing
0	Level 9 assists given, or continuous Level 7 or 8 assists given, or unable to initiate, continue, or complete subtask or task	Risks to safety of such severity were observed that task was stopped or taken over to prevent harm	Unacceptable (standards not met)	Subtasks are consistently performed w/lack of precision and/or economy of effort & action so that task progress is unattainable

Process-outcome data are linked to task actions and are rated for the precision, economy of effort, and completeness with which a subtask is performed. Therefore, each time a prompt is provided, the practitioner uses the data grids to note the level of assistance provided (independence), as well as to note whether the assist was given to improve task safety or the adequacy of the task outcome.

PASS SUMMARY SCORES

Independence is rated for each subtask of a PASS task, and the Independence summary score for any task consists of the mean of all task subtask ratings. Safety for each PASS task is a single summary score that reflects total subtask safety. Adequacy is also a single summary score that reflects the combined quality and process data. If quality and

Table 7-3

Example of PASS Independence Data Grid for Two Medication-Management Subtasks

Independence data

Subtask	Verbal supportive	Verbal nondirective	Verbal directive	Gestures	Task/environment modification	Demonstration	Physical guidance	Physical support	Total assist
Assist Level →	1	2	3	4	5	6	7	8	9
1 <u>Reports next time</u> medication to be taken <u>correctly</u> (based on testing time, matches directions on label)	√√√	√							
2 <u>Distributes pills from first pill bottle</u> into <u>correct</u> time slots <u>for the next 2 days</u> (all pills & all slots indicated, days indicated)	√√√	√√√	√√						

process yield different scores, the lower of the two scores is used. Use of the lowest score was chosen so that patients are not put in a situation of risk through practitioner overestimation of task safety and adequacy.

Psychometric Properties of the PASS

POPULATIONS

The PASS was originally designed for an adult population. However, the PASS has been used to document functional status and change in adolescents and adults from various diagnostic populations, including depression, bipolar disorder, dementia, schizophrenia, developmental delay, spinal cord injury, multiple sclerosis, head trauma, stroke, heart failure, cardiac arrest, heart transplant, artificial heart, osteoarthritis, and macular degeneration. It has also been used with healthy older adult populations in the United States and Canada.

RELIABILITY AND VALIDITY

Reliability

Test-retest reliability was established by administering the PASS to 20 older adults, 4 subjects from each of the following diagnostic populations: osteoarthritis, heart failure, dementia, and depression, as well as healthy controls. For both the PASS-Clinic and PASS-Home, the reliability intervals were 3 days. PASS-Clinic test-retest reliability was Independence, r = .92; Safety, 89% agreement; and Adequacy, r = .82. PASS-Home test-retest reliability was Independence, r = .96; Safety, 90% agreement; and Adequacy, r = .97. Therefore, the PASS demonstrated good to excellent measurement stability. Inter-observer reliability was established by administering the PASS to 25 older adults from the same diagnostic categories. A total of five different practitioners participated in dyads. Percent agreement among 21 raters for the PASS-Clinic was Independence, 92%; Safety, 93%; and Adequacy, 90%. PASS-Home inter-observer agreement among 26 raters was Independence, 96%; Safety, 97%; and Adequacy, 88%. Therefore, decision consistency among practitioners observing the same patient perform everyday tasks was good to excellent. PASS-Clinic and PASS-Home tasks also had good to excellent interobserver reliabilities.

Validity

Content validity of the PASS is based on the interview schedules of the OARS Multidimensional Functional Assessment Questionnaire: Activities of Daily Living,[11] the Comprehensive Assessment and Referral,[12] the rating scales for Physical Self-Maintenance and Instrumental Self-Maintenance,[13] and the Functional Assessment Questionnaire.[14] The self-report items from these tools were adapted and converted into performance-based items consisting of specific tasks, subtasks, and performance criteria.

Evidence of the construct validity of the PASS is gleaned from multiple investigations. Construct validity of the unidimensionality of the Independence, Safety, and Adequacy scales of the PASS was established using exploratory factor analysis, specifically Cattell's scree test.[15] For all three constructs, examination of the scree plots revealed the presence of a dominant construct that met the unidimensionality assumption for each construct.[16] Construct validity of the 26 core tasks was confirmed in several studies. For older adults with depression, Rasch analysis was used to identify task-difficulty differences between inpatients and outpatients, and those who were readmitted to an inpatient facility versus those who were not readmitted within one year.[16] For older adult females with depression, Rasch analysis revealed that all PIADL, CIADL, PSC, and FM (in that order) were more difficult for those who required inpatient treatment (n = 60, mean age = 73.7 + 7.1, 93% Caucasian) than those who required outpatient treatment (n = 59, mean age = 75.7 + 4.1, 81% Caucasian). Although Rasch analysis revealed no significant differences in the difficulty level of inpatients with depression who were readmitted (n = 15; 13 females; mean age = 73.6 + 7.8, 100% Caucasian)/non-readmitted (n = 43; 37 females; mean age = 72.84 + 7.0, 91% Caucasian) within 1 year of discharge, those who were readmitted consistently demonstrated greater difficulty in task performance at discharge, especially in the CIADL and PIADL domains. Likewise, for female patients with depression, those with slower cognitive processing speeds (n = 76, mean age = 74.2 + 5.9, 84 % Caucasian) on the Trails B (a neuropsychological test of cognitive flexibility) showed significantly worse performance in CIADL, PSC, PIADL, and FM (in that order) than those patients with depression and faster cognitive processing speeds (n = 23, mean age = 75.5 + 4.7, 100% Caucasian).[16]

In a comparison of female heart failure patients (n = 55, mean age 78.3 + 5.2, 84% Caucasian) with female healthy older adults (n = 57, mean age = 78.7 + 2.8, 86% Caucasian), at baseline and at the 6-month follow-up, task performance for those with heart failure was less independent and adequate but equally safe as that of the healthy older adults. At baseline, those with heart failure showed mild depression, whereas at the 6-month follow-up, both groups exhibited mild depression.[17] In a similar study comparing older adult females who had osteoarthritis of the knee (n = 56, mean age 81.2 + 2.9, 86% Caucasian) with the same healthy older adult group, performance of the osteoarthritis group was significantly less independent and adequate for FM, PSC, and IADL, and also significantly less safe for FM.[18]

SENSITIVITY TO CHANGE

In 274 older females (mean age = 78.8 + 5.1, 86% Caucasian), the PASS detected significant (p < .001) change in independence of performance over 6 months for FM, PSC, CIADL, PIADL, and the overall constructs of Independence and Adequacy. Safety did not evidence change because subjects remained consistently safe in spite of deteriorating independence and adequacy. In a preliminary study of 217 stroke survivors (94 females; mean age = 64.4 + 15.4; 93.5 % Caucasian), the PASS was able to detect change in function between 24 hours post-stroke and 5 days, 3 months, 6 months, 9 months, and 12 months post-stroke for all three constructs (ie, Independence, Safety, Adequacy) and all four domains (ie, FM, PSC, CIADL, PIADL) of function. Significant changes (p < .05 or greater) were found for Independence, Safety, and Adequacy, as well as FM and CIADL. The PASS PSC and PIADL domain tasks measured improvement over time, but the changes were not significant.

METHOD EFFECT

In addition to the objective PASS-Clinic and PASS-Home, there are also subjective self-report (PASS-SR), proxy-report (PASS-PR), and clinical judgment (PASS-CJ) versions of the PASS, each with acceptable psychometric properties. The PASS-SR and the PASS-PR include the same 26 core PASS tasks, but they also address the concepts of habit and skill. Patients (or their proxies) are asked "Do you manage your medications *routinely* without assistance?" (habit), as well as "Can you manage your medications without assistance?" (skill). Rogers and Holm[19] examined perceived habits (PASS-SR), perceived skills (PASS-SR), and demonstrated skills (PASS-Home) in 59 older females (mean age = 75.7 + 4.1, 81% Caucasian) being treated for depression. Overall, the subjects' self-reported skills were greater than their demonstrated skills, which in turn were greater than their self-reported habits. Thus, the performance-based objective skill measure (PASS-Home) yielded greater disability than the subjective skill measure (PASS-SR), which has many implications for intervention planning.

Another methodological study examined five methods of collecting functional status data in patients with osteoarthritis of the knee.[20] The PASS-Home was used as the gold standard, because it assesses the "lived in" environment, and functional status on the PASS-Home was compared with functional status ratings on the PASS-SR, PASS-PR,

PASS-CJ, and PASS-Clinic. Overall, the subjective self-report and proxy-report methods had the greatest concordance with performance in the home; however, depending on the task and domain, discordance was often 31% to 54%, indicating that even at best, assessment methods are not interchangeable.

OTHER STUDIES

Other research on the use of the PASS or PASS items with cognitively and physically impaired older adults has been reported at conferences,[21-24] and in the literature.[25] Research on the relationship of the PASS with neuropsychology measures has also been reported in the literature.[26-28]

Clinical Utility of the PASS

Because the PASS is criterion-referenced, each task can stand alone. This allows practitioners to select tasks that are relevant for each patient's lifestyle. This is key to a patient-centered approach. Additionally, if there is an everyday task vital to a patient's lifestyle that is not included in the 26 PASS core tasks, the task development template can be used to develop a new task. The interactive assessment strategy used in the PASS also allows practitioners to identify the point of task breakdown as well as assistance strategies that result in a better functional outcome. This information is valuable for both intervention and discharge planning. Finally, the greater proportion of PASS tasks consist of IADL tasks. This makes the PASS unique among functional assessment tools because it enables practitioners to address task performance that is necessary for successful community living.

Summary

The PASS is a reliable and valid performance-based observational tool for assessing everyday tasks necessary for living in the community. The PASS yields scores for independence, safety, and adequacy of performance. Because it is criterion-referenced, practitioners can select to administer the total tool, or only those items relevant to the patient. The use of interactive assessment when administering the PASS enables practitioners to identify the point of task breakdown as well as types of assistance that enable improvement in task performance. Self-report, proxy-report, and clinical judgment versions of the PASS are also available.

References

1. Rogers JC, Holm MB. *Performance Assessment of Self-Care Skills (3.1)*. Pittsburgh, PA: Authors; 1984. (Available from M. B. Holm, 5018 Forbes Tower, University of Pittsburgh, Pittsburgh, PA, 15260, or mbholm@pitt.edu).
2. Finlayson M, Havens B, Holm MB, Van Denend T. Integrating a performance-based observation measure of functional status into a population-based longitudinal study of aging. *Can J Aging*. 2003;22:185-195.
3. Fuerstein R, Rand Y, Hoffman MB. *The Dynamic Assessment of Retarded Performers: The Learning Potential Assessment Device—Theory, Instruments and Techniques*. Baltimore, MD: University Park Press; 1979.
4. Missiuna C. Dynamic assessment: a model for broadening assessment in occupational therapy. *Can J Occup Ther*. 1987;54:17-21.

5. Tzuriel D, Haywood HC. The development of interactive-dynamic approaches to assessment of learning potential. In: Haywood HC, Tzurial D, eds. *Interactive Assessment*. New York: Springer-Verlag; 1991:3-37.

6. Vygotsky LS. *Mind in Society: The Development of Higher Psychological Processes*. Cambridge, MA: Harvard University Press; 1978.

7. Haywood HC, Tzuriel D, Vaught S. Psychoeducational assessment from a transactional perspective. In: Haywood HC, Tzurial D, eds. *Interactive Assessment*. New York: Springer-Verlag; 1991:38-63.

8. Gold MW. Stimulus factors in skill training of the retarded on a complex assembly task: Acquisition, transfer, and retention. *Am J Ment Def*. 1972;76:517-526.

9. Lent JR, McLean BM. The trainable retarded: the technology of teaching. In: Haring NG, Schiefelbush RL, eds. *Teaching Special Children*. New York: McGraw-Hill; 1976: 197-231.

10. Gold MW. *Try Another Way Training Manual*. Champaign, IL: Research Press; 1980.

11. Pfeiffer E. *Multidimensional Functional Assessment: The OÀRS Methodology*. Durham, NC: Center for the Study of Aging and Development; 1975.

12. Gurland B, Kuriansky J, Sharpe L, Simon R, Stiller P, Birkett P. The Comprehensive Assessment and Referral Evaluation (CARE). *Int J Aging Hum Dev*. 1977;8;9-42.

13. Lawton MP, Moss M, Fulcomer M, Kleban MH. A research and service oriented multilevel assessment instrument. *J Gerontol*. 1982;37:91-99.

14. Pfeffer RI. The Functional Activities Questionnaire. In: McDowell I, Newell C, eds. *Measuring Health: A Guide to Rating Scales and Questionnaires*. 2nd ed. New York: Oxford Press; 1987:92-95.

15. Cattell RB. The screen test for the number of factors. *Multivariate Beh Res*. 1966;1:245-276.

16. Chisholm D. Disability in Older Adults with Depression (unpublished doctoral dissertation). Pittsburgh, PA: University of Pittsburgh; 2005.

17. Raina KD. Disability in older women with heart failure (unpublished doctoral dissertation). Pittsburgh, PA: University of Pittsburgh; 2005.

18. Rogers JC, Holm MB, Beach S, Schulz R, Starz T. Task independence, safety, and adequacy among nondisabled and OAK-disabled older women. *Arthritis Care Res*. 2001;45:410-418.

19. Rogers JC, Holm MB. Daily living skills and habits of older women with depression. *Occup Ther J Res*. 2000; 20:68S-85S.

20. Rogers JC, Holm MB, Beach S, et al. Concordance of four methods of disability assessment using performance in the home as the criterion method. *Arthritis Rheum (Arthritis Care Res)*. 2003;49:640-647.

21. Holm MB, Rogers JC. Functional assessment outcomes: differences between settings. *Arch Phys Med Rehabil*. 1990;71:761.

22. Holm MB, Rogers JC. Functional performance differences between the health care setting and the home. *Gerontologist*. 1990;30:327A.

23. Holm MB, Rogers JC. In-home safety for persons with cognitive impairment. *Gerontologist*. 1990;30:217A.

24. Shook J, Beck C. Caring for cognitively and physically impaired nursing home residents: is there a difference in the assistance needed from staff? *Gerontologist*. 1989;29:293A.

25. Skurla E, Rogers C, Sunderland T. Direct assessment of activities of daily living in Alzheimer's disease. A controlled study. *J Am Geriatr Soc*. 1988;36:97-103.

26. Goldstein G, McCue M, Rogers JC, Nussbaum PD. Diagnostic differences in memory test based predictions of functional capacity in the elderly. *Neuropsychol Rehabil*. 1992;2:307-317.

27. McCue M, Rogers JC, Goldstein G. Relationships between neuropsychological and functional assessment in depressed and demented elderly. *Rehabil Psychol*. 1990;35:91-99.

28. Rogers JC, Holm MB, Goldstein G, Nussbaum PD. Stability and change in functional assessment of patients with geropsychiatric disorders. *Am J Occup Ther*. 1994;48:914-918.

8

THE COMPREHENSIVE OCCUPATIONAL THERAPY EVALUATION (COTE)

Sara J. Brayman, PhD, OTR/L, FAOTA

"The art of remediation is the matching of capacity with expectation." Gail Fidler, Dialogues with Gale Fidler, Texas Woman's University, February, 1991, Dallas, TX.

Introduction

The *Occupational Therapy Practice Framework, Domain and Process*[1] describes the focus and delivery of occupational therapy services. Because the focus of the profession is on patient engagement in occupation, practitioners must also be concerned with the factors that underlie that engagement. The domain of occupational therapy is facilitating the patient's engagement in the areas of occupation (Activities of Daily Living, Instrumental Activities of Daily Living, Work, Play, Leisure, and Social Participation). This is viewed as the "overarching outcome of the occupational therapy process."[1(p615)] The process that occupational therapists employ involves evaluation, intervention, and outcomes. The Comprehensive Occupational Therapy Evaluation (COTE) is an instrument that assists therapists in evaluating some patient factors, performance skills, and patterns that impact engagement in occupation.

The COTE is a rating scale that provides a "thumbnail" picture of a person's occupational performance. It was originally designed as a means to delineate occupational therapy's role in a treatment milieu within an inpatient psychiatric setting and to provide a standard and objective means of reporting patient behaviors observed by occupational therapists. This scale enables the therapist to report a large volume of diverse and pertinent information quickly in a consistent format using defined terminology. This chapter includes a description of the original scale and a listing of the behaviors and their definitions.

The COTE was developed in 1975 by five occupational therapists, a psychiatrist, and a psychologist practicing at the Greenville Hospital System in Greenville, South Carolina. The instrument was designed to address four objectives. The first objective concerned the focus of the instrument—to identify the behaviors that occurred in and were particularly pertinent to the practice of occupational therapy. The behaviors included in the COTE Scale reflected occupational therapy's traditional emphasis on occupational performance. Occupational therapy often provides the only opportunity for patients to practice behaviors necessary to interact with objects in the environment and to perform daily life tasks. Daily life requires that individuals interact with others and master the tasks necessary to function in their occupational environment. Many of the behaviors included in the COTE were identified in 1954 by Ayres as being important factors in successful participation and production in a work setting.[2] These behaviors, which included punctuality, organization, initiative, responsibility, dependability, attention to detail, neatness, interest, and concentration, served as the basis for this instrument.

The second objective guiding the development of the COTE was to define the behaviors in a manner that would allow the observations of different occupational therapists to correspond. Each of the behaviors included on the COTE was defined and subdivided into five levels of performance. These definitions, complete with the description of each level of performance were printed on the instrument. This immediate reference was included to decrease misinterpretation by both the reader and the therapist and to eliminate the use of vague descriptions.

The third objective related to finding an efficient and effective tool to communicate a great deal of information to the physician and other members of the treatment team. Therapists were overwhelmed by the amount of documentation required by the facility and the payers, and by the excessive time needed to complete the paperwork. This resulted in documentation that contained little useful information about patient performance. Narrative notes often reflected single events occurring during therapy, rather than ongoing patient behaviors. The physicians valued occupational therapy and wanted more information about how their patients performed during occupational therapy. The COTE imposes a structure for reporting observations made during the occupational therapy process.

The fourth objective guiding the development of the scale was to provide an efficient means of retrieving data needed for treatment planning and evaluating treatment results. Since therapists used numbers to rate behaviors on the COTE, progress or changes in behaviors could be easily noted and measured.

The content of the COTE has changed little since its development in 1975. Some of the behaviors have been redefined, and one item, conceptualization, which addresses the ability to abstract, has been added to the list of behaviors. The COTE was originally designed as a grid with cells for therapists to record daily behaviors over the several days of hospital stay. The grid format now includes only space to record initial and follow-up records of behavior.

Behaviors Assessed by the COTE Scale

Twenty-six behaviors are included in the COTE. These are divided into three areas: 1) general behaviors, 2) interpersonal behaviors, and 3) task behaviors. All behaviors are rated on a 5-point scale. The eight behaviors included in part one of the scale provide information about the patient's overall performance patterns. These patterns are not uniquely observable by OT but are included to provide some general information about the patient's overall personal habits and routine.

The six behaviors listed in part two involve performance skills related to communication/interaction. These behaviors are included because the occupational therapy environment provides opportunities for the patient to interact with others during structured and unstructured activities. Patients may behave differently during OT than they do at other times. Part three of the COTE scale consists of 12 behaviors that relate to performance skills, an area central to occupational therapy. The COTE's emphasis on task behaviors emphasizes the importance of performance in occupation.

PART ONE: GENERAL BEHAVIORS

Behaviors in part one provide for an overall impression of the patient's general level of performance patterns. These performance patterns include behaviors that influence function. The definitions of terms for the COTE scale are in Appendix C.

"Behavior IA Appearance" reflects how the person is doing at self-care. The factors selected to assess appearance are considered to be within the patient's control within a clinical or community setting. These include neatness, cleanliness, and appropriate attire. Appearance is rated according to the number of factors involved.

"Behavior IB Non-Productive Behavior" includes such behaviors as rocking, playing with hands, or talking to self. When patients engage in non-productive behaviors, their opportunity for successful performance in areas of occupation becomes compromised. Non-productive behavior may be an indicator of a dominating habit resulting in a dysfunctional performance pattern.

"Behavior IC Activity Level" may be two-directional. A level of activity is problematic when it is so high or low that it attracts the attention of others, disrupts performance, or prevents participation. Activity level is rated according to its effect on participation.

"Behavior ID Expression" includes the many elements that can provide indications of a patient's feelings. Some of these elements are body language, volume and tone of voice, facial expression, posture and bearing, and the degree of animation displayed. Expression is rated according to its appropriateness to the situation.

"Behavior IE Responsibility" is a measure of the patient's personal accountability. This behavior is reflected by attendance patterns, adherence to known rules, care of equipment and supplies, and adherence to behavioral contracts. Responsibility is measured according to the degree it is assumed.

"Behavior IF Attendance" is a behavior that reflects an individual's commitment and motivation to participate. The amount of encouragement needed for attendance is the basis for rating this behavior.

"Behavior IG Reality Orientation" addresses the patient's awareness of person, time, place, and situation. The behavior rating is based on the number of factors of which the patient is aware.

"Behavior IH Conceptualization" is a higher-level cognitive function that represents the patient's level of learning and response to situations. It is rated on a continuum that reflects responses that range from concrete to abstract.

PART TWO: INTERPERSONAL/COMMUNICATION SKILLS

Interpersonal relationships affect performance in all social activities. Effective performance in areas of occupation often depends upon effective social interaction. Occupational therapy provides both structured and nonstructured opportunities for these interactions to occur.

"Behavior II A Independence" shows how independently the patient can function in occupational therapy. While OT may include structured activity, opportunities exist in each session for a patient to be independent. Independence is rated according to the number of independent actions observed.

"Behavior II B Cooperation" indicates how well the patient cooperates with the intervention program. Indicators used for rating this behavior are compliance and opposition to the program and the therapist as demonstrated by the patient's ability to follow directions.

"Behavior II C Self-Assertion," like "Behavior 1B Non-Productive Behavior," is two-directional; behaviors can vacillate between passivity and dominance with self-assertion lying midway.

"Behavior II D Sociability" refers to a performance skill related to communication and interaction. This behavior is demonstrated by how well the patient socializes with the staff and other patients during the therapy session. This behavior is rated by whether or not the patient can participate, initiate, or respond to social interactions.

"Behavior II E Attention-Getting Behavior" reflects the amount of time that the patient spends seeking attention. Examples include recreated questions, frequent requests for assistance, and overt requests for approval or merely doing nothing in order to get attention.

"Behavior II F Negative Response from Others" is an indicator of the patient's effect on the therapists and other patients. Examples of this behavior include asking or demanding special privileges, or interactions with fellow patients that result in negative responses. This behavior is rated according to the number of negative responses evoked from other persons during the session.

PART THREE: BEHAVIORS RELATED TO PERFORMANCE SKILLS

Behaviors in part three of the COTE (Appendix B) reflect occupational therapy's emphasis on performance skills and patterns that lead to engagement in occupation. Occupational therapy provides a unique opportunity to observe a patient's behavior during the activities that reflect the challenges of daily life. The occupational therapist can select numerous types of activities that require performance skills not readily observable in group or individual "talk" therapy. The occupational therapist can select numerous activities or contexts in order to provide an opportunity to observe a patient's performance skills. Examples of various contexts and activities are included here only to illustrate or clarify how these performance skills are rated on the scale. They are not included as prescriptive methods required in order to assess a given performance skill.

"Behavior III A Engagement" reflects the commitment made to performance in occupations or activities as a result of self-choice motivation and meaning. This is a significant behavior as no task can be accomplished unless it is begun. The patient's participation in a magazine-collage activity can illustrate the degree of engagement and would be scored as follows:

0—After receiving directions, the patient chooses a magazine, gathers scissors and glue, and selects items for the collage. The items selected are cut out, arranged, and glued as directed.

1—The patient performs as above but requires gentle encouragement to begin.

2—The patient participates in the activity but requires encouragement by name to begin and then further encouragement to continue the activity.

3—The patient needs frequent support and encouragement at each step of the activity.

4—The patient is unable to participate in the activity.

"Behavior III B Concentration/Attention" is an important patient factor and can be measured by the patient's ability to sustain engagement in activities and occupations. This mental function is measured by the amount of time spent attending to the activity at hand. For example, when working on a budget-balancing activity, the patient's performance would be rated as follows:

0—The patient is able to attend to the activity, work throughout the session, and resume after interruptions.

1—The patient has difficulty resuming the activity after interruption, exhibiting some non-productive behaviors.

2—The patient is able to participate in the task for only half of the session and is unable to resume the activity after interruption without therapist intervention.

3—The patient is easily distracted and is able to concentrate on the activity less than one quarter of the session, requiring therapist reminders to resume.

4—The patient loses concentration in less than 1 minute and lapses into non-productive behavior.

"Behavior III C Coordination" is a performance skill that relates to using more than one body part to interact with task objects in a manner that supports task performance. This skill is an indicator of a motor skill that demonstrates how well the body and brain function together. Coordination can serve as a measurable monitor of the patient's response to medication or other treatments. Glazing a ceramic stein is an activity in which coordination can be easily noted.

0—The patient applies underglaze or stain and conforms to the fine detailed feature of the bisque ware.

1—The patient has some difficulty but can glaze neatly in large areas.

2—The patient can stay within the guide except in very precise areas.

3—The patient can only manage a one-color overglaze because of unsteady hands.

4—The patient is unable to manipulate the brush.

"Behavior III D Following Directions" reflects the ability to respond to an activity demand in order to carry out the desired activity. The occupational therapist may use games such as charades to assess the patient's ability to follow directions. This behavior would be scored as follows:

1—The patient actively plays charades, and, once the game is learned, responds to and uses standard game symbols without reinforcement.

2—The patient needs assistance and reinforcement regarding the procedures; reminders about rules or symbols may be needed each time the patient takes a turn.

3—The patient requires guidance from the therapist at each step of the activity.

4—The patient is unable to participate in the activity.

"Behavior III E Activity Neatness/Attention to Detail" reflects opposite ends of a continuum related to how well a patient can accomplish a task and to the quality of that task. Either can be readily observed while the patient is engaged in a tile-trivet activity. Rate one, not both. These behaviors are scored as follows:

(A) Activity Neatness

0—Given directions, a large box of assorted tiles, a trivet, and glue, the patient creates a pleasing design by selecting, placing, and gluing the tiles neatly in place within the 30-minute session.

1—The design is disorderly or excessive glue is dribbled on the surface of the tiles. However, the activity is completed within the allotted time.

2—The design may be haphazard, and the surface of the tiles may be spotted with glue.

3—The patient's work is sloppy; glue may be spilled onto hands and work surfaces and applied on the wrong side of the tiles

4—The therapist has to intervene during this activity, as the patient requires close supervision and is apt to streamline the task by pouring large quantities of glue onto the trivet before dumping the tiles onto it.

(B) Attention to Detail

0—Given directions, a large box of assorted tiles, a trivet, and glue, the patient creates a pleasing design by selecting, placing, and gluing the tiles neatly in place within the 30-minute session.

1—Tiles are selected carefully and placed on the trivet with precision. A full 60 minutes is used to accomplish the task.

2—Excessive time is used to create the design or select the tiles. However, once these steps are accomplished, the remainder of the task is completed in the allotted time.

3—Two sessions are required to complete the activity. Each tile is painstakingly placed, and the patient may even use tools to assure proper alignment of the tiles.

4—The patient takes many sessions to complete the task, if it is completed at all. The tiniest tiles available are selected. Calipers may be used to set and space the tiles on the trivet.

"Behavior III F Problem Solving" is a patient factor that represents a higher level of cognitive functioning. It requires the patient to plan and carry out actions in response to a challenge. A group puzzle activity provides the opportunity to observe this patient factor. The patients are each given a package containing all but one piece of a jigsaw puzzle plus one odd piece that belongs to another puzzle. Each patient is directed to bargain with other patients and trade puzzle pieces so that each person's puzzle can be assembled. This performance skill would be rated as follows:

0—Given instructions, the patient quickly recognizes the odd puzzle piece and approaches others to trade it and secure the missing piece in order to complete the puzzle.

1—The patient systematically assembles the puzzle, notes the missing piece and the extra piece, and seeks advice from the therapist. The patient attempts to locate the missing piece by going from person to person trying all odd pieces until the puzzle is completed.

2—The puzzle is assembled by trial and error. After discovering that a puzzle piece is missing, the patient goes from person to person, trying all odd pieces until a match is found.

3—The patient is able to put together the puzzle with effort. Repeated attempts are made to fit the odd piece into the puzzle. The patient does not recognize that the odd piece does not belong in the puzzle.

4—The patient is unable to assemble the puzzle.

"Behavior III G Complexity and Organization of Tasks" can be rated using multilevel activities such as leather lacing. Each style of lacing carries its own degree of complexity. For example, lacing with a double buttonhole stitch requires more organization and is far more complex than lacing with a whip stitch.

0—Given instructions, the patient is able to accomplish the double buttonhole stitch, and when given directions, can begin, end, and splice the lacing without difficulty.

1—The patient can do the lacing but cannot figure out how to splice, begin, or end it, even with detailed instructions.

2—The patient can do the lacing but has difficulty keeping the twist out of the lace. The lacing is accomplished one stitch at a time and requires cuing from the therapist

3—The patient can only do simple stitching, such as the running stitch or the whip stitch, and needs reinforcement from the therapist.

4—The patient cannot manage the task.

"Behavior III H Initial Learning" is evaluated when the patient is performing an activity that is unfamiliar and requires instruction. Assembling a link belt can provide an excellent opportunity in which to observe this phenomenon.

0—The patient follows all written or verbal instruction and begins assembly of the belt without assistance from the therapist.

1—The patient requires additional instruction and assistance from the therapist before beginning to assemble the belt. After the therapist inserts the first two links, the patient is able to continue independently.

2—The patient is unable to do doublewide belts but can accomplish a singlewide variety with minimal assistance from the therapist.

3—The patient is unable to assemble the link belt without moderate assistance from the therapist.

4—The patient is unable to accomplish any part of the task.

"Behavior III I Interest in Activity" illustrates the patient's willingness to try new or different activities. One way to rate a patient's interest is by observing participation in a group parachute activity

0—The patient participates with enthusiasm.

1—The patient is willing and does participate, though is somewhat guarded at first. After a brief time, participation is enthusiastic.

2—The patient participates only by being present, otherwise demonstrating no interest or commitment to the activity.

3—The patient may join in the activity for the first five minutes, but then stands or sits outside the circle and watches the others participate.

4—The patient does not participate and is unwilling to be a spectator.

"Behavior III J Interest in Accomplishment" indicates whether the patient can set goals and work toward them by taking the steps needed to complete the activity. This behavior requires the expenditure of physical and mental energy. Craft activities, such as decoupage, require many separate steps and a commitment to complete them. This behavior is rated as follows:

0—The patient carefully selects a to be decoupaged, prepares the wooden surface appropriately, and sands between coats. An effort is made to ensure that everything is done correctly and that the completed project will be pleasing.

1—The patient wants to do the activity and initially makes the investment, although interest wanes before the project is completed. The first steps of the activity are done with care, but the last steps are hastily finished.

2—The patient expresses interest in the activity but seems to want to get finished as quickly as possible. No substantial investment in the activity is demonstrated, although the patient expresses a desire to complete the task.

3—The patient does the activity only with substantial therapist encouragement. No investment or commitment to complete the activity is exhibited.

4—The patient demonstrates no interest or pleasure in the activity and does not complete it. The project may be discarded or abandoned when the patient prepares to leave the session.

"Behavior III K Decision Making" is a patient factor that is an integral part of daily living. This higher-level cognitive function refers to an individual's ability to process knowledge in order to select a course of action. Decision making is dependent on the number and kinds of choices and degree of support available. This behavior is rated as follows:

0—After collaboration with the therapist regarding the goals for treatment, the patient chooses an activity from a variety of available alternatives and proceeds independently.

1—After collaboration with the therapist regarding the goals for treatment, the patient selects an appropriate activity, occasionally seeking the therapist's reassurance.

2—The patient makes decisions about the activity but often seeks reassurance from the therapist.

3—The patient selects an activity from two alternatives.

4—The patient cannot or will not make a decision.

"Behavior III L Frustration Tolerance" can be an indicator of the patient's ability to persevere in activities when each phase does not come easily. The ability to tolerate frustration reflects the ability to adapt and make accommodations or adjustments. This behavior can be seen when patients are asked to assemble wooden or plastic models.

0—The patient assembles the wooden pieces of the model, carefully planning each step of the assembly. The model is completed even with minor difficulties such as a missing part or dried glue.

1—The patient becomes frustrated with minor glitches but is able to make the necessary adjustments.

2—The patient becomes frustrated with any unanticipated difficulty such as a missing part or dried glue.

3—The patient becomes frustrated by all aspects of assembly, but attempts to continue the activity.

4—The patient is unable to complete the task.

Case Study 1: Marie

The format of the COTE is useful in developing a treatment plan. The COTE readily displays areas of strengths and weaknesses and can help the therapist identify treatment priorities. The following example reflects the use of the COTE in an initial evaluation of the behaviors of a 49-year-old woman who is a patient in a community mental health facility. This patient was escorted to the occupational therapy area by the therapist. She sat quietly on the sofa, seemingly unaware of the activities around her. She responded only when approached and answered direct inquiries, but did not volunteer information or initiate conversation. After discovering the patient's needs and wants and identifying the factors that would support her ability to engage in the desired areas of occupation, the therapist completed an occupational profile, which provided information about the patient's occupational history, her roles, and her reason for seeking service. The therapist directed the patient to sit at a table with two other patients who were working on craft activities. The therapist then introduced a basic craft activity, a tile trivet, to assess the patient's task behaviors. The patient was directed to select tiles of any three colors, place a small amount of glue on each tile, and glue it to the trivet in any pattern or design that she selected.

The patient needed to be encouraged three times to begin selecting tiles. She was unable to determine a design or pattern for the tiles and began gluing only after the therapist had suggested a design. She was able to manipulate the tiles and the glue bottle, and she placed the tiles face side up on the trivet. However, some tiles were placed and glued somewhat haphazardly. She was unable to complete the task and demonstrated no interest in the activity or in the activities going on around her.

While recording this patient's performance on the COTE scale, the therapist was identifying some of the patient's problem areas. The patient's major difficulties were found to be in the areas of independence, self-assertion, sociability, and concentration. Based on her history and her performance in occupational therapy, the therapist discussed the patient's performance with her. The therapist and the patient collaborated in the development of treatment goals to increase independence, socialization, self-assertion, and self-esteem.

Case Study 2: Charlie

A 38-year-old man was seen by the occupational therapist in a community halfway house for men recently released from prison. He was neat and well-groomed and on time for the therapy session. He responded eagerly to the occupational therapist about his desire to move from the halfway house and live independently. After interviewing the patient and completing the occupational profile, the occupational therapist learned that Charlie had limited knowledge or experience in managing his personal finances. Together, Charlie and the therapist determined that he would need to prepare a budget in order to manage his income and take care of his anticipated monthly expenses. In order to accomplish this goal, Charlie needed to identify the expenses that he could anticipate, and determine a budget.

With the therapist's encouragement, the patient was able to start a list of some of the items that would compose his monthly expenses. He listed rent, cigarettes, and utilities but then seemed to lose interest in the task. The therapist redirected him, and he added food and transportation to his list. He was unable to estimate a dollar amount for any of the items on his list and could not identify a way to find out about costs. Charlie indicated that he didn't know where to start and seemed to divert his attention to the television in an adjacent room. The therapist redirected him by suggesting that he begin to scan the yellow pages to find listings for apartments. Charlie was able to identify several housing options but became discouraged after two voice mail responses, and he closed the telephone book and discontinued his exploration. He stated that he would never be able to afford to live in a nice place and be independent. The therapist redirected Charlie and he resumed his telephone search.

The therapist used the COTE scale to assess Charlie's behaviors and identified problems in "Behavior IH Conceptualization," "IIB Independence," "IIIA Engagement," "IIIB Concentration," "IIIF Problem Solving," "IIIG Complexity and Organization of the Task," and "IIIL Frustration Tolerance."

The therapist reviewed the completed COTE with the patient and provided him with some concrete examples of his behaviors. They discussed how the behaviors were barriers to achieving his occupational goals and collaborated on strategies to address them.

Reliability and Validity

Interrater reliability of the initial COTE was determined by computing percent agreement between the ratings of two therapists, with five different therapists involved. Ratings within 2 degrees of each other were considered acceptable, and the percent agreement for 55 patients ranged from 76% to 100% and averaged 95%. Percent agreement for exact agreements ranged from 36% to 84% and averaged 63%. A subsequent review of interrater reliability was done by personal correspondence with the director of occupational therapy of a large general hospital. Reliability data were reported on seven cases and agreement ranged from 96% to 100%.

This author used the COTE scale as a tool to assess the competence of occupational therapists and occupational therapy assistants in observing and documenting patient behaviors. The results were curious. The percent agreement between experienced occupational therapists and new occupational therapists was not as high as the percent agreement between experienced therapists and experienced occupational therapy assistants. Nor was the percent agreement between experienced occupational therapy assistants and new occupational therapy assistants or new occupational therapists as high as it was between new therapists and new assistants.

Validity was determined by randomly selecting the charts of five discharged patients from a group of 400. Total scores for the first and last days in occupational therapy were compared. The scores averaged 31 and 17, respectively, and the drop in the score agreed with the observations of other professionals in the acute hospital setting. A similar review comparing initial and discharge scores showed average admission scores of 33.5, with a discharge score of 22.25 and an average variance of 10.8.

In a study conducted by an occupational therapy student in the psychiatric unit of a medical university hospital, it was observed that a patient's total COTE scores decreased from the first to the last day in occupational therapy. To ensure validity of each day's ratings, the student scored the patients on a new scale each day to avoid the influence of the previous day's score. The average score for the first day of occupational therapy was 20, with a range of 0 to 28. The average decrease in scores was 11 points, with a range of 0 to 57. Again, similar results in a different setting support the validity of this instrument.

Format

The COTE is designed as a checklist with a grid to display numerical scores for each behavior. The COTE originally provided a means for daily documentation of patient performance over the span of the hospital stay. The grid format was used to display daily profiles, which were helpful in identifying changes in patient performance during the course of treatment. Sixteen spaces were allocated to record ratings of each behavior on each day of the patient's hospital stay. This document was used by the team and the patient to review progress, plan further intervention, or process performance.

The marked decrease in lengths of stay no longer affords the opportunity to examine and respond to a sequelae of changes in behavioral profiles. Hospital stays now average less than 4 days, barely enough time for medication regimens to be established or for the members of the treatment team to gain rapport with the patient. However, the grid format does allow the opportunity to easily compare and contrast patient admission and discharge behaviors, thus providing information about functional outcomes.

Although designed as a reporting tool for an inpatient psychiatric setting, the COTE readily lends itself to use in community settings such as mental health centers, supported living centers, and shelters. Often patients seen in these sites exhibit behaviors similar to those of patients seen during the time the COTE was developed.

The actual COTE document was designed so that the parameters of each behavior were printed on the back. This was done in response to a physician's request for clarification of the reports. The document also provides space for the therapist to record goals, treatment plans, and other pertinent information. The structure of the document can be tailored to meet the specific demands of the therapist and or facility.

Application

The COTE creates a structure for organizing and recording diverse patient behaviors that may affect the ability to successfully perform in chosen areas of occupation. These behaviors may then be addressed in therapy. Because the list of behaviors is expansive and addresses multiple performance areas of occupation, the rater is compelled to consider performance skills and patterns and the demands of activities, as well as the patient factors that are involved in performance. This can contribute to a more comprehensive view of the patient performance and provide valuable information to guide the intervention plan.

The grid can be used to simplify comparison of variances in patient performance from one session to another in order to monitor the effects of a new medication, change in context, or treatment intervention. The numerical scores, which can be easily monitored, provide hard data that is useful in documenting outcomes for payers and quality improvement.

Quality management/improvement initiatives are data driven, and the comparison between admission and discharge behaviors offers measurable performance-outcome data. The emphasis of COTE on function is compatible with accreditation standards and patient-centered care. For example, since entries on the COTE are numerical rather than narrative, outcome criteria can be expressed numerically. To illustrate, discharge criteria for a patient with a diagnosis of depressive neurosis may be: 1) able to socialize with more than one person at a time, 2) able to follow three-step directions, and 3) able to function independently in therapy. The data retriever would be directed to look for scores of 0-1 in behaviors 2A (independence), 2D (sociability), and 3D (following directions) entered on the last day of hospitalization. If the scores relating to those behaviors are higher than 0 or 1, then the treatment objectives in occupational therapy were not met.

Another focus of quality management/improvement is to improve the efficiency of service delivery. In hospitals with increasingly shorter hospital stays and rapid turnover of patients (which increase productivity standards and result in greater demands for clarity in notes and records), documentation must be made more effective and efficient. Community settings also demand increased efficiency in service delivery. It takes far less time to complete a COTE than to write a meaningful narrative note. The structure of this instrument guides therapists' reports so that patients' functional performance is documented.

The COTE provides a strong foundation for discussion of patient goals and treatment priorities. For example, during a routine peer review process, colleagues examine patient records to determine the appropriateness of interventions provided to patients. Because the behavioral assessment is straightforward and the parameters guiding the assessment are evident, therapists can make judgments based on similar information. Discussions regarding differences in goals, intervention approaches, and expected outcomes can be based on performance data. A peer review of records also allows therapists to discuss goals and intervention priorities. A comparison of the COTE with treatment plans can also be useful in assessing whether patient goals and treatment plans appropriately reflect patient performance.

The COTE provides an excellent mechanism for teaching students and new therapists how to observe and document patient behaviors. Because many different behaviors are addressed on this instrument, the supervising therapist can identify learning needs through concurrent evaluations with the new therapist or student.

The COTE also serves as a useful intervention tool when collaborating with patients in setting goals, developing strategies for intervention, or monitoring progress. Discussing the COTE score with the patient allows the therapist to explain how the patient's behaviors affect occupational performance. Using the profile outlined on the COTE, the patient and therapist can collaborate on an appropriate treatment plan. Patients may even identify areas of difficulty that have not been observed in therapy. The language used to delineate each behavior is simple, does not contain jargon, and often provides concrete examples that are helpful for patient and therapist alike.

The COTE can assist the therapist in defining occupational therapy services in psychiatry and community settings. Its format allows for efficient recording of a patient's general, interpersonal, and task behaviors. This behavioral rating scale is not dependent on a specific area of occupation, activity, intervention, or context. The behaviors included on the scale are related to occupational performance and are defined in straightforward manner as they relate to patient functional performance in any occupation, activity, or setting.

Summary

The profession of occupational therapy has experienced renewed emphasis on patient participation in occupation and is moving toward helping therapists " …more clearly affirm and articulate occupational therapy's unique focus on occupation and daily life activities and the application of an intervention process that facilitates an engagement in occupation to support participation in life."[1] The COTE scale guides the occupational therapist's assessment of behaviors that reflect the context, patient factors, and activity demands as they relate to the performance skills and performance patterns necessary for the patient to engage in occupation to support participation in daily life.

References

1. The American Occupational Therapy Association. Occupational Therapy Practice Framework: domain and process. *Amer J Occup Ther.* 2002;56:610-639.
2. Ayres AJ. A form used to evaluate the work behavior of patients. *Amer J Occup Ther.* 1954;8:73-74.

COMMUNITY ADAPTIVE PLANNING ASSESSMENT

Harriett Davidson, MA, OTR
Kathlyn L. Reed, PhD, OTR, MLIS, FAOTA

"...adaptation at the level of an individual person is based on inborn physiological mechanisms as well as on human capacities for memory and intention....The concept of adaptation thus prompts therapists to think not only about change, but also about continuity in the lives of our clients." Spencer JC, Davidson HA, White VK. Continuity and change: past experience as adaptive repertoire in occupational adaptation. Am J Occup Ther. 1996;50:527.

Introduction

After addressing the immediate needs of the patient, the primary task of the occupational therapist becomes planning, with the patient, his or her future and return to community living. Such planning should include consideration of how the occupational therapist can assist the patient to integrate back into community life and should include the patient in the process. Current practice is expected to be collaborative and client-centered,[1] with a focus on "assisting people to engage in daily life activities that they find meaningful and purposeful."[2(p610)] An assessment tool to assist in future planning for mental health populations should address the patient's perspective, occupational performance, and participation within expected contexts, including community life. Such a tool should be structured for the collaborative process, with attention to the therapist's clinical reasoning in procedural, interactive, and conditional areas.[3]

The Community Adaptive Planning Assessment (CAPA) was developed to be used in a variety of practice settings and to enable future planning following major life changes, whether such changes result from illness, injury, social disorganization, or other events requiring major adaptive transitions. Occupational therapists have always concerned themselves with the whole human being in mental health practice.[4] The authors of the CAPA have taken the view that an assessment based on occupational adaptation as a process should be useful in a variety of practice settings, independent of whether the major focus is on psychosocial or physical dimensions. While many assessments in occupational therapy are designed for persons with specific diagnoses or occupational problems, the current practice philosophy of occupational therapy affirms: "Psychosocial dimensions of human performance are fundamental to all aspects of occupation and occupational therapy, with every patient, and across all practice settings."[1(p669)]

Therapists may be met with the challenge of having a patient referred to them for a physical illness or injury only to realize there is a more urgent need to address the patient's concomitant psychosocial disorders. The challenge of enacting a practice that is holistic is fraught with "ambiguities and contradictions"[5(p269)] and requires that the therapist have a clear view of the interaction between the person, the context, and the occupation. Support for holistic occupation-based assessment and intervention such as that guided by the CAPA is found in three examples from current literature: (1) the *Occupational Therapy Practice Framework*, which provides a model for such practice,[2] (2) the assumption that occupation changes the way the brain works,[6] and (3) the blending of physical and psychosocial concerns of practice in the current literature of occupational therapy, eg, common approaches to occupational impairments resulting from pain, and neuromotor and cognitive dysfunction.[7]

The assessment process should permit the gathering of rich qualitative as well as quantitative data, allowing for reasonable plans for the future. Current occupational therapy literature describes the use of narratives and emphasizes the importance of helping patients connect their past "life stories" to their present life situations and to their futures.[8-10] Helping patients imagine a meaningful future supports hopefulness[11] and has been identified as "a foundation through which persons can activate their resilience and will to survive major life difficulties."[11-13]

Assuring patients' active participation in the goal-setting process is a professional responsibility demanded by ethical principles and regulatory agencies and is linked to the degree patients participate in the therapeutic process.[14] Involving the patients in setting clinical goals has been addressed in the literature[13,15,16] and, to a lesser degree, in planning for the postintervention period. The value of the narrative approach in goal-setting is emphasized for patients with cognitive and motivational difficulties, such as individuals in mental health settings.[17]

An additional consideration when planning an assessment in occupational therapy is the purpose for which it will be used.[15] Although there are a number of classifications for assessments in health-related fields, a widely accepted classification identifies discriminative measures (which differentiate between people when no external criterion is available), predictive measures (which classify people according to predefined categories), and evaluative measures (which are designed to measure change over time).[18] The CAPA is designed to have an evaluative emphasis, as it is intended to examine performance that is responsive to change and can be used to determine whether or not change is occurring.

Below is a set of assumptions underlying the development of the CAPA, the elements found to support such a process, a description of the development of the tool and ways it has been used, and a short discussion of additional work that needs to be done.

Criteria for Evaluating Community Planning and Integration Instruments

ASSUMPTIONS

1. The environmental context is equal to or more powerful a determinant in shaping the lives and functioning of persons with disabilities as is their individual impairments.[19,20]

2. The focus of evaluation is on conceptualizing goals and strategies, rather than on completing complex measurements based on collected data. Embedded in this assumption is the belief that the patient has the ability to engage in this future planning process, either individually or in concert with family members and friends. The therapist is asked specifically to estimate the patient's ability to participate in the planning and follow-through process and to estimate the need for external support to do so. If the patient is unable to participate, then the CAPA becomes a tool for planning with a caretaker or family member.[13]

3. Consideration is given to four major traditions of evaluation: experimentation, behavior observation, survey, and ethnography (participant observer). The qualitative aspects of measurement designed to capture the "insider's perspective," or meaning, of the occupational experience are stressed as the method of choice for the CAPA. However, the patient is asked to rate four factors on a 10-point scale, and the therapist is asked to estimate a number to represent the patient's future ability to follow through with the implementation of plans.

Concepts That Guided Construction of the CAPA

Longitudinal orientation that connects the future to past experience by:

a. Organizing evaluation data of the patient's past experience in terms of short-term adaptation (about 1 calendar year), including:

   1. adaptive strategies (coping)

   2. adaptive resources (family and friends, knowledge and use of community, work skills, work history, finances, educational attainment, housing situation, knowledge and use of transportation options, leisure interests)

   3. adaptive repertoire (typical patterns, routines, and roles).

b. Organizing evaluation data of patient's past experience in terms of long-term (life-long) adaptation, including:

   1. adaptive strategies (resilience, hardiness, sense of coherence)

   2. adaptive resources

   3. adaptive repertoire.

c. Organizing evaluation data of patient's future plans and planning (future orientation).

d. Organizing evaluation data so that patient and therapist can see connection (continuity) between past experiences and anticipated future directions (life stories, narrative).

    e. Considering the overall constellation of occupations regularly practiced by the patient (habits, routines, roles).

Focus on occupational performance by:

    a. Organizing evaluation data of patient's skills in problem solving (motor, process, communication/interaction skills)

    b. Organizing occupational functions/areas at the level of the individual (activities of daily living [ADL], instrumental activities of daily living [IADL], education, work, leisure, play, social participation)

    c. Using a *top-down* approach stressing a focus on occupation and occupational performance as opposed to a focus on performance components.

Consideration of performance contexts by:

    a. Organizing specific environmental contexts in which the occupations occur (cultural, physical, social, personal, spiritual, temporal)

    b. Considering the negotiability of such contexts.[20]

Focus on patterns of occupational performance by:

    a. Using a narrative approach,[21] whereby the patient and therapist discover the past patterns through the patient's storytelling

    b. Discovering the changing meanings that accompany the changing patterns

    c. Identifying the adaptive repertoire (the past patterns that the patient can use to shape future patterns while incorporating needed change).[10]

Examine the meaning of occupations by:

    a. Considering the value of occupations from the patient's perspective

    b. Considering the satisfaction with time spent and importance of continuing the occupation, as seen by the patient.

Engage the patient in the collaborative process by:

    a. Incorporating the therapist's qualitative judgment (clinical reasoning, clinical decision making) about the extent to which the patient is able to follow through on implementing plans independently

    b. Considering the kinds of support and resources (such as social, community, financial, educational housing, transportation, leisure/recreation, and accessibility resources) that the patient needs in the future.

Comparison With Other Assessments That Meet Some of the Identified Patient Needs

The development of the CAPA coincided with an era of increased interest in narrative approaches, greater focus on the importance of environments, and a strong commitment to a client-centered approach. During this same time period, a number of other occupational therapists were developing other assessments that measure some of the same elements of occupational adaptation as does the CAPA. The Occupational Performance History Interview (OPHI-II)[22] is intended to measure aspects of occupational adaptation through life history narrative describing adaptation over time (occupational competence, identity, and behavior settings). It addresses past and present adaptive patterns, examines occupational meaning, and engages the patient in the assessment process; it charts the adaptive trajectory and describes the findings in terms of relative adaptation. It does not fine-tune the examination of the potential losses and gains involved with goal setting and decision making, and it does not examine the specific occupations and environmental influences in relation to adaptation as does the CAPA.

The Canadian Occupational Performance Measure (COPM)[23] is a client-centered method of gaining a patient's perspectives for treatment planning, for establishing treatment goals, and for measuring the effects of treatment. The therapist using the COPM asks the patient to rate satisfaction and performance in problem areas of ADL, work, play, and leisure in a way similar to that of using the CAPA. However, the therapist using the COPM does not examine occupations that are rewarding or support systems that may benefit or inhibit performance.

The Occupational Role History[24] is designed as a screening that uses a semi-structured interview to gather data that identify skills and patterns of performance in occupational roles, both past and present, as well as the balance between those roles. Interpretation and organization of future planning are left up to the therapist's clinical judgment, whereas the CAPA provides more opportunity to obtain in-depth patient input.

Other assessments that provide information about important aspects of occupational adaptation but do not provide a whole picture include: The Role Checklist,[25] The Social Support Inventory for People with Disability (SSIPD),[26] The Reintegration to Normal Living Index (RNLI),[27] and The Community Integration Measure (CIM).[28] Table 9-1 compares how these assessments address the elements of occupational adaptation considered important in the CAPA.

Development of the CAPA

The idea of examining adaptive patterns for community and adaptive responses to facilitate community living emerged as a part of the research tradition in occupational adaptation at Texas Woman's University. An extensive search and analysis of available literature and assessments convinced Spencer and Davidson that an instrument enabling the therapist to collaborate with the client to examine adaptive patterns for community living was not available. Work began in the mid-1980s with the Neighborhood Environments Project, a forerunner of the CAPA in which qualitative data were collected through interviews and videotapes of elderly community-dwelling persons from a variety of cultural and ethnic backgrounds living in Houston. The project included elderly persons of white, black, Hispanic, Chinese, and Vietnamese origins. The involvement of graduate students from matched culture and ethnic backgrounds allowed the interviews to be conducted in the preferred or primary language of the interviewee and then translated into English for analysis. Though this work was unpublished, qualitative analysis of the data resulted in the description of alternative patterns that elderly individuals used to continue satisfying social participation in the community as they aged.

Table 9-1

Comparison of the Areas Assessed in Select Occupational Adaptation Instruments

	Longitudinal orientation	Focus on occupational performance	Grounded in the community	Consideration of performance contexts	Focus on patterns of occupational performance	Examination of meaning of occupations	Engagement in collaborative process
CAPA	x	x	x	x Supportiveness of environment	x	x	x
OPHI-II	x	x	x	x	x	x	x
ORH	x	x	x		x		x
COPM	x	x Lists problems	x			x Importance of problem occupations	x
Role Checklist	x	x	x			x	x
CIM			x				
RNLI			x				
SSIPD				x			

Three adaptive patterns used by these individuals were identified from this study: an independent pattern, an interdependent-with-family pattern, and an interdependent-with-neighbors pattern. In addition, the data led to the construction of the first version of the instrument. Version I of the CAPA (originally named the Community Adaptive Patterns Assessment) was developed to represent the idea that each person uses a repertoire of typical adaptive patterns within his or her community or local world[10] and examined participation within occupations in terms of (1) activity patterns, (2) mobility patterns, and (3) roles and relationships, including social support exchanges. It was designed to document former adaptive patterns prior to the onset of a disability or major life transition, to identify potential losses in one or more of the three adaptive patterns anticipated, and to suggest alternative adaptive strategies that might be implemented to increase the adaptive repertoire to meet important needs of the patient. Version I generated scores that were weighted based on the importance and frequency of identified occupations.

The practical usability of Version I was evaluated by a group of professional master's therapy students with 30 patients who had had a stroke, were in acute care, had short-term and long-term rehabilitation, and were in home health service delivery settings. Revisions were made based on the analysis of data from patients, students, and therapists. Trustworthiness of the data was examined by interviewing a patient's family members and the patient together. Particularly in families or cultures in which decisions were jointly made, the process of comparing differing perspectives was found to lead to increased trustworthiness.[13] A team of experienced therapists recruited nationally through the American Occupational Therapy Foundation (AOTF) evaluated the use of the CAPA for clinical effectiveness in discharge planning during rehabilitation, with follow-up 3 months later in the community.

The trustworthiness of the information gathered was evaluated by comparison with information gathered from family members. Trustworthiness, or accuracy or believability, is a concept usually associated with qualitative measures and is related to reliability and validity in quantitative measures. Elements of trustworthiness include credibility, transferability, dependability, and confirmability; these are ensured by such strategies as prolonged engagement, triangulation, member checks, peer debriefing, and following audit trails. Trustworthiness is considered particularly important in the evaluation of individuals with central nervous system or mental health disorders. In a study of patients with strokes, two therapists each interviewed eight patients and their spouses separately, both at discharge and at a 3-month follow-up. Comparisons of information between the family member and patient yielded a high level of agreement, even from those who might not be expected to report accurately because of cognitive limitations.

Clinical effectiveness involves "whether a qualitative tool provides relevant and important information organized in a way that helps shape interventions that have valuable outcomes for the patient."[13(p26)] To examine whether use of the CAPA for discharge planning could help identify meaningful and attainable goals and then to determine whether the patient actually implemented the goals upon return to the community, content analysis was done on the outcome data for these 16 patients. Categories that emerged included:

1. Goal met as originally documented.
2. Goal met to some extent, but participant realizes some limitations.
3. Goal to be achieved required a new solution.
4. Goal not yet achieved but still viable.

5. Accommodation achieved through a new but related goal satisfying to participant or family member.

6. Accommodation through a new but related goal not satisfying to participant or family member.

7. Goal not met and abandoned.

Analysis revealed that planning using the CAPA resulted in the achievement of most community-oriented goals (83% of occupational goals were implemented in one of the forms identified; 87% of mobility goals were implemented; 71% of relationship goals were implemented).

Following the evaluation of these studies, and with consultation from expert analysts, Version II of the CAPA was prepared. The usability of this version was evaluated by professional and post-professional master's students with 75 patients from a variety of rehabilitation settings.

Some revisions were then made, and a structured reporting format was added. As work with the assessment continued to evolve, a modified version became known as the Collaborative Adaptive Planning Assessment to emphasize the collaborative nature of the assessment, involving planning with the patients, their family members, and other members of the team (see Appendix D).

Studies of the Usability of the CAPA

Spencer, Hersch, Eschenfelder, Fournet, and Murray-Gerzik[29] used the CAPA in a study describing the adaptive processes of elderly persons being treated on a transitional unit for de-conditioning before they returned to their community. The CAPA provided the data for an adaptation-based intervention that was compared to a protocol-based intervention (using standard protocols of the setting). The researchers found support for the use of the CAPA for an individualized intervention based upon meaningful occupational performance and contexts.

A second study at Texas Woman's University involved examining the process of adaptation to a hand injury using both qualitative and quantitative measures. In a published case study, Anderson and Spencer[30] demonstrated the usefulness of the CAPA in fully engaging a patient with a hand injury in finding meaning in the rehabilitation process. Following the partial amputation of three fingers, dissatisfied with his occupational therapy program, and described by his therapist as a pain management problem who "does not want to work," the patient was transferred to a new clinic. There the therapist, using the CAPA, helped the patient link his occupational history with a recovery grounded in meaningful activity (playing the guitar) and negotiate his environment to again play the guitar.

Description of the CAPA

The purpose of the CAPA is to establish a collaborative planning process between service providers and patients at times of major life changes, which might include the onset of disability, a change in disability status, or changes in the environment. The focus is on the overall constellation of occupations in people's daily lives, providing an opportunity for examination and creative problem solving about balancing expected losses (things the person may no longer be able to do following this major event) and expected gains (new ways to continue meaningful occupations or finding new occupations that are important).

The CAPA is used first to examine broad areas of occupation and determine whether changes are expected within any of these areas. If changes are expected, then the CAPA is used to examine major occupations within each broad area to identify expected losses and possible gains and to document goals for the future.

For each major occupation of the individual, the interview process is designed to gather information about:

1. Occupation (activities the individual includes in this occupation and the amount of time dedicated to the performance)

2. Persons (persons with whom the occupation is done and the roles of individuals involved)

3. Context (physical, cultural, social, and personal aspects of the environment in which the occupation is done and how the person gets to the setting)

4. Value (ways in which the occupation is valued by the key persons involved).

The CAPA was designed to record information on separate cards, which could then be arranged in various ways for data comparison and intervention planning.

A separate occupation card is used for each occupation. Each card has three columns:

1. Previous Status, or how the patient performed the selected occupation before the onset of the problem that is being addressed in therapy

2. Expected Changes, or the expected losses following the onset of the problem and intervention for that problem

3. Outcomes, a place to document the extent to which the future planning goals were met based upon follow-up information.

The left-hand column of each card indicates basic information sought about each occupation: (1) time satisfaction (satisfaction with time spent with each occupation), (2) participation satisfaction (satisfaction with the amount of active participation in each occupation), (3) negotiability rating (satisfaction with the ability to perform within the context),[31] and (4) importance rating (importance of continuing with the occupation).

In addition to yielding narrative data, the CAPA provides optional rating scales for each of the four areas (1-10, with 10 representing the highest measure of response and 1 the least).

An occupational hierarchy is used for a more detailed examination of specific occupations within each performance area. The structure for documentation is provided on the occupation cards for occupation, persons, environment, and values, each with a place for past, present, and future data (Table 9-2).

The collaborative planning process is present- and future-oriented and involves an acknowledgment of need to examine the skills and experiences from the patient's past (adaptive repertoire), the possible future limitations or needed changes, and the possible gains. This involves reflection and discussion, with the therapist as an expert in the realities of what might be possible based upon professional knowledge and the patient as an expert on his or her own past and hopes for the future. This collaboration has been termed "a dialectic between limits and possibilities."[11(p192)]

The evaluation of outcomes takes place at follow-up and includes documentation of the following possible outcomes:

Table 9-2

Structure and Content for Documentation of Occupation Cards of CAPA

	Past	**Present**	**Future**
Occupation	How done before	Collaborative identification of potential losses and potential gains	Evaluation of outcomes
Persons			
Environment			
Value			

1. Goal met as planned.
2. Goal met with changes (modifications).
3. Goal still in progress.
4. Goal abandoned.

Administration

The therapist who is using the CAPA must have a level of comfort with the qualitative method of data collection, with the interactive reasoning process described by Mattingly,[3] and with the concepts of occupational adaptation. In addition, the therapist needs to have a clear idea of the intended yield, the focus of the data to be gathered (ie, the concepts of continuity and change, of occupational adaptation, of goal setting, and of the past-present-future orientation). The collaborative nature of the interview suggests that the patient must understand the importance of engaging in the exploration of areas, even in the face of the ambiguity of current functional status, and must be willing to face the possibility of future gains as well as losses.

The therapist must be wise in selecting the optimal time for dealing with the questions asked and must recognize that the patient's acknowledgement of some "expected changes" may come at the price of a sense of loss, which must then be dealt with so that discouragement or despair does not result. The therapist may also choose to gather information for the CAPA over time because issues occur during the ongoing intervention and discharge planning.

The interview process begins with the collection of personal information that is relevant to the planning process. If the therapist has already gathered this information, it may simply be entered on the CAPA form. One of the questions in the CAPA asks about the patient's reported coping style. The therapist may want to verify the coping style by using observations of the patient in occupational situations. The therapist begins the CAPA by examining the patient's occupational areas generally. Then, if it is determined that there are problems in one or more of the occupational areas, the therapist moves to a more detailed examination of a specific area. The therapist must use judgment in the focus for each of the occupations, spending time on those occupations in which major losses are to be anticipated. Interview questions are designed to match the structure of the occupation cards but need not be worded precisely like the assessment, as this is a qualitative tool with a semi-structured format (see Appendix E).

The summary report should integrate information according to the following format, with variations as needed for specific purposes. It should:

1. Synthesize key information from the individual occupation cards and scores on the quantitative rating scales.
2. Note the patient's ability to manage overall occupations.
3. Describe the social network and personal geographic territory (contexts).
4. Identify those occupations easiest and most difficult to give up.
5. Document how well the patient was able to engage in the collaborative process.
6. Note an impression of the amount of support the patient might need to implement plans and to see connections between therapy and future plans (see Appendix D for the complete format for reporting).

Application to Mental Health Populations (When It Is Appropriate to Use)

In short-term interventions, mental health patients (as is true of any patients with acute illness) may be unable to participate fully in the collaborative process because of the severity of their symptoms or the effects of their medications. The CAPA includes a place for the therapist's estimate of the patient's level of ability to engage in the planning process and the anticipated need of support for participation in the intervention. The therapist includes this information in goal setting and planning. A family member or caretaker may become a member of the collaborative team, as long as it is acceptable to the patient. The CAPA can also be used at a later time when the patient can more fully participate. Information from the initial administration of the CAPA can be provided at a follow-up meeting.

Case Study

Lucille Thomas is a 47-year-old wife and mother who had been diagnosed with bipolar disorder some years ago. She was seen in an inpatient psychiatric setting for an exacerbation of her symptoms. Her medication was adjusted, she participated in functional groups in occupational therapy, and her symptoms abated. A brief interview revealed the following information: shortly before Lucille's admission, her husband, Richard, had experienced a right, lower extremity (LE), below-knee amputation, and, soon afterwards, a CVA with mild residual dysfunction. He had been employed as a truck driver, and though he was seen in rehabilitation, he was still unable to drive and was uncertain about his occupational future. Lucille's primary role was that of homemaker; there was one son, living within a 100-mile radius, who seldom had contact with her. The occupational therapist recognized the potential for another exacerbation of Lucille's symptoms, as her current circumstance represented a major adaptive transition for her. In the past, stressors had resulted in a need for hospitalization. Until her husband's illness, she had been quite dependent upon him for social support, household maintenance, income, and transportation, since she did not drive. Therefore, in preparing for discharge, the therapist interviewed Lucille using the CAPA.

Lucille's daily round of activities included cooking and doing some household chores, reading, and knitting. Because of previous difficulties with driving, she did not hold a license and depended upon her husband for transportation when shopping, going to church, and occasionally visiting with friends. On initial assessment, the therapist asked Lucille to describe her satisfaction and participation in her valued occupations. She scored them as 3 or 4 out of a possible 10 (though she reported that before the onset of her current symptoms she would have scored them higher). The environmental negotiability ratings for the occupations were scored 2s and 3s. In addition, her husband had enjoyed camaraderie with fellow truck drivers, and now he spent most of his time with his wife, placing additional stress upon her to be a good companion and caretaker. Her potential losses of roles included losing an "able" husband, social support system, and wage-earner. The therapist and Lucille explored possible gains from the circumstances, and Lucille discovered: (1) the possibility to become reacquainted with her son, from whom she had become estranged, by asking him to come visit and help with badly needed household repairs; (2) the possibility that she could take on new roles in the home as she came to recognize that her occupations had become restricted and diminished in meaning; and (3) the benefits of risking asking friends to drive her places sometimes, thus enlarging her social support system. With the husband's assistance, Lucille set goals for: (1) asking the son to repair the porch steps, (2) learning how to care for the plants in the husband's vegetable garden, and (3) contacting a friend about driving her to the grocery store. In a 3-month follow-up, Lucille had contacted her son. Although he primarily spent time with the husband, he and Lucille were able to be on speaking terms. Lucille also had discovered pleasure in working in the garden, even though some of the vegetables did not live. And lastly, she had found one friend with whom she went shopping weekly. She was reporting higher scores in environment negotiability and also person and participation satisfaction, and had not experienced an increase in symptoms of her bipolar disorder. See Table 9-3 for a full description of the Occupation Card for Household Management: Grocery Shopping.

Table 9-3

Occupation Card for Household Management for Lucille

Occupation Card

Occupation/Activity: Household management: grocery shopping

* Fill out one for each major occupation

	Previous Status	Expected Changes	Outcomes
1. Occupation			
Time satisfaction 1 2 3 4 5 6 7 8 9 10 *Ask the client to rate, on a scale from 1 to 10. Month 1: 3/10 Month 3: 7/10	Has lost her license. Formerly had a planned schedule when husband drove her to the grocery store. "I can't count on him anymore." Month 3: Husband still not driving. **Adaptation** Month 1: Taxi temporary solution; requires more time and work to schedule, and is expensive. Exploration of resources among friends and church members for driver. Month 3: Contacted friend about a regular schedule for shopping.	**Losses** Month 1: Unable to obtain license at this time. Husband no longer able to drive.	Month 1: Goal: To develop alternative ways to do grocery shopping. Outcome: Taking taxi, but unsatisfactory to self and husband. Schedule not managed; uncertainty about drive. Month 3: Outcome: Still takes extra time to coordinate schedules, but friend is driving. Summary: Goal met.
2. Persons Participation satisfaction 1 2 3 4 5 6 7 8 9 10 Month 1: 3/10 Month 3: 7/10	Month 1: Social support limited to husband. Formerly relied only on husband for transportation and money for grocery shopping.	**Losses** Month 1: Loss of husband to drive her ("I miss the time we spent together shopping.") and worried about money, as he was not working. Husband questioning his own role as husband and wage earner, as he is not working. Does not like taxi driver. "I am still hoping my husband can drive me soon."	Month 1: Goal: to explore alternative sources for transportation and social support. To actively seek alternative support system. To obtain reliable driver and develop friendship. To maintain cordial relationships with friend who drives. Summary: Has talked to several members of church.

Table 9-3, continued
Occupation Card for Household Management for Lucille

Occupation Card

Occupation/Activity: Household management: grocery shopping

* Fill out one for each major occupation

	Previous Status	Expected Changes	Outcome
		Adaptation	Goal met as
		Month 1: Define loss of	modified. Has
		husband as a driver as	extended goal to
		a temporary change	include husband in
		that she can manage.	home chores in
		Acknowledge the value	other ways so he
		of considering longer-	maintains his role
		term alternative plans.	identity.
		Month 3: Acknowledge	
		need for stronger support	
		system.	
3. Environment	Month 1: Limited	**Losses**	Month 1: Goal:
	negotiability. Difficulty	Month 1: Needed to go	To develop strategy
Negotiability rating	with unfamiliar environ-	to an unfamiliar store	for managing
1 2 3 4 5 6 7 8 9 10	ments. Formerly shopped	that was closer to home.	shopping at an
	at only one grocery store,	Month 2: Needed to	unfamiliar grocery
	which was familiar and	shop more econom-	store. To develop
Month 1: 2/10	personnel were friendly.	ically, since husband	skill in economic
	Husband always drove	was not currently	grocery shopping.
	her there.	working.	
Month 3: 7/10		Month 3:	Month 3: Goal:
			To continue role
		Adaptation	as grocery shopper
		Month 1: Work with	without husband
		husband and therapist	as driver.
		on scanning the	
		shelves and seeking	Summary: Work
		needed information	is continuing on
		in new grocery settings.	meeting goal.
		Scanning newspapers	
		and shelves for	
		comparative shopping.	
		Month 3: Accepting the	
		possibility that she can	
		negotiate grocery	
		shopping environments	
		without husband's	
		presence.	

Table 9-3, continued
Occupation Card for Household Management for Lucille

Occupation Card

Occupation/Activity: Household management: grocery shopping
* Fill out one for each major occupation

	Previous Status	Expected Changes	Outcome
4. Value Importance rating 1 2 3 4 5 6 7 8 9 10 Month 1: 7/10 Month 3: 8/10	Month 1: Grocery shopping is important to her because it supports her role as a cook, which is important to her only meaningful role as wife and homemaker.	**Losses** Month 1: Loss of time spent with husband, who drove, as this gave meaning to this occupation for her. Threat of loss of husband's salary meant she could not always buy the food they both enjoyed. Month 3: Threat to meaning of the whole occupation (sharing with husband, ability to afford choice foods). **Adaptation** Month 1: Find other ways to share time with husband. Explore meal preferences with husband that had changed since onset of his disability. Month 3: Acknowledge the restrictions in her own social participation, and be willing to find satisfaction in new roles.	Month 1: Goal: To acknowledge why this occupation was so important to her. To discover ways to prepare pleasurable food at lower cost. Month 3: Goal: To participate in valued activities with friends. Summary: Original goal was expanded to include broadened social participation. Goal met as modified.

Summary

The studies done to date with the CAPA indicate clinical usefulness, trustworthiness, and clinical effectiveness in selected populations—primarily the elderly and individuals with long-term disabling conditions that involve physical disorders with concomitant psychosocial and cognitive concerns. Though there is evidence from the work of others[32,33] that community-dwelling individuals with severe mental health problems are able to report their experiences and values, future work should explore further the strategies for engaging patients with severe cognitive or behavioral disorders in the collaborative process. In addition, because of the importance of the narrative data and the time necessary for collection of such information, we recommend further exploration of the use of the CAPA with consultation models of practice.

Acknowledgment

Jean Spencer, PhD, OTR, FAOTA, is acknowledged as the primary author and publisher of the CAPA, and we dedicate this chapter to her memory.

References

1. American Occupational Therapy Association. Psychosocial aspects of occupational therapy. *Am J Occup Ther.* 2004;58:669-672.
2. American Occupational Therapy Association. Occupational therapy practice framework: domain and process. *Am J Occup Ther.* 2002;56:609-639.
3. Mattingly C. The narrative nature of clinical reasoning. In: Mattingly C, Fleming MH, eds. *Clinical Reasoning: Forms of Inquiry in a Therapeutic Practice.* Philadelphia, PA: FA Davis; 1994:239-269.
4. Hemphill-Pearson B, Hunter M. Holism in mental health practice. *Occupational Therapy in Mental Health.* 1997;13:35-49.
5. Finlay L. Holism in occupational therapy: elusive fiction and ambivalent struggle. *Am J Occup Ther.* 2001;55:268-276.
6. Lohman H, Royeen C. Posttraumatic stress disorder and traumatic hand injuries: A neuro-occupational view. *Am J Occup Ther.* 2002;56:527-537.
7. Cara E, MacRae A. *Psychosocial Occupational Therapy: A Clinical Practice.* 2nd ed. Clifton Park, NY: Thomson Delmar Learning; 2005.
8. Helfrich C, Kielhofner G. Volitional narratives and the meaning of therapy. *Am J Occup Ther.* 1994;48:319-326.
9. Helfrich C, Kielhofner G, Mattingly C. Volition as narrative: understanding motivation in chronic illness. *Am J Occup Ther.* 1994;311-317.
10. Spencer J, Davidson H, White VK. Continuity and change: past experience as adaptive repertoire in occupational adaptation. *Am J Occup Ther.* 1996;50:526-534.
11. Spencer J, Davidson H, White V. Helping clients develop hopes for the future. *Am J Occup Ther.* 1997;51:191-198.
12. Fine SB. Resilience and human adaptability: who rises above adversity? 1990 Eleanor Clarke Slagle lecture. *Am J Occup Ther.* 1991;45:493-503.
13. Spencer JC, Davidson HA. The Community Adaptive Planning Assessment: a clinical tool for documenting future planning with clients. *Am J Occup Ther.* 1998;52:19-30.
14. Melville LL, Baltic TA, Bettcher TW, Nelson, DL. Patients' perspectives on the Self-Identified Goals Assessment. *Am J Occup Ther.* 2002;54:650-659.
15. Ottenbacher KJ, Cusick A. Discriminative versus evaluative assessment: some observations in goal attainment scaling. *Am J Occup Ther.* 1993;47:349-354.
16. Trombly CS, Radomski MV, Davis ES. Achievement of self-identified goals by adults with traumatic brain injury: phase 1. *Am J Occup Ther.* 1998;52:810-818.
17. Kielhofner G, Barrett L. Meaning and misunderstanding in occupational forms: a study of therapeutic goal setting. *Am J Occup Ther.* 1998;52:345-353.
18. McDowell I, Newell C. *Measuring Health.* 2nd ed. New York, NY: Oxford University Press; 1996.
19. McColl MA. Measuring community integration and social support. In: Law M, Baum C, Dunn W, eds. *Measuring Occupational Performance: Supporting Best Practice in Occupational Therapy.* 2nd ed. Thorofare, NJ: SLACK Incorporated; 2005:301-312.
20. Spencer JC. Evaluation of performance contexts. In: Crepeau EB, Cohn ES, Schell BAB, eds. *Willard and Spackman's Occupational Therapy.* 10th ed. Philadelphia, PA: Lippincott Williams & Wilkins; 2003:982-1004.

21. Spencer J, Krefting L, Mattingly C. Incorporation of ethnographic methods in occupational therapy assessment. *Am J Occup Ther.* 1993;47:303-309.
22. Kielhofner G, Mallinson T, Forsyth K, Lai J-S. Psychometric properties of the second version of the Occupational Performance History Interview (OPHI-II). *Am J Occup Ther.* 2001;55:260-267.
23. Law M, Baptiste S, Carswell A, McColl MA, Polatajko H, Pollock N. *The Canadian Occupational Performance Measure.* 3rd ed. Ottowa: Canadian Association of Occupational Therapists; 1998.
24. Florey LL, Michelman SM. Occupational Role History: a screening tool for psychiatric occupational history. *Am J Occup Ther.* 1982;36:301-308.
25. Oakley F, Kielhofner G, Barris R, Reicher RF. The Role Checklist: development and empirical assessment of reliability. *Occup Ther J Res.* 1986;6:157-169.
26. McColl MA, Friedland J. Development of a multidimensional index for assessing social support in rehabilitation. *Occup Ther J Res.* 1989;9:218-234.
27. Wood-Dauphinee S, Opzoomer A, Williams JI, Marchand B, Spitzer WO. Assessment of global function: The Reintegration to Normal Living Index. *Arch Phys Med Rehab.* 1988;69:583-590.
28. McColl MA, Davies D, Carlson P, Johnston J, Minnes P. The Community Integration Measure: Development and preliminary validation. *Arch Phys Med Rehab.* 2001;82:429-434.
29. Spencer J, Hersch G, Eschenfelder V, Fournet J, Murray-Gerzik M. Outcomes of protocol-based and adaptation-based occupational therapy interventions for low-income elderly persons on a transitional unit. *Am J Occup Ther.* 1999;53:159-170.
30. Anderson C, Spencer J. An environmental approach to evaluation and treatment in an upper extremity injury clinic. In: Letts L , Rigby P, Stewart D, eds. *Using Environments to Enable Occupational Performance.* Thorofare, NJ: SLACK Incorporated; 2003:207-218.
31. Bates P. The self-care environment: Issues of space and furnishings. In: Christiansen C, ed. *Ways of Living: Self-Care Strategies for Special Needs.* Rockville, MD: American Occupational Therapy Association; 1994:423-457.
32. Brown C, Hamera E, Long C. The Daily Activities Checklist: a functional assessment for consumers with mental illness living in the community. *Occup Ther Health Care.* 1996;10:33-44.
33. Hachey R, Boyer G, Mercier C. Perceived and valued roles of adults with severe mental health problems. *Can J Occup Ther.* 2001;68:112-120.

10

VOCATIONAL ASSESSMENTS USED IN MENTAL HEALTH

Cindee Quake-Rapp, PhD, OTR

"No other technique for the conduct of life attaches the individual so firmly to reality as laying emphasis on work; for his work at least gives him a secure place in a portion of reality, in the human community." Freud S. Civilization and Its Discontents. *New York: W. W. Norton & Company; 1989.*

Introduction

Two-thirds of persons with mental illness would like to be competitively employed, although 85% of those participating in public mental health systems are not.[1,2]

The President's New Freedom Commission on Mental Health emphasizes the importance of work in the recovery for persons with mental illness.[3] The role of the occupational therapist in assessing vocational potential is to adopt a client-centered approach based on meaningful occupation, to ensure that employment goals are based on individual preferences. Occupational therapists incorporate occupational analysis in the process of job development, and provide follow up assistance in an environment moving toward supported employment.[4]

Assessment of vocational potential should focus on social and vocational functioning and the integration of the individual with mental illness into the community. Occupational therapists must assess factors that are shown to be significant predictors of vocational potential for persons with mental illness. This chapter will identify research-based predictors of vocational potential of persons with mental illness and how these predictive variables can be used as a reference when designing and evaluating outcomes of vocational rehabilitation programs.

History of Mental Health Services Involving Work-Related Occupations

The use of "work" as a therapeutic intervention was introduced in 1772 by physician and psychiatrist Philippe Pinel. Pinel believed that the use of occupational therapy and theatrics was more successful than punishment, incarceration, or bleeding.

He staged a mock trial for a tailor who thought he was going to be executed by the guillotine, acquitting him of his imaginary crime. In addition, the tailor was involved in work therapy through mending patients' clothes. The recognition by Pinel that "meaningful occupation" coupled with kindness was successful in treating persons with mental illness led to the Moral Treatment movement of the early 1800s in Europe.[5] Moral treatment was based on the belief that providing an environment that closely resembled the real world with emphasis on literature, physical exercise, and work alleviated stress and improved occupations of daily living for persons with mental illness.

By the mid-1800s, asylums were built in Europe and America to house and treat the mentally ill. It became apparent that the nonrestrained patients did not have meaningful ways to occupy their time. Work programs and recreational activities were implemented where patients were involved in occupations related to farming, dairy, greenhouses, and ground crews. Asylums prided themselves on their beautiful landscaping and grounds maintained by patients. Both patients and the institution benefited from this symbiotic relationship that provided a transition from the hospital to the community.[6]

By the turn of the 19th century, humane and restorative treatment declined, and old procedures such as restraining patients reoccurred. Overcrowding developed because institutions had no established criteria for admitting patients and became dumping grounds for unwanted people in society. By the early 1950s, psychotropic medications reduced the length of stay in asylums, and the Community Mental Health movement began the massive deinstitutionalization and social integration of the 1960s.

State and federal policies of the 1960s and 1970s emphasized human rights of persons with mental illness, and in 1972, a federal court ruled that patients in mental health facilities could not work without pay. Gone were the dairy farms, agricultural pursuits, and pristine grounds of institutions that could not afford to pay patients or increase staff to occupy the patients' abundant free time.[6]

Deinstitutionalization dramatically increased the homeless population, including the one-third who are mentally ill. Mental illness became a social welfare problem: housing and employment became community problems without adequate federal and state support. Mental health practice focused on stabilization of symptoms and protection of persons with mental illness from the stressors of adult roles and community life. Vocational rehabilitation involved lengthy train-and-place models where patients were placed in highly protected and segregated settings such as sheltered workshops, prevocational training units, and transitional employment managed by the mental health agency.[7] State vocational rehabilitation agencies used paper-and-pencil tests and psychological evaluations for assessing the vocational potential of clients despite considerable evidence that direct placement in a job was the best predictor of eventual vocational success.[8,9] Train-and-place models promoted low expectations and long-term dependency on the mental health system, and were not effective transitions to competitive employment.[7] During the 1980s, supported employment was developed as a "place-and-train model," replacing the old adage of extensive prevocational training prior to finding a job.[10] The Rehabilitation Act Amendments of 1986 define supported employment as rapid placement in a competitive work setting while providing necessary training and follow-up support on the job. Over two decades of research has identified supported employment as a specific evidence-based practice for persons with severe mental illness.[11-13] The 1992 Rehabilitation Act Amendments emphasized employment as the primary goal of rehabilitation and mandated presumptive employability—meaning applicants are presumed to be employable unless proven otherwise. The amendments state that eligible individuals must be provided choice and increased control in determining the vocation rehabilitation goals and objectives, determining services, providers of services, and methods to provide and/or secure services.

Predictors of Vocational Potential for Persons With Mental Illness

Tsang et al conducted a meta-analysis of controlled studies on significant predictors of employment outcomes in persons with mental illness.[14] Based on prior research, the authors found that premorbid functioning, work history, and social skills are consistent predictors of employment outcomes. Cognitive functioning and family relationships were also significant predictors, although not extensively studied. Additional predictors of vocational outcomes found in the literature include self-concept in the worker role, amount of job development services, supported employment versus traditional vocational services, and community support.[7,15]

In best practice supportive employment, lengthy prevocational assessment is not considered effective because it discourages people who desire competitive employment. The initial assessment is done quickly by gathering a patient-centered occupational profile[16] on previous work experiences, job preferences, education, current adjustment, and other job-related factors such as transportation needs and family support.[7] Ongoing work-based vocational assessment is a continuous process that measures work experiences in competitive real world jobs rather than relying on a battery of prevocational assessments. In determining the occupational profile of a person with mental illness, one must identify his or her needs, wants, and concerns regarding engagement in occupations of work. Information should be gathered on premorbid functioning in work, leisure, and social skills before the onset of mental illness. Premorbid occupational performance in job acquisition, work skills, work adjustment, and other life experiences are significant predictors of employment outcomes.[14] A group of people with schizophrenia who had a prior or current employment history was shown to have significant improvement in work-related skills when compared to a group that had never been employed.[17] Table 10-1 provides examples of how to obtain an occupational profile.

The following occupational performance assessments can aid in information gathering for the occupational profile and range from 7 to 30 minutes to administer.[18]

Occupational Performance Assessments

CANADIAN OCCUPATIONAL PERFORMANCE MEASURE (COPM)

The COPM[19] is a client-centered outcome measure designed for use by occupational therapists to measure change in a patient's self-perception of occupational performance

Table 10-1
Examples of Information Gathering for an Occupational Profile

Occupational History

Obtain information from patient concerning:

- current roles
- responsibilities
- future roles
- lifestyle issues
- work history
- medical history
- necessary and chosen occupations

Patterns of Living

Interview patient about daily routines:

- sleeping
- eating habits
- dressing behavior
- personal hygiene
- socialization behavior with siblings, peers, and other adults
- response to stimulation
- habits

Interests

Interview patient about:

- preferred occupations
- time spent engaging with occupations
- interests in leisure pursuits
- interest in activities of daily living (ADLs) and (IADLs)
- interest in socializing with others

Needs

Interview patient about concerns and issues regarding their interpretation of their employment needs.

- temporal needs
- environmental needs
- external support needs
- security needs
- activity level needs

Priorities

Interview patient to determine what their priorities are for employment.

Concerns

Interview patient to determine what concerns they have regarding their potential or ongoing employment.

over time. It is designed for any patient population. The COPM is standardized, with a semi-structured interview and a structured scoring method. According to the authors, differences between assessment and reassessment over time are the most meaningful scores of this instrument.

OCCUPATIONAL PERFORMANCE HISTORY INTERVIEW II (OPH-II)

The OPH-II[20] is a client-centered historical interview that focuses on a person's life history, the impact of disability, and future directions that the person would like to follow in life. The OPH-II is designed for patients that can respond to a narrative history interview.

OCCUPATIONAL SELF-ASSESSMENT (OSA)

The OSA[21] self-report format identifies essential components of the occupational profile, such as the patient's values, priorities, and goals. The OSA addresses the patient's perception of his or her occupational performance and how his or her environment influences occupational performance. Examples of activities included on the OSA are:

1. Handling responsibility
2. Managing finances
3. Leisure pursuits
4. Environmental support—physical and social

Situational Assessment

When selecting an instrument or tool for assessing the occupational performance of work or work potential, the occupational therapist should address vocational assessment as an ongoing collaborative process of systematic observation and analysis. Situational assessment is the best clinical predictor of future work performance and rates a person's work-adjustment skills in the setting that most resembles the work that will be done. The ability of a person with a mental illness to function in one environment is not predictive of his or her ability to function in another environment.[14] Situational assessment involves repeated observations and rating of job behaviors and attitudes in actual or simulated work environments over time. Typical situational assessments include work quality and quantity, performance on specific work tasks, attitude, and interpersonal relations with coworkers and supervisor.[22] Situational assessments are an effective way to assess areas that have a demonstrated link to employment outcomes such as social and motor skills. Studies reveal that vocational assessment conducted in a real or simulated work setting with people performing real work tasks reliably predicts subsequent community employment.[23,24]

Social Interaction Skills

According to Marsh and Bond,[25] people with severe mental illness display limitation in the most basic instrumental activities of daily living (IADL), such as greeting people on the street or paying for a purchase in a store. Tsang et al found that work-related social skills can be categorized into job-securing social skills and job-retaining social skills.[14] The first tier of social survival skills encompasses grooming, politeness, and personal appearance. The second tier consists of handling general and specific work-related situations such as the ability to interact appropriately with supervisors, colleagues, and subordinates. The third tier encompasses the benefits that a person can obtain from possessing social survival skills and handling work-related situations such as getting a job, maintaining a job, and perceiving satisfaction and achievement from the job. The ability to get along with others and function socially is a significant predictor of future employment outcomes.[14] Occupational performance assessments often include social interaction and adjustment questions.

ASSESSING SOCIAL SKILLS OF PEOPLE WITH SCHIZOPHRENIA

Tsang and Pearson designed a two-part measure[26] that was developed and validated on a model for assessing social skills for seeking and maintaining a job for people with schizophrenia.[27] The instrument consists of a 10-item self-administered checklist and a role-play exercise. The role-play exercise involves participation in a job interview and request to leave work due to an urgent need. The self-administered checklist provides feedback on the patient's perceived competence in handling work-related social situations.[28]

SOCIAL ADJUSTMENT SCALE SELF-REPORT

The Social Adjustment Scale Self-Report[29,30] has 54 questions that measure worker role performance over a 2-week period of time. Questions include such items as work for pay; unpaid work; work as a student; social and leisure activities; relationships with extended family, spouse, and one's children; relationships with the family unit; and perception of economic functioning. Questions within each area include:
1. Performance at expected tasks
2. Friction with people
3. Aspects of interpersonal relationships
4. Feelings
5. Satisfactions

SOCIAL ADAPTATION SELF-EVALUATION SCALE

The Social Adaptation Self-Evaluation Scale is a 21-item self-report that detects discrete differences in social motivation and behavior that may not be discerned in psychiatric assessment.[31,32] This assessment addresses a patient's self-perception and motivation toward an action rather than on objective performance. Questions are asked about the patient's occupation (if the patient is employed), or a home-related activity (if he or she is not employed).

SOCIAL PROBLEM-SOLVING INVENTORY (SPSI)

The SPSI[33] consists of 70 items designed to assess self-appraisal of multiple dimensions of the problem-solving process. The SPSI identifies adaptive coping mechanisms for specific problematic situations encountered in everyday life. The following subscales are included in the inventory:
1. Cognition subscale
2. Emotion subscale

3. Behavior subscale
4. Problem definition and formulation subscale
5. Generation of alternative solutions subscale
6. Decision-making subscale
7. Solution implementation and verification subscale

Self-Concept in Worker Role

The most useful paper-and-pencil test predictors of future vocational outcomes are tests that measure a person's ego strength or self-concept in the role of worker.[14] Self-concept and perception of the worker role are crucial factors for successful engagement with work.

WORKER ROLE INTERVIEW (WRI)

The WRI[34] identifies psychosocial and environmental factors that influence return to work. The WRI is a semi-structured interview used to identify psychosocial and environmental factors as part of the initial evaluation for the injured worker, the worker with a chronic disability, and the worker with poor or limited work histories.

SELF DESCRIPTION QUESTIONNAIRE III

The SDQIII[35] is a 136-item instrument designed to measure self-concept and specific global areas for young adults (aged 18 and older) that measures 11 factors. The 13 SDQIII scales are:

1. Physical ability
2. Physical appearance
3. Opposite sex relationships
4. Same sex relationships
5. Honesty/trustworthiness
6. Parent relationships
7. Emotional stability
8. Self-esteem
9. Verbal, math, and academic
10. Problem solving
11. Religion/spirituality factors

Job Development Services

According to Cook, client-centered job development should be tailored to patient preferences.[22] Research identifies that patients have better outcomes when services are designed to coincide with personal preferences. The more vocational services that persons with mental illness receive, the better the employment outcomes they achieve, especially those receiving job development services.[22] Cook identified the following effects of job development and job support on competitive employment outcomes for persons with mental illness:[36]

1. Persons who receive job development services were five times more likely to secure competitive employment compared to persons who did not receive job development.

2. Persons with no prior work history had limited chances of obtaining competitive employment without job development.

3. People involved with integrated clinical and vocational services had better employment outcomes.

Supported Employment Versus Traditional Vocational Services

Best practice vocational rehabilitation services should integrate clinical and employment services, provide ongoing job support, and match the job with the patient's individual preferences. In addition, rapid job placement into competitive employment is more effective than traditional vocational services for consumers with both good and poor work histories.[7,11,12,36]

People with mental illness need ongoing support that is not time-limited.[36] Moll, Huff, and Detwiler identify the compatibility of occupational therapy and supported employment as follows:[4]

1. Value of meaningful occupation

2. Patient-centered approach

3. Goals based on individual preferences

4. Job placement based on function and skill level

5. Identification of job modifications that promote successful outcomes

6. Expertise in environmental assessment and fit between person, environment, and occupation

7. Understanding and advocacy of the American with Disabilities Act

Occupational therapists must shift their focus from vocational assessment and skill development to developing and accessing support in the work environment. Moll, Huff, and Detwiler suggest that therapists network with employers to develop or match jobs, and market patients to prospective employers.[4] Occupational therapists are ideally trained to integrate evidence-best supportive employment principles when providing vocational services.

References

1. Mueser KT, Salyers MP, Mueser PR. A prospective analysis of work in schizophrenia. *Schizophr Bull.* 2001;27:281-296.

2. Rogers ES, Walsh D, Masotta L, et al. *Massachusetts Survey of Client Preferences for Community Support Services, Final Report.* Boston, MA: Boston University Center for Psychiatric Rehabilitation; 1991.

3. New Freedom Commission on Mental Health. *Achieving the Promise: Transforming Mental Health Care in America, Final Report.* Rockville, MD; 2003. DHHS Pub. No. SMA-03-3832.

4. Moll S, Huff J, Detwiler L. Supported employment: evidence for a best practice model in psychosocial rehabilitation. *Can J Occup Ther.* 2003;70:298-310.

5. Humane treatment for the mad? *Physicians Weekly.* 1999;16:1.

6. The Ridge. The history of mental illness. Ohio University. 2001. Available at: http://cscwww.cats.ohiou. edu/~ridges/history.html. Accessed January 22, 2006.

7. Becker DR, Drake RE. *Supported Employment for People With Severe Mental Illness: A Guideline Developed for the Behavioral Health Recovery Management Project.* New Hampshire-Dartmouth Psychiatric Research Center; 2004:1-15.

8. Bond GR, Dincin J. Accelerating entry into transitional employment in a psychiatric rehabilitation agency. *Rehabil Psychol.* 1986;32:143-155.

9. Roessler R, Boone S. Evaluation diagnoses as indicators of employment potential. *Vocational Eval Work Adjustment Bull.* 1982;15:103-106.

10. Wehman P, Moore MS. *Vocational Rehabilitation and Supported Employment.* Baltimore, MD: Paul Brookes; 1988.

11. Bond GR. Supported employment: evidence for an evidence-based practice. *Psychiatr Rehabil J.* 2004;27:345-359.

12. Bond GR, Becker DR, Drake RE, et al. Implementing supported employment as an evidence-based practice [abstract]. *Psychiatr Serv.* 2001;52:313-322.

13. Twamley EW, Dilip J, Lehman AF. Vocational rehabilitation in schizophrenia and other psychotic disorders: a literature review and meta-analysis of randomized controlled trials. *J Nerv Ment Dis.* 2003;191:515-523.

14. Tsang H, Lam P, Bacon NG, Leung O. Predictors of employment outcomes for people with psychiatric disabilities: a review of the literature since the mid '80s. *J Rehabil.* 2000;66:19-31.

15. Cook JA, Jonikas JA, Solomon, ML. Models of vocational rehabilitation for youths and adults with severe mental illness: implications for America 2000 and ADA-Americans with disabilities act. *Am Rehabil.* Autumn, 1992. Available at: http://www.findarticles.com/p/articles/mi_m0842/is_n3_v18/ai_12766848. Accessed January 22, 2006.

16. American Occupational Therapy Association. *Occupational Therapy Practice Framework: Domain and Process.* Bethesda, MD: AOTA; 2001.

17. Anthony WA, Rogers ES, Cohen M, Davis R. Relationships between psychiatric symptomatology, work skills, and future vocational performance. *Psychiatr Serv.* 1995;46:353-358.

18. Law M, Baum CM, Dunn W. Occupational performance assessment. In: Christiansen CH, Baum CM, eds. *Occupational Therapy: Performance, Participation, and Well-Being.* Thorofare, NJ: SLACK Incorporated; 2005:345.

19. Law M, Baptiste S, Carswell A, McColl MA, Polatajko H, Pollock N. *The Canadian Occupational Performance Measure.* 3rd ed. Toronto, Ontario: CAOT Publications ACE; 1998.

20. Kielhofner G, Mallinson T, Crawford C, et al. *Occupational Performance History Interview II (OPHI-II),* Version 2.1. Chicago, IL: Model of Human Occupation Clearinghouse; 2004.

21. Baron K, Kielhofner G, Iyenger A, Goldhammer V, Wolenski J. *Occupational Self Assessment (OSA),* Version 2.1. Chicago, IL: Model of Human Occupation Clearinghouse; 2002.

22. Cook JA. Research based principles of vocational rehabilitation for psychiatric disability. Veterans Industry. 2003. Available at: http://www1.va.gov/vetind/page.cfm?pg=6. Accessed January 22, 2006.

23. Bond GR, Fried-Meyer MH. Predictive validity of situational assessment at a psychiatric rehabilitation center. *Rehabil Psychol.* 1987;32:99-112.

24. Cook JA, Solomon ML, Jonikas JA, Frazier M. *Thresholds Supported Competitive Employment Program for Youth with Severe Mental Illness. Final Report to the US Dept of Education.* Washington, DC: Office of Special Education and Rehabilitation Services; 1990. Grant G008630404.

25. Marsh DT, Bond GR. New directions in the psychological treatment of serious mental illness. *Contemp Psychol.* 1995;40:787-792.

26. Tsang H, Pearson V. Reliability and validity of a simple measure for assessing the social skills of people with schizophrenia necessary for seeking and securing a job. *Can J Occup Ther.* 2000;67:250-259.

27. Pearson V, Tsang H. A conceptual framework for work related social skills in psychiatric rehabilitation. *J Rehabil.* 1997;62:61-67.

28. Tsang H. Applying social skills training in the context of vocational rehabilitation for people with schizophrenia. *J Nerv Ment Dis.* 2001;189:90-98.

29. Weissman MM, Olfson M, Gameroff MJ, Feder A, Fuentes M. A comparison of three scales for assessing social functioning in primary care. *Am J Psychiatry.* 2001;158:460-466.

30. Weisman MM, Bothwell S. Assessment of social function by patient self-report. *Arch Gen Psychiatry.* 1976;33:1111-1115.

31. Bosc M. Assessment of social functioning in depression. *Compr Psychiatry.* 2000;41:63-69.

32. Bosc M, Dubini A, Polin V. Development and validation of a social functioning scale, the social adaptation self-evaluation scale. *Eur Neuropsychopharmacol.* 1997;7:57-70.

33. D'Zurilla TJ, Nezu A. Development and preliminary evaluation of the social problem-solving inventory. *Psychol Assess: J Consult Clin Psychol.* 1990;85(2):156-163.
34. Braveman B, Robson M, Velozo C, et al. *Worker Role Interview (WRI),* Version 10.0. Chicago, IL: Model of Human Occupation Clearinghouse; 2005.
35. Marsh HW. *Self Description Questionnaire III.* Sydney, Australia: SELF Research Centre, University of Western Sydney; 1998.
36. Cook JA. Executive summary of findings from the employment intervention demonstration project (EIDP). University of Illinois at Chicago. 2005. Available at: http://www.psych.uic.edu/eidp/eidpfindings.htm. Accessed January 22, 2006.

PART V:
BEHAVIORAL ASSESSMENTS

ASSESSMENTS USED WITH THE MODEL OF HUMAN OCCUPATION

Jessica Kramer, MS, OTR/L
Gary Kielhofner, DrPH, OTR/L, FAOTA
Kirsty Forsyth, PhD, OTR

"Good assessment is critical to understanding clients and their needs. Moreover, assessment is a prerequisite to making good decisions about the goals and strategies of therapy...From the perspective of MOHO theory, comprehensive assessment means that a therapist will at minimum raise and seek answers to questions pertaining to the client's occupational adaptation, volition, habitation, performance capacity, and environmental impact." Kielhofner G. A Model of Human Occupation: Theory and Application. 4th ed. Baltimore, MD: Lippincott, Williams & Wilkins; 2007:155.

Introduction

The occupational therapy process begins with evaluation whereby a therapist generates an occupational profile along with an analysis of a patient's occupational performance.[1] In order to do this, a therapist must understand the patient's occupational history, interests, values, and perspective regarding problems of occupational functioning, and then identify factors influencing successful occupational performance. Occupational therapists can ensure this evaluation process is "top-down" and evidence-based by using a well-researched, occupation-based conceptual practice model to guide data collection and interpretation. The Model of Human Occupation (MOHO)[2] is an occupational therapy practice model that therapists can use to systematically identify performance skills and patterns, environments, and individual patient factors that are impacting occupational adaptation, by using the model's "technology for application."[3(p20)] The instruments used with this model have undergone rigorous psychometric development to ensure that the information they provide is dependable and useful in a clinical context.

This chapter will first review MOHO concepts, then discuss MOHO-based assessment tools appropriate for use in mental health contexts. These assessments are key to generating an occupational profile, identifying problems in skills, and developing an explanation of the patients' circumstances. It should be noted that the brief review of MOHO concepts in this chapter is only an introduction. Use of MOHO instruments requires at least a basic knowledge of MOHO and is augmented when one has a solid grasp of this model. Readers are referred to *A Model of Human Occupation: Theory and Application*,[2] where both the theory and the assessments are covered in more depth.

MOHO Concepts

OCCUPATIONAL ADAPTATION AND DIMENSIONS OF DOING

Individuals are actors that engage in occupations in a variety of contexts over time. Identifying with specific roles, engaging in interesting activities, being connected with the temporal patterns of life, meeting responsibilities, and fulfilling personal expectations and values are all aspects of our lives as occupational beings. According to MOHO, when individuals maintain patterns of occupational participation within the environments that reflect their sense of who they are as occupational beings, the end result is a sense of *occupational adaptation*. Occupational adaptation involves the "construction of a positive occupational identity and achieving occupational competence over time."[2(p121)] Occupational identity and competence are influenced by our experiences, including illness and impairment, and these experiences may require individuals to reframe their sense of who they are or what occupations they enact in their daily lives. Several MOHO assessments explore a patient's sense of occupational competence and occupational identity (Table 11-1).

Engaging in occupations involves three levels of doing: *occupational participation, occupational performance,* and *occupational skill*.[2] These concepts describe different levels at which one can examine doing.[4]

Occupational participation refers to engagement in work, play, or activities of daily living (ADL) that are desired and necessary for well-being according to a person's socio-cultural context. Occupational participation is influenced by environmental and cultural contexts, as well as by individual patient factors, such as motivation and motor capacities. Occupational participation may include maintaining a home, being an employee, or being a member of a social community.

The actions required to participate at this broad level make up the next level of doing—occupational performance. Examples of occupational performance associated with occupational participation include preparing a meal, making a sale to a customer, and playing a game of cards.

Performing occupations such as these requires a discrete set of purposeful actions that arise during our engagement in goal-directed activities. These observable actions, or skills, are a function of the interaction between the environment and an individual's personal characteristics. Motor, process, communication, and interaction skills[1,2,5] associated with making a sale to a customer include manipulating money, sequencing actions to ring up the purchase on the register, and speaking with the customer. Readers may recognize that MOHO's conceptualization of skill is used in the *Occupational Therapy Practice Framework*.[2]

MOHO assessments evaluate a patient's participation, performance, and skill so that the therapist can best identify the level of doing that is causing a patient difficulty.

Table 11-1
Levels of Doing

Levels of Doing	Example
Occupational Participation	Salesperson
Occupational Performance	Make a sale to a customer
Occupational Skills	• Speak with customer
	• Sequence actions to use register
	• Manipulate money

Adapted from Kielhofner G. *A Model of Human Occupation: Theory and Application.* 4th ed. Baltimore, MD: Lippincott, Williams & Wilkins; 2007: 105.

Individual Client Factors

In addition to describing the process of occupational adaptation and articulating the different levels of doing associated with engagement in occupation, MOHO also explains how individual patient factors impact a person's participation in occupations.

VOLITION

Humans are the product of an evolutionary process that has given them a drive to engage in action.[2] This drive for occupation underlies volition. Throughout life, engaging in occupations results in certain thoughts and feelings about doing. These thoughts and feelings comprise:

- An individual's sense of personal effectiveness while performing an activity (personal causation)
- The importance and worth attached to that activity (values)
- Enjoyment and satisfaction from engaging in that activity (interests)

Thoughts and feelings related to personal causation, interests, and values intersect to produce a person's volitional orientation to doing. These thoughts create a dynamic and ongoing volitional process of anticipating, choosing, experiencing, and interpreting participation in certain occupations.[2] During the volitional process, an individual:

- Anticipates what engagement in the activity will be like
- Chooses to begin or terminate an activity based on interests, values, and sense of control
- Experiences that engagement in a variety of ways (fulfilling, anxiety-producing)
- Interprets and makes sense of his or her actions and experiences

The volitional process is ongoing and shapes an individual's future engagement in occupations.

HABITUATION

Recurrent patterns of engagement and interaction support daily routines and customs that help organize a person's life. These habituated patterns of action are regulated by habits and roles. "Habits preserve a way we have learned to do something from earlier performance in a given environment,"[2(p65)] and allow performance to be more efficient and more effective. Habits can impact how a routine activity is performed, regulate how time is used, and produce styles of behavior that characterize an individual's performance. For example, a habituated pattern of taking public transportation enables a person to quickly get to a familiar place, while taking medication at the same time every day decreases the chances of missing a dose.

Having an internalized role is the incorporation of a socially or personally defined status and related actions and attitudes. Roles help determine the manner and content of our actions and the types of things that are done—they partition our time. Typical roles in western culture for teenagers include being a member of a family, a student, and a friend, while adults may have roles as a spouse, a parent, and a worker. Some roles have a clearly defined status, such as the role of a homeowner; this role entails keeping the house structurally sound, paying the bills, and creating a welcoming space. Other roles, however, are less formalized or do not have a recognized social status, such as the role of a member of a day program.

PERFORMANCE CAPACITY

Participation in occupations is supported by the state of one's physical and mental components, as well as the subjective experience of living within one's body. Occupational therapists use a variety of conceptual practice models to measure, classify, and describe the state of physical and mental components in order to explain problems of function. However, MOHO considers how an individual's subjective experience of living in the body influences how the person performs and interacts with the world. Attempting to understand a person's "view from the inside"[2(p83)] can be especially powerful when working with patients who experience positive psychotic symptoms, such as hallucinations and delusions.

THE ENVIRONMENT

All aspects of the environment, including man-made and natural spaces, objects, other community members, and local customs offer either an opportunity or a barrier to participating in meaningful and culturally relevant occupations. MOHO recognizes that the environment is comprised of both physical and social elements. The physical environment includes spaces and objects; spaces can be both built and natural, while objects include things that people interact with or use while engaging in a variety of activities. Social groups and occupational forms make up the social aspect of the environment. Social groups can be formal or informal, and have related expectations for behavior within that group. Occupational forms include the actions and manners that characterize a certain activity and are connected to the meaning of the activity.

Each aspect of the environment can provide resources or opportunities for engagement in occupations, or can demand and constrain specific actions. Each environment impacts an individual in a different way, depending on that person's volition, habitation, and performance capacity.

SUMMARY

The process of occupational adaptation, participation and performance, individual patient factors, and the environment, as articulated by MOHO, allows an occupational therapist to understand how a variety of factors influences a person's engagement in occupations. Next, this chapter will review the MOHO-based assessments that therapists can use to systematically identify and document the factors impacting successful participation for patients with mental health difficulties.

Interview Assessments

Interview assessments enable a therapist to establish therapeutic rapport and gain a greater understanding of a patient's history and concerns. Two commonly used MOHO interview assessments include the Occupational Performance History Interview (OPHI-II) and the Occupational Circumstances Assessment Interview and Rating Scale (OCAIRS).

OCCUPATIONAL PERFORMANCE HISTORY INTERVIEW (OPHI-II)

Using the OPHI-II

The OPHI-II[6] is a semi-structured historical interview that provides a patient with an opportunity to both reflect upon and actively construct meaning from past and current occupational participation. Therapists guide the OPHI-II interview process, using questions to elicit narratives (stories) from the patient. These narratives enable individuals to "integrate their past, present, and future into a coherent whole,"[6(p9)] and can take several forms. Some narratives refer to changes in life direction or focus on "turning" events. A person's perceptions of the impact of these turning events may shift as time passes and as life unfolds.[7] Other stories reveal an individual's motives or causation, and help to explain how circumstances were resolved.[8] Through such stories, people are able to enact narratives in their everyday lives. Narratives in response to questions about the meaning of particular events can result in metaphors that help make sense of complex and difficult situations.[8] The information the therapist and patient gather during the interview is then used to complete three rating scales and plot a life history.

Questions in the OPHI-II interview guide and the OPHI-II items are grouped according to three MOHO concepts: Occupational Identity, Occupational Competence, and Occupational Settings (Environment). Each of these concepts has a rating scale that includes a 4-point rating of occupational functioning and items about past and current occupational participation. The past ratings capture previous experiences that an individual can draw upon during current periods of occupational challenges, while the current ratings enable the identification of factors that are presently impacting occupational functioning. The *Occupational Identity Scale* captures a person's sense of self as an occupational being and level of self-awareness through the following items:

- Has personal goals and projects
- Identifies a desired occupational lifestyle
- Expects success
- Accepts responsibility
- Appraises abilities and limitations
- Has commitments and values

- Recognizes identity and obligations
- Has interests
- Felt effective (in the past)
- Found meaning/satisfaction in lifestyle (in the past)
- Made occupational choices (in the past)

The *Occupational Competence Scale* reflects one's ability to maintain a routine, actualize an identity, and meet demands and responsibilities. The competence items include:
- Maintains satisfying lifestyle
- Fulfills role expectations
- Works toward goals
- Meets personal performance standards
- Organizes time for responsibilities
- Participates in interests
- Fulfilled roles (in the past)
- Maintained habits (in the past)
- Achieved satisfaction (in the past)

The *Occupational Settings Scale* captures the influence of the physical and social environment on a person's occupational participation. This scale encompasses a range of everyday environments in which individuals participate in work, play, or ADL, as reflected in the items:
- Home-life occupational forms
- Major productive role occupational forms
- Leisure occupational forms
- Home-life social groups
- Major productive role social groups
- Leisure social groups
- Home-life physical space, objects, and resources
- Major productive role physical space, objects, and resources
- Leisure physical space, objects, and resources

While the ratings on the items help to identify factors contributing to problems in occupational adaptation, therapists can also use the OPHI-II keyforms to obtain instantaneous patient measures to monitor progress and evaluate intervention success.

Paper-and-pencil keyforms for each rating scale, developed using Rasch measurement,[9] convert the ordinal patient ratings to interval measures, and provide the therapist with an individual patient measure and error. When a therapist is unable to rate a patient on an item, due to its irrelevance to a person's particular situation or lack of adequate information, the therapist can visually inspect the patterns of ratings, using the keyform to approximate a patient measure. Figure 11-1 is an example of an OPHI-II keyform.

The final step in completing the OPHI-II is the plotting of the patient's life history narrative. Drawing out a plot line that reflects the narratives elicited from the patient during the interview provides a graphic portrayal of the patient's life history. The resulting nar-

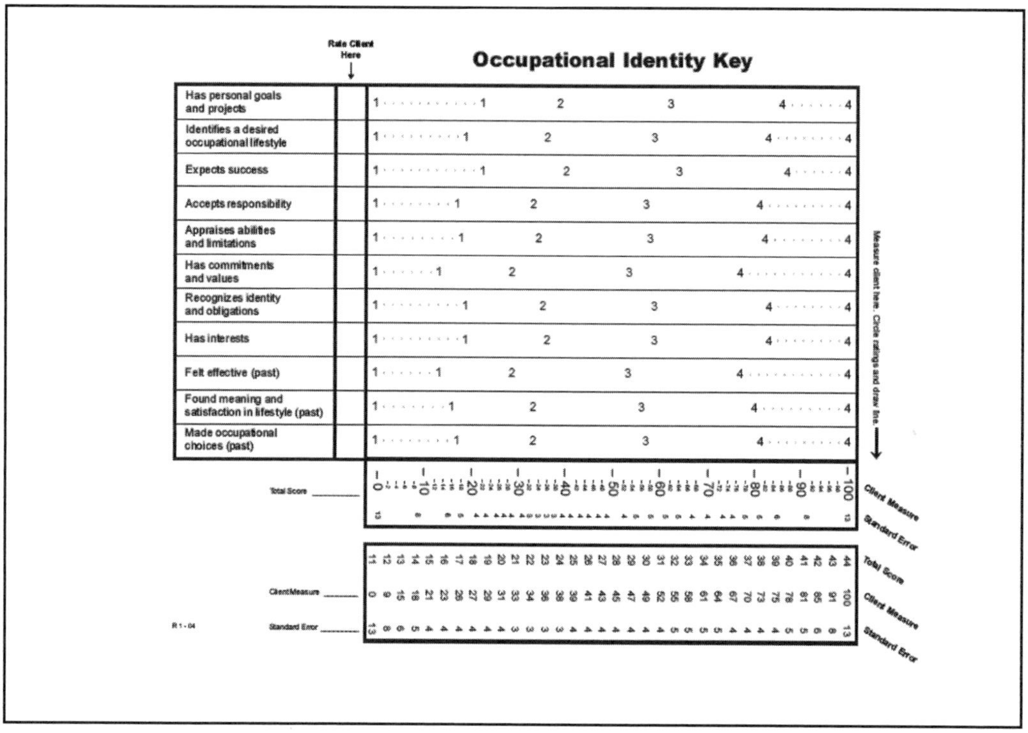

Figure 11-1. OPHI-II Keyform for the Identity Scale. Reprinted with permission from MOHO Clearinghouse.

rative slopes are helpful when planning intervention goals, and patients report finding them very motivational and helpful for understanding life histories.[10]

Research and Development of the OPHI-II

The OPHI-II has undergone 25 years of development. Investigations on the first version of the OPHI confirmed that the instrument had acceptable inter-rater and test-retest reliability[11,12] and construct validity.[13] Revisions were made in order to improve the interview process.[14] Psychometric analysis of the OPHI using Rasch measurement theory[9] revealed that there were three underlying constructs of occupational adaptation; as a result, the three subscales of occupational competence, occupational identity, and the occupational environment were created.[15] An international study of the OPHI-II (using six different language versions) provided evidence of the internal consistency and construct validity of the three rating scales of the OPHI-II.[16] This international sample also provided the calibrations for the development of the OPHI-II keyforms.[17]

The OPHI-II was used in a variety of situations to better understand and address the mental health needs of patients. A study using the OPHI-II in a secure forensic setting revealed that patients felt bored and dissatisfied, and desired further engagement in occupations.[18] The OPHI-II interview explicated the identity of homeless adolescent mothers and found the identity was influenced by the person's development, role choices, and future desire to engage in the mother role.[19] The OPHI-II was also used to better understand the experiences of those living with chronic fatigue syndrome,[20,21] caregivers of persons diagnosed with schizophrenia,[22] and persons living with HIV/AIDS.[23-25] In addition, aspects of the OPHI, particularly the narrative slope, predict future function as well as service outcomes.[25,26]

THE OCCUPATIONAL CIRCUMSTANCES ASSESSMENT INTERVIEW AND RATING SCALE (OCAIRS)

Using the OCAIRS

The OCAIRS is another semi-structured interview that provides both qualitative (interview responses) and quantitative (ratings on items) information about a patient's life and occupational participation. The newest version of the OCAIRS,[27] a revision of the original OCAIRS developed by Kaplan and Kielhofner,[28] provides three semi-structured interview formats targeted to the needs of different patient groups. Each of these interview formats, designed for use in physical rehabilitation, mental health, and forensic mental health, are administered and therapists then use the information to rate patients on 12 items, using a shared 4-point rating scale. The OCAIRS items include:

1. Roles
2. Habits
3. Personal causation
4. Values
5. Interests
6. Skills
7. Short-term goals
8. Long-term goals
9. Interpretation of past experiences
10. Physical environment
11. Social environment
12. Readiness for change

Although the assessment yields information similar to that obtained by the OPHI-II, the OCAIRS interview can, with practice, be completed in 20 to 30 minutes. Detailed interview questions for each format also make the OCAIRS an excellent tool for learning interviewing skills. Like the OPHI-II, the OCAIRS can systematically identify factors impacting occupational participation, while providing the therapist with an opportunity to understand a patient's perception of current circumstances.

Each OCAIRS item is rated according to how it facilitates, allows, inhibits, or restricts occupational participation; each rating has descriptive statements to assist the therapist in making a rating decision. While the descriptors are not a shortcut to understanding MOHO and the process of occupational change, they enable the therapist to spend time reflecting on the patient, rather than on researching the intended meaning of the item. Ultimately, the therapist makes a rating based on the available patient information and the item's overall impact on the patient's occupational participation. Based on the findings from the evaluation process, the therapist can use the OCAIRS summary form to indicate the need for occupational therapy intervention.

Research and Development of the OCAIRS

The current OCAIRS format and content reflect research conducted on the previous versions of the assessment.[29-34] Collectively, these studies found that the OCAIRS had evidence of good inter-rater reliability. OCAIRS scores also have shown to discriminate between patients who are in need of occupational therapy services and those who are not, as well as between those with varying severities of psychiatric disorder.[31,32] The OCAIRS is a commonly used assessment instrument in both specialized and general psychiatric care, and is recognized internationally as a cross-cultural assessment of occupational functioning.[35-38]

Case Study 1: Using the OCAIRS

Bert was a 58-year-old man who retired early due to rheumatoid arthritis (RA). He came to the attention of his community mental health center because his daughter was "worried he is becoming depressed." An occupational therapy referral was initiated because Bert was not engaging in everyday activity, and this was affecting his mental well-being. On initial contact, Bert appeared to be withdrawn and was apathetic. He was conversational, once engaged, so the therapist reasoned that it was appropriate to use the OCAIRS to obtain the needed information about his occupational participation.

Bert described himself as previously a social man who felt productive within his worker role as an owner of a restaurant. He retired due to his physical health and found this transition very difficult. He now described himself as "useless" and had no focus to his day. Bert had given up many activities: he used to be an active grandfather and spent time with his grandchildren on a weekly basis; he used to ballroom dance with his wife until it became too painful; he used to work long hours at the restaurant, which made him feel productive.

Currently, Bert couldn't identify any roles or responsibilities, which had led to an empty routine. He sat on the couch most of the day feeling ineffective. He felt that he couldn't complete any activities and had lost all his confidence. He was able to identify strong values around family, being productive, and socializing. He also has strong interests in playing golf and ballroom dancing, although he no longer participated in these. He stated that his physical skill had been slowly deteriorating for over 10 years due to RA. He now described himself as feeling "low" and having a "clouded mind," and found it hard to concentrate on anything. He could not identify any short- or long-term goals. He discussed his previous life experiences in a very positive way, and said he always saw himself as a "fighter," able to handle most situations. His physical environment supported his lack of physical skills and special equipment was evident within the environment. His wife was supportive of her husband, although he described her as "fussing"; he felt "guilty" that he couldn't do more around the house to help out.

The OCAIRS gave a picture of a man who didn't make an easy adjustment into retirement due to physical impairments, and was now facing mental health challenges (Figure 11-2).

Early occupational therapy intervention sessions focused on building Bert's values and using these values as levers to support his volition, and on identification of activities that would bring him some satisfaction and enjoyment. Graded support to participate in valued occupational forms provided the therapeutic structure that allowed Bert to regain some of his lost personal causation, and provided a foundation for him to start to take back some of his lost roles and responsibilities.

OCAIRS Rating Key

F: Facilitates	Facilitates participation in occupation
A: Allows	Allows participation in occupation
I: Inhibits	Inhibits participation in occupation
R: Restricts	Restricts participation in occupation

Summary of Client's Scores:

Roles	Habits	Personal Causation	Values	Interests	Skills	Short-term goals	Long-term goals	Interpretation of past experiences	Physical environment	Social environment	Readiness for change
F	F	F	**F**	F	F	F	F	**F**	**F**	F	F
A	A	A	A	A	A	A	A	A	A	A	A
I	I	I	I	I	I	I	I	I	I	**I**	**I**
R	**R**	**R**	R	**R**	**R**	**R**	**R**	R	R	R	R

Need for Occupational Therapy:

	4	Shows positive occupational participation, no need for OT
	3	Need for minimal intervention/consultative OT services
	2	Need for OT intervention indicated to restore/improve participation
✓	1	Need for extensive OT intervention indicated to improve participation. Referral for follow-up services also recommended.

Figure 11-2. Bert's ratings on the OCAIRS. Reprinted with permission from MOHO Clearinghouse.

Observational Assessments

THE VOLITIONAL QUESTIONNAIRE (VQ)

Using the VQ

Volitional assessments, such as checklists and interviews, require an individual to have the cognitive abilities and skills to reflect upon and complete the assessment. However, interests, values, and a person's sense of causation can be explicated when the occupational therapist understands how the volitional process works, and observes a person engaged in both familiar and unfamiliar occupations. Through systematic observation guided by theory, therapists can use the Volitional Questionnaire (VQ)[39] to assess the volition of individuals who are unable to communicate their sense of volition due to significant limitations in cognitive, verbal, or physical ability.

The VQ yields two types of information: an understanding of a person's inner motives and corresponding sense of personal causation, interests, and values, and information about how specific environments enhance or attenuate that sense of volition. The VQ observation can occur during a formal or informal observation period, such as a therapy session, or during a routine activity, such as meal time. The observation can last from 5 to 30 minutes, and therapists are encouraged to use professional skills and provide visual, verbal, or physical support as needed. The level of support required to engage in the activity is then considered when rating the items.

The VQ items seek to reveal how confident someone feels doing an activity, how important the activity is, and how enjoyable the activity is, and include:

- Shows curiosity
- Initiates actions/tasks
- Tries new things
- Shows pride
- Seeks challenges
- Seeks additional responsibilities
- Tries to correct mistakes
- Tries to solve problems
- Shows preferences
- Pursues an activity to completion/accomplishment
- Stays engaged
- Invests additional energy/emotion/attention
- Indicates goals
- Shows that an activity is special or significant

The therapist considers whether the patient demonstrates the item spontaneously, with minimal or maximal support, or not at all, using the 4-point rating scale. In addition to rating the items, the therapist also considers the spaces, objects, social groups, and activity forms within the environment during the observation. When conducting an observation in more than one setting, if volitional ratings differ across the settings, the therapist should consider how the environmental characteristics differ across the settings. In this way, the therapist is able to identify the interests and values of a patient who is unable to verbally share this information and, simultaneously, describe the environments that are most supportive and motivating for the patient. This information supports a more client-centered intervention planning and goal-setting process.

Research and Development of the VQ

Research on the psychometric properties of the VQ has confirmed the theory of volitional development first proposed by Reilly.[40] Volitional development begins with the exploration stage, in which an individual tries to do things in order to discover capacities, interests, and values. In the next stage, the competence stage, an individual begins to practice these capacities and to work toward goals. When new challenges are sought and accomplished, an individual is demonstrating the final stage, volitional achievement. Repeated studies have confirmed that VQ items fall along this volitional continuum,[41,42] indicating that the assessment has good content validity. In addition, the VQ has the sensitivity to detect differences between patients with different levels of volition.[42] However,

Li and Kielhofner's[42] study revealed that therapists were not using the VQ rating scales in a consistent manner. Therefore, therapists using the VQ should not only familiarize themselves with MOHO concepts, but should also be familiar with the "Remotivation Process," an intervention based on the VQ and volitional development.[43]

ASSESSMENT OF COMMUNICATION AND INTERACTION SKILLS (ACIS)

Using the ACIS

The ACIS is a formal observational tool designed to measure an individual's performance in occupational forms within a social group.[44] The instrument allows occupational therapists to determine a patient's strengths and weaknesses in interacting and communicating with others in the course of daily occupations. The ACIS was developed for use in a wide range of settings.

ACIS observations are carried out in contexts that are meaningful and relevant to the patient's life. Because social situations cannot be standardized, the ACIS does not adjust scores for the type of social group or task in which the person is observed. Rather, a format exists for classifying the context of observation and its degree of approximation to the kind of everyday social situations in which the patient performs or wants to perform. The ACIS contains a single scale that consists of 19 skill items divided into three communication and interaction domains: physicality, information exchange, and relations. The items are rated on a 4-point scale with a focus on the impact of the skills on both the progression of the social interaction and the occupational form, as well as on the impact on other persons with whom the patient interacts. The ACIS items include:

- Contents
- Gazes
- Gestures
- Maneuvers
- Orients
- Postures
- Articulates
- Asserts
- Asks
- Engages
- Expresses
- Modulates
- Shares
- Speaks
- Sustains
- Collaborates
- Conforms
- Focuses
- Relates
- Respect

The ACIS is supported by a detailed manual designed to instruct and guide the therapist in its use.[44] The manual provides criteria, supported by examples, for applying the rating to each item. The therapist begins by interviewing the patient (or a significant other) in order to ascertain appropriate and meaningful contexts in which to observe the patient. To administer the ACIS, the therapist observes patients' communication and social interaction while engaging with others to complete an occupational form. The observing therapist can be the group leader or a participant. Therefore, the ACIS can be administered during a therapeutic group.

The total administration time for the ACIS varies from 20 to 60 minutes. Observation time ranges from 15 to 45 minutes. The rating is completed following conclusion of the session. Completing the ratings takes from 5 to 20 minutes, depending on the number of qualitative comments the therapist wishes to enter into the form. It may be possible to observe more than one person during an observation session; however, the dependability of doing so has not yet been examined in research.

Research and Development of the ACIS

Simon[45] found modest inter-rater reliability with the first version of the ACIS. Salamy[46] revised the ACIS and found evidence that the items worked well together to constitute a single scale of communication/interaction. The reseacher's findings also indicated the need for further revision. Subsequently, Forsyth[47] made extensive revisions in the ACIS scale. In a study of persons who had a wide range of psychosocial impairments, findings suggest the revised scale items work together to form a single valid measure of communication/interaction skills.[48] Moreover, consistency was found between and within a large sample of raters. Further research examining the dependability of the ACIS is currently underway.

Case Study: Using the ACIS

John was a 17-year-old student diagnosed with a nonspecific mental health condition and in the care of a psychiatrist. The school identified social skills as an immediate challenge. The occupational therapist assessed John using the ACIS, and made recommendations concerning his disruptiveness and aggression.

The occupational therapist observed John in the classroom, during recess, and during lunchtime (all natural contexts in which John was expected to perform in the school). Ratings based on these three observations are shown in Figure 11-3, and reflect the composite of these observations. John demonstrated mostly adequate skills in the area of information exchange. In contrast, he had problems with physicality and relations.

In the area of physicality, John had the following skill problems. When he was excited or angry, he tended to use physical forms of contact (eg, hugging, kissing, shoving, and grabbing) that made others uncomfortable or upset. He often failed to make eye contact, except when he was angry. In the latter situation, he would "stare down" the person with whom he was angry. John had a tendency to stand too close to people, making them uncomfortable. He appeared to have little awareness of others' reactions to his behaviors. In fact, when others withdrew in reaction to some of his inappropriate physical interaction, he would continue or intensify the offending behavior. For example, he would try to move closer and closer to someone who was uncomfortable with his proximity, or shove someone harder when he or she tried to ignore him after a first push.

John also had problems with engaging others. He often initiated interactions in ways that made others uncomfortable. He often failed to respect social norms, such as picking up and using others' possessions and going ahead of others in line. He also had diffi-

Competent (4):	Competent performance that supports communication/ interaction and yields good interpersonal/ group outcomes. Examiner observes no evidence of a deficit
Questionable (3):	Questionable performance that places at risk communication/interaction and yields uncertain interpersonal/group outcomes. Examiner questions the presence of deficit.
Ineffective (2):	Ineffective performance that interferes with communication/ interaction and yields undesirable interpersonal/ group outcomes. Examiner observes a mild to moderate deficit.
Deficit (1):	Deficit performance that impedes communication/ interaction and yields unacceptable group outcomes. Examiner observes a severe deficit (risk of damage, danger, provocation, or breakdown of interpersonal group relations).

Physicality

Contacts	4	3	2	**1**
Gazes	4	3	2	**1**
Gestures	**4**	3	2	1
Maneuvers	4	3	**2**	1
Orients	4	3	2	**1**
Postures	4	3	2	**1**

Information Exchange

Articulates	4	**3**	2	1
Asserts	4	3	**2**	1
Asks	4	**3**	2	1
Engages	4	3	2	**1**
Expresses	4	3	**2**	1
Modulates	4	3	**2**	1
Shares	4	**3**	2	1
Speaks	**4**	3	2	1
Sustains	**4**	3	2	1

Relations

Collaborates	4	3	2	**1**
Conforms	4	3	2	**1**
Focuses	4	3	**2**	1
Relates	4	3	**2**	1
Respects	4	3	2	**1**

Figure 11-3. John's ratings on the ACIS. Reprinted with permission from MOHO Clearinghouse.

culty asserting himself. John seemed to be unaware of how to make requests and tended to "bully" others when he wanted something. As with his difficulties in the physical domain, John seemed to engage in these behaviors with limited understanding of how his behavior was received by others. John was clearly motivated to interact with others and liked their attention when he received it. His difficulty in getting his social needs met in ways that fit the needs or expectations of others meant that he was often engaged in tense interactions with others who were fleeing, avoiding him, or reacting angrily to his transgressions. Therefore, much of John's social interaction was marked by strain, conflict, and negative affect. The assessment revealed that, while John was motivated to engage in positive interactions, he lacked the skill to be able to accomplish his desires. He did not so much disregard others, as he had difficulty in being able to "see" his own behavior and "read" its impact on others.

Based on the assessment, the therapist supported John in graded engagement in school occupational forms with a focus on social skills. The therapist tried to enable John to be more aware of his own social actions and the impact on others. The therapist first reviewed with John videotapes of him in the classroom, guiding him to watch himself and to watch others' reactions to him. In order to assist John in being better able to read others' reactions to his behavior, the therapist and John practiced identifying and labeling the various facial expressions and gestures of others. These exercises were aimed at helping John identify how people felt inside, based on how they appeared to him. The therapist also provided specific training in the skills in which he had shown the most difficulty. For example, he practiced how to initiate interactions with others, how to assert himself without becoming aggressive, and how to make socially acceptable physical contact.

Self-Report Assessments

THE OCCUPATIONAL SELF ASSESSMENT (OSA) AND THE CHILD OCCUPATIONAL SELF-ASSESSMENT (COSA)

Using the OSA and the COSA

Although the field of occupational therapy has embraced the value for client-centered practice,[1,49] therapists still report that such a practice is difficult to implement.[50,51] The use of client-centered evaluation tools can help make client-centered practice easier to implement.[52] The OSA and COSA were developed to assess the MOHO concepts of occupational competence and value for occupation through client self report. The OSA[53] was developed for use with clients aged 18 and older, and the COSA[54] can be used with clients as young as 8 years old.

The OSA and the COSA use a two-part self-report. Clients are presented with a list of items that represent a range of everyday activities. The 21 items on the OSA include "Taking care of the place I live," "Identifying and solving problems," and "Getting along with others"; the COSA's 25 items cover typical activities in school, home, and in the community, including "Get my chores done," "Finish my work in class on time," and "Calm myself down when I am upset." First, clients use a 4-point scale to rate how well they do each activity. This rating is an indicator of the client's sense of occupational competence. Next, clients use a 4-point scale to rate how important the activity is to them.

Myself	I have a big problem doing this	I have a little problem doing this	I do this ok	I am really good at doing this	Not really important to me	Important to me	Really important to me	Most important of all to me
Keep working on something even when it gets hard	☹ ☹	☹	☺	☺ ☺	☆	☆ ☆	☆ ☆ ☆	☆ ☆ ☆ ☆
Calm myself down when I get upset	☹ ☹	☹	☺	☺ ☺	☆	☆ ☆	☆ ☆ ☆	☆ ☆ ☆ ☆
Make my body do what I want it to	☹ ☹	☹	☺	☺ ☺	☆	☆ ☆	☆ ☆ ☆	☆ ☆ ☆ ☆

Figure 11-4. Excerpt from the COSA Rating Form. Reprinted with permission from MOHO Clearinghouse.

The rated level of importance reflects the value for the occupation, which is an aspect of occupational identity. Items and rating scales use simple language to facilitate the client's understanding; additionally, the COSA rating scale includes visual cues for each response (smiling and frowning faces for competence, and stars for importance) (Figure 11-4).

After the client completes the ratings, the therapist and the client can review the responses to identify areas that are a priority to the client. In addition, the therapist and patient can visually scan the report form to identify large gaps between ratings of competence and importance. Items that are considered more difficult to do, but are rated as highly important for the patient, indicate an area that can be addressed during occupational therapy intervention.

Research and Development of the OSA and COSA

A series of studies on both the OSA and COSA indicate reliable and valid measures of client competence and value for occupation. A series of international studies[55,56] (G. Kielhofner, unpublished data, 2005) indicates that the OSA items work in a valid and reliable manner across cultural, diagnostic, and language differences. The most recent study confirms that the OSA is a sensitive measure that can be used over time as an outcome measure (G. Kielhofner, unpublished data, 2005). As a result, the OSA has paper keyforms, like the OPHI-II, which therapists and clients can use to obtain client measures and errors for outcome evaluation.

The COSA also was found to be a valid and reliable assessment tool.[57,58] The 4-point ratings scales can be used in a reliable and valid manner by children ages 8 to 17, and modifications to the administration procedures to ensure access do not impact the reliability of assessment.[58] Items on the COSA are valid measures of competence and value for occupation, although several items require further testing and development to confirm the psychometric properties,[58] and research to develop paper keyforms is also in progress.

Case Study 3: Using the COSA

Sam was an 11-year-old Caucasian male with a diagnosis of Attention Deficit Hyperactivity Disorder (ADHD) and Pervasive Developmental Delay nonspecific (PDD NOS), who was admitted to a diagnostic assessment center and hospital diversion program as a step down from a 7-week acute inpatient hospitalization. At time of admission, Sam was accompanied by his biological mother, who had full legal custody. Sam was admitted due to uncontrollable impulsive behavior, which included being verbally and physically assaultive. Medications to manage Sam's attention deficit had been unsuccessful due to adverse reactions, such as skin rashes, the development of tics, and significant adverse behavioral changes. Sam was currently not on medication.

Sam's family consisted of his biological mother. His parents were never married, but he had regular contact with his father. His parents had a history of drug and alcohol abuse; there was no reported physical or sexual abuse. Sam was an only child. Prior to his recent acute admission, Sam had been living at home with his mother and attending a collaborative school for children with special needs. His mother was very interested in having Sam come home; however, she felt his behavior needed to be in better control.

Sam was familiar with the occupational therapist, and eager to leave the unit to participate in the COSA, which was described to him as a tool to better understand what activities were important to him and the areas in which he would like more help. Sam requested a reward of going outside once he completed the assessment. Sam was interviewed in an office space off the unit. He sat in a desk chair, which he spun around throughout the interview. When Sam was required to answer a question, he would stop and point to the appropriate face or star to answer the question. At the completion of the assessment, although eager to go outside, Sam stood up, turned to the occupational therapist, and said, "I think this is a very good test." See Figure 11-5 for Sam's responses on the COSA.

Due to Sam's impulsivity, he often had difficulty following classroom rules, yet his answers on the COSA showed that he clearly valued the rules. Sam had difficulty organizing and regulating his arousal system to independently complete his homework in the evening. Sam also reported difficulty in making others understand his ideas, which often resulted in increased frustration and, consequently, behavioral outbursts. His ability to persevere when tasks were difficult could also be compromised, contributing to potential behavioral problems.

Sam recognized that he had trouble controlling his anger and making friends. He demonstrated difficulty in recognizing nonverbal signals from his peers and required explicit instruction on how to interpret others' reactions in order to control his own responses to their behavior.

The following goals were developed in a follow-up discussion with Sam:

- Sam will follow classroom rules with one reminder for 1 week.
- Following instruction in organizational strategies and self-regulation strategies, Sam will independently complete his assigned homework for 1 week.
- Sam will initiate a cooperative play activity with a peer on the unit daily for 1 week.
- Sam will demonstrate improved anger management skills by improving his ability to express his ideas and remaining restraint-free for 1 week.

Myself	I have a big problem doing this	I have a little problem doing this	I do this ok	I am really good at doing this	Not really important to me	Important to me	Really important to me	Most important of all to me
Keep my body clean				X				X
Dress myself				X				X
Eat my meals without any help				X				X
Buy something myself				X				X
Get my chores done				X				X
Get enough sleep				X				X
Have enough time to do things I like			X				X	
Take care of my things				X				X
Get around from one place to another				X				X
Choose things that I want to do				X				X
Keep my mind on what I am doing				X				X
Do things with my family				X				X
Do things with my Friends				X				X
Do things with my Classmates		X						X
Follow classroom rules	X							X
Finish my work in class on time			X					X
Get my homework done	X							X
Ask my teacher questions when I need to			X					X
Make others understand my ideas	X							X
Think of ways to do things when I have a problem				X				X
Keep working on something even when it gets hard		X						X
Calm myself down when I am upset			X					X
Make my body do what I want it to do				X		X		
Use my hands to work with things				X				X
Finish what I am doing without getting tired too soon				X				X

Figure 11-5. Sam's responses on the COSA. Reprinted with permission from MOHO Clearinghouse.

The therapist recommended the following intervention strategies to support Sam in achieving his goals:

- Classroom rules will be represented with pictures and words and will be reviewed with the entire class at the beginning of the day, and prior to transitions, to assist Sam in improving his performance in following rules.

- Sam will be provided individual instruction in how to organize his daily homework. In addition, he will learn strategies to regulate his particular arousal system to maximize his ability to sustain his performance.

- Sam will participate in a social skills group with an emphasis on anger management. Sam will also learn strategies to engage his peers in appropriate play activities to improve his ability to form friendships.

- Consultation with unit staff and teachers will be provided to ensure follow-through with programs and to provide Sam with regular feedback on his performance and progress toward goals.

Assessments That Use a Variety of Data-Gathering Methods

THE MODEL OF HUMAN OCCUPATION SCREENING TOOL (MOHOST)

Using the MOHOST

Developed by a therapist practicing in a bustling, acute care mental health unit, the MOHOST[59] is an occupation-based screening tool that allows a therapist to identify patient strengths and needs while formally documenting occupational therapy knowledge that often goes unrecognized. The MOHOST is a flexible assessment that allows a therapist to gather information in a variety of ways, including observation, patient and caregiver interviews, consultation with interdisciplinary staff, and chart reviews. The MOHOST is intended to be used with a variety of patients in a variety of settings.

The 24 MOHOST items are arranged into six main concept areas based on MOHO. They are:

1. Motivation for occupation
2. Pattern of occupation
3. Communication and interaction skills
4. Process skills
5. Motor skills
6. Environment

Of special note are the terms used to describe these MOHO concepts. Instead of using terms like "volition" and "habituation," the MOHOST uses more familiar words to convey MOHO ideas to patients, families, and other professionals. The 4-point rating scale indicates how occupational participation is facilitated or restricted by patient or environmental factors. To further facilitate the implementation of MOHO therapeutic reasoning, and to maintain the therapist's focus on occupation throughout the evaluation process, the MOHOST manual provides links to other MOHO assessments that therapists can use in their practice to gain a more in-depth understanding of their patients' occupational profile and needs.

Research and Development of the MOHOST

The first study conducted on the MOHOST, which included data from the United States and the United Kingdom, revealed that the MOHOST items and rating scale can discriminate between patients with differing levels of occupational participation.[60] The study found that MOHOST items validly represent the construct of occupational participation, and that therapists are able to use the MOHOST in a valid manner across a variety of intervention settings that included community-based, forensic, and acute mental health settings. Further research and development of the MOHOST is needed to ensure this clinically useful tool is also psychometrically sound.

Case Study 4: Using the MOHOST

Sophie was referred to a community team by her general practitioner. An initial assessment was completed and written up in two formats—a narrative home visit report and a MOHOST Form. The narrative home visit report provides a detailed account of Sophie's needs, and is complemented by the MOHOST Form, which gives a brief summary of the occupational therapist's observations (Figure 11-6).

The referral was received from Sophie's general practitioner. The referral stated that Sophie was now reporting "difficulties with coping and mobility." It also stated that Sophie has early dementia and had a previous medical history of osteoarthritis and congestive heart failure. This report was a compilation of information gathered on a home visit (Sophie, Sophie's husband, and occupational therapist present) and a telephone contact with Sophie's daughter.

Sophie was previously a very active person. She worked behind the bar of a local pub for 20 years before her retirement 5 years ago. She enjoyed the social aspect of her job and felt that a lot of the "regulars" at the pub were like friends. Since retirement, she has felt isolated. She was extremely house proud, always had high standards for cleanliness, and ran the household very efficiently. It was important for Sophie to always present herself well. She took great care in her appearance, liked to be "well turned out" and had her hair set once a week. She enjoyed spending time with her daughter and family. She was particularly close to her granddaughter and they had previously spent time together every Saturday out in the community. She also enjoyed board games and knitting. She used to volunteer at a local sheltered housing complex, where she made soup and meals. She was also involved in church events and ran charity events for the women's guild.

Sophie's husband and daughter both confirmed that Sophie's activity levels fell when she retired 5 years ago. There has been a gradual deterioration over a 12-month period. She has been sitting in her chair all day, doing very little since her recent hospital admission 6 months ago. Sophie's daughter feels that her current low mood is due to social isolation since retiring and having reduced mobility ascending/descending stairs due to painful and swollen feet.

During the occupational therapist's visit to her home, Sophie was observed to be responsive and cooperative; she reported that her mood had been low for 6 months and that she no longer took any interest in activities that were once meaningful. Sophie identified the source of her low mood to include: 1) her inability to mobilize outdoors, 2) her recent hospital admission (6 months ago), and 3) a flood in the apartment above. She stated that she is not doing any activities that were previously meaningful to her.

MOHOST Rating Key

F: Facilitates	Facilitates participation in occupation
A: Allows	Allows participation in occupation
I: Inhibits	Inhibits participation in occupation
R: Restricts	Restricts participation in occupation

Summary of Client's Ratings:

Motivation for Occupation				Pattern of Occupation				Communication & Interaction				Process Skills				Motor Skills				Environment: Home			
Appraisal of ability	Expectation of success	Interest	Choices	Routine	Adaptability	Roles	Responsibility	Non-verbal Skills	Conversation	Vocal Expression	Relationships	Knowledge	Timing	Organization	Problem-Solving	Posture & Mobility	Co-ordination	Strength & Effort	Energy	Physical Space	Physical Resources	Social Groups	Occupational Demands
F	F	F	F	F	F	F	F	**F**	**F**	**F**	F	**F**	**F**	**F**	F	F	F	F	F	F	F	**F**	F
A	A	A	A	A	A	A	A	A	A	A	A	A	A	A	A	A	**A**	A	A	A	A	A	**A**
I	I	**I**	I	I	**I**	I	I	I	I	I	**I**	I	I	I	**I**	**I**	I	**I**	**I**	I	I	I	I
R	**R**	R	**R**	**R**	R	**R**	**R**	R	R	R	R	R	R	R	R	R	R	R	R	**R**	**R**	R	R

Figure 11-6. Summary of Sophie's MOHOST Ratings. Reprinted with permission from MOHO Clearinghouse.

Sophie needed a walker to get around. She was observed moving about her apartment independently and safely using this frame. She had not gone outside for the past 12 months due to inability to ascend/descend stairs. She was observed to have swollen feet with hyper-extended big toes, which Sophie stated were painful. She wears glasses, although she stated that she is able to read without them. She reported deteriorated eyesight since a cataract operation. She stated that she had hearing aids, which she was not wearing on the visit. She was answering questions appropriately and followed the conversations, which indicated she could hear people talking adequately.

Sophie lives in a two-bedroom, first floor apartment. External access is by two steps into the building, 100 yards of paved corridor, then 16 steps that are broken halfway up with a landing (with a rail on right side ascending). The apartment is well-maintained and has central heat and a telephone line.

Sophie stated she has had home care services for the last 3 months, 3 times per day, 7 days a week. Sophie stated she had not been enjoying the company of her granddaughter recently. Sophie lived with her husband and he stated he is in good health. He stated that he was frustrated with his wife's lack of engagement in activities and her perception that he hasn't been completing tasks to her standards. Sophie's daughter and her husband live close by. They both work full-time, but Sophie's daughter attends every evening to support Sophie. Sophie had asked friends to no longer come around; she stated she doesn't want them to see her unkempt.

Sophie's husband stated that Sophie rises at 9 am when the home care assistant arrives. She goes through her morning routine, then has breakfast at 9:30 am. She sits in the lounge chair watching TV all day and evening. The homecare assistant comes again at 1 pm to carry out domestic tasks. She then arrives at 10 pm to support Sophie with her nighttime routine. Sophie stated she is not happy with this routine but can't "be bothered to do anything."

Sophie's self-care routine happens entirely within her bedroom. Sophie does not strip wash at the bathroom sink, use the shower, or use a perch stool due to lack of confidence in her balance. Sophie stated that to wash herself she has an established routine and sits on the bedside commode. To carry out this routine, the homecare assistant arranges needed objects to support lack of mobility and provides verbal encouragement. Sophie and her daughter both stated that she has the skills to dress herself independently on the commode. Grooming was very important to Sophie and she stated she is unable to set her hair and no longer has access to the hairdresser.

Sophie was observed on the visit to: independently transfer on/off 16-inch high commode using a walker safely, and independently transfer on/off 16-inch high toilet, using a 2-inch raised toilet seat and right wall grab rail safely. Bed transfer was not observed and Sophie did not want to attempt a shower transfer as she is not currently using the shower and is comfortable with her current arrangement of strip washing at bedside.

The kitchen was observed to have a gas cooker with overhead grille, microwave, electric kettle, continuous surfaces, and a table and chairs. Although Sophie previously enjoyed cooking for the sheltered housing volunteer position, her husband now does all the cooking and hot drinks. She stated that she has "no interest" in cooking, although she does occasionally help prepare meals with her husband. She felt she wouldn't be able to do this independently. They had a diet of toast in the morning, banana and bread for lunch, and a cooked meal in the evening. Sophie stated that she doesn't eat the vegetables because her husband doesn't prepare them well enough. Sophie's husband felt that Sophie still had the skill to cook, but that she was not motivated to do so. He was frustrated by his wife's lack of engagement with cooking. During the occupational therapy evaluation, the therapist asked Sophie to make tea. Sophie stated she wouldn't be able to complete the activity. She did, however, manage to make the hot drink independently. With respect to motor skills, she was slow and unsteady at times; however, she physically managed without intervention. She demonstrated some stiffness and reduction in strength. She appeared to lack energy and sat at regular intervals during the activity. With respect to process skills, Sophie managed to use knowledge, and plan and organize the activity. She did, however, have difficulty problem solving.

Sophie could identify interests in which she engaged in the past. She specifically identified the social aspect of these interests as being enjoyable and satisfying. Sophie now appeared to have reduced leisure opportunities. She could identify specific television programs that she enjoyed watching. She received a weekly visit at home from the church. She could not identify anything else that brought her enjoyment. Sophie's daughter was particularly concerned that Sophie was not engaging in leisure activities. Her daughter stated she felt that this is the key for supporting her mother to "re-engage in life again."

Sophie was unable to identify any goals for the future. Sophie felt very pessimistic about her ability to return to a meaningful life. She stated she feels "hopeless" about the future. Sophie's current situation is not supportive of her mental or physical health. Although Sophie wanted to change her circumstances, she was not ready to independently change and therefore required further extended occupational therapy input.

Based on these observations and the resulting MOHOST ratings, the therapist generated the following goals for Sophie's occupational therapy intervention:

- Sophie will identify one previous interest she would like to engage in, and participate in this activity once a week.
- Sophie will assist her husband in the kitchen to prepare dinner by fixing vegetables every evening.
- Sophie will wash and set her hair with adaptations and assistance as needed.

Other MOHO Assessments

In addition to the assessments discussed here, several other MOHO instruments can be used in mental health practice. The Modified Interest Checklist, used to gather data related to interests, was used in a variety of situations and settings: to discriminate between adolescents with different occupational needs,[61] with adults in inpatient psychiatric units,[62] and with older adults with dementia.[63] Another assessment, the Occupational Questionnaire, can be used to identify activity patterns for clients with a variety of occupational participation needs, from depression[64] to HIV/AIDS.[65] These assessments can be downloaded from the MOHO Clearinghouse website at www.moho.uic.edu.

Summary

MOHO is an occupational therapy conceptual practice framework that explains patient and environmental factors that impact successful occupational adaptation. This model is a highly developed model represented in over 300 publications. The evidence base of this model is substantial, including over 100 published studies. In mental health, occupational therapists can use MOHO concepts and MOHO-based assessment tools during the evaluation process to generate an occupation profile of their patients and gain an in-depth understanding of their patients' occupational needs.

For further information, therapists are encouraged to refer to the MOHO text[2] or visit the MOHO website at www.moho.uic.edu to search the MOHO database to support their evidence-based practice.

References

1. American Occupational Therapy Association. Occupational therapy practice framework: domain and process. *Am J Occup Ther.* 2002;56:609-639.
2. Kielhofner G. *A Model of Human Occupation: Theory and Application.* 4th ed. Baltimore, MD: Lippincott, Williams & Wilkins; 2007.
3. Kielhofner G. *Conceptual Foundations of Occupational Therapy.* 3rd ed. Philadelphia, PA: FA Davis; 2004.
4. Haglund L, Henriksson C. Activity: From action to activity. *Scandinavian Journal of Caring Sciences.* 1995;9:227-234.
5. Fisher A. *Assessment of Motor and Process Skills.* 3rd ed. Ft. Collins, CO: Three Star Press; 1999.
6. Kielhofner G, Mallinson T, Crawford C, et al. *The Occupational Performance History Interview-II* (version 2.1). Model of Human Occupation Clearinghouse, Department of Occupational Therapy, College of Applied Health Sciences, University of Illinois at Chicago; 2004.
7. Kielhofner G, Borell L, Freidheim L, et al. Crafting occupational life. In: Kielhofner G, ed. *Model of Human Occupation: Theory and Application.* 3rd ed. Baltimore, MD: Lippincott Williams & Wilkins; 2002:124-144.

8. Helfrich C, Kielhofner G, Mattingly C. Volition as narrative: An understanding of motivation in chronic illness. *Am J Occup Ther.* 1994;48:311-317.

9. Wright B, Masters G. *Rating Scale Analysis.* Chicago, IL: MESA Press; 1982.

10. Apte A, Kielhofner G, Paul-Ward A, Braveman B. Therapists' and clients' perceptions of the occupational performance history interview. *Occupational Therapy in Health Care.* 2005;19:173-192.

11. Kielhofner G, Henry A. Development and investigation of the occupational performance history interview. *Am J Occup Ther.* 1988;42:489-498.

12. Kielhofner G, Henry A, Walens W, Rogers E. A generalizability study of the Occupational Performance History Interview. *Occupational Therapy Journal of Research.* 1991;11:292-306.

13. Lynch K, Bridle M. Construct validity of the Occupational Performance Interview. *Occupational Therapy Journal of Research.* 1993;13:231-240.

14. Kielhofner G, Mallinson T. Gathering narrative data through interviews: empirical observations and suggested guidelines. *Scan J Occup Ther.* 1995;2:63-68.

15. Mallinson T, Mahaffey L, Kielhofner G. The occupational performance history interview: Evidence for three underlying constructs of occupational adaptation. *Can J Occup Ther.* 1998;65:219-228.

16. Kielhofner G, Mallinson T, Forsyth K, Lai JS. Psychometric properties of the second version of the Occupational Performance History Interview (OPHI-II). *Am J Occup Ther.* 2001;55:260-267.

17. Kielhofner G, Dobria L, Forsyth K, Basu S. The construction of keyforms for obtaining instantaneous measures from the Occupational Performance History Interview Rating Scales. *OTJR: Occupation, Participation & Health.* 2005;25:23-32.

18. Farnworth L, Nikitin L, Fossey E. Being in a secure forensic psychiatric unit: every day is the same, killing time or making the most of it. *British Journal of Occupational Therapy.* 2004;67:430-438.

19. Levin M, Helfrich C. Mothering role identity and competence among parenting and pregnant homeless adolescents. *Journal of Occupational Science.* 2004;11:95-104.

20. Gray ML, Fossey EM. Illness experience and occupations of people with chronic fatigue syndrome. *Australian Occupational Therapy Journal.* 2003;50:127-136.

21. Taylor R, Kielhofner G. An occupational therapy approach to persons with chronic fatigue syndrome: part two, assessment and intervention. *Occupational Therapy in Health Care.* 2003;17:63-87.

22. Chaffey L, Fossey E. Caring and daily life: occupational experiences of women living with sons diagnosed with schizophrenia. *Australian Occupational Therapy Journal.* 2004;51:199-207.

23. Braveman B. A qualitative exploration of the sub-scales of the Occupational Performance History Interview [doctoral dissertation]. University of Illinois at Chicago, Chicago, IL; 2002.

24. Braveman B, Helfrich CA. Occupational identity: exploring the narratives of three men living with AIDS. *Journal of Occupational Science.* 2001;8:25-31.

25. Kielhofner G, Braveman B, Finlayson M, Paul-Ward A, Goldbaum L, Goldstein K. Outcomes of a vocational program for persons with AIDS. *Am J Occup Ther.* 2004;58:64-72.

26. Henry AD. Predicting psychosocial functioning and symptomatic recovery of adolescents and young adults with a first psychotic episode: a six-month follow-up study. Unpublished doctoral dissertation, Boston University; 1994.

27. Forsyth K, Deshpande S, Kielhofner G, et al. The Occupational Circumstances Assessment Interview and Rating Scale (version 4.0). MOHO Clearinghouse, Department of Occupational Therapy, College of Applied Health Sciences, University of Illinois at Chicago: Chicago, IL; 2005.

28. Kaplan K, Kielhofner G. *Occupational Case Analysis Interview and Rating Scale.* Thorofare, NJ: SLACK Incorporated; 1989.

29. Brollier C, Watts JH, Bauer D, Schmidt W. A concurrent validity study of two occupational therapy evaluation instruments: the AOF and OCAIRS. *Occupational Therapy In Mental Health.* 1989;8:49-59.

30. Haglund L, Henriksson C. Testing a Swedish version of OCAIRS on two different patient groups. *Scandinavian Journal of Caring Sciences.* 1994;8:223-230.

31. Haglund L, Thorell L, Walinder J. Assessment of occupational functioning for screening of patients to occupational therapy in general psychiatric care. *Occupational Therapy Journal of Research.* 1998;4:193-206.

32. Haglund L, Thorell L, Walinder J. Occupational functioning in relation to psychiatric diagnoses; schizophrenia and mood disorders. *Journal of Psychiatry.* 1998;52:223-229.

33. Kaplan K. Objectifying Clinical Judgment: Content Validity and Inter-rater Reliability of the Occupational Case Analysis Interview and Rating Scale [unpublished masters thesis]. Virginia Commonwealth University; 1983.

34. Lai J, Haglund L, Kielhofner G. Occupational case analysis interview and rating scale. *Scandinavian Journal of Caring Sciences.* 1999;13:276-73.

35. Haglund L. Assessments in general psychiatric care. *Occupational Therapy in Mental Health.* 2000;15:35-47.

36. Haglund L. Occupational therapists agreement in screening patients in general psychiatric care for OT. *Scand J Occup Ther.* 1996;3:62-68.

37. Neville-Jan A, Bradley M, Bunn C, Gehri B. The Model of Human Occupation and individuals with co-dependency problems. *Occupational Therapy in Mental Health.* 1991;11:73-97.

38. Roitman DM, Ziv N. Application of the Model of Human Occupation in a geriatric population in Israel: two case studies. *Israeli Journal of Occupational Therapy.* 2004;13:E24-28.

39. De las Heras CG, Geist R, Kielhofner G, Li Y. *The Volitional Questionnaire* (version 4.0). Model of Human Occupation Clearinghouse, Department of Occupational Therapy, College of Applied Health Sciences, University of Illinois at Chicago: Chicago, IL; 2003.

40. Reilly M. *Play as Exploratory Learning.* Beverly Hills, CA: Sage; 1974.

41. Chern J, Kielhofner G, de las Heras C, Magalhaes L. The volitional questionnaire: psychometric develop-ment and practical use. *Am J Occup Ther.* 1996;50:516-25.

42. Li Y, Kielhofner G. Psychometric properties of the volitional questionnaire. *Israeli Journal of Occupational Therapy.* 2004;13:E85-98.

43. De las Heras CG, Llerena V, Kielhofner G. *Remotivation Process: Progressive Intervention for Individuals with Severe Volitional Challenges* (version 1.0). Model of Human Occupation Clearinghouse, Department of Occupational Therapy, College of Applied Health Sciences, University of Illinois at Chicago: Chicago, IL; 2003.

44. De las Heras CG, Geist R, Kielhofner G, Li Y. *The Volitional Questionnaire* (version 4.0). Model of Human Occupation Clearinghouse, Department of Occupational Therapy, College of Applied Health Sciences, University of Illinois at Chicago: Chicago, IL; 2003.

45. Simon S. The development of an assessment for communication and interaction skills [unpublished master's thesis]. University of Illinois at Chicago: Chicago, IL; 1989.

46. Salamy M. Construct validity of the Assessment for Communication and Interaction Skills [unpublished master's thesis]. University of Illinois at Chicago: Chicago, IL; 1993.

47. Forsyth K. Measurement properties of the Assessment of Communication and Interaction Skills (ACIS) [unpublished master's thesis]. University of Illinois at Chicago: Chicago, IL; 1996.

48. Forsyth K, Lai J, Kielhofner G. The assessment of communication and interaction skills (ACIS): measure-ment properties. *British Journal of Occupational Therapy.* 1999;62:69-74.

49. Canadian Association of Occupational Therapists. *Enabling Occupation: An Occupational Therapy Perspective.* Ottawa, ON: CAOT Publications; 1997.

50. Sumsion S, Smyth G. Barriers to client-centredness and their resolution. *Can J Occup Ther.* 2000;67:15-21.

51. Wilkins S, Pollock N, Rochon S, Law M. Implementing client-centred practice: why is it so difficult to do? *Can J Occup Ther.* 2001;68:70-79.

52. Restall G, Ripat J, Stern M. A framework of strategies for client-centred practice. *Can J Occup Ther.* 2003;70:103-112.

53. Baron K, Kielhofner G, Iyenger A, Goldhammer V, Wolenski J. *The Occupational Self Assessment (OSA)* (Version 2.1). Model of Human Occupation Clearinghouse, Department of Occupational Therapy, College of Applied Health Sciences, University of Illinois at Chicago: Chicago, IL; 2002.

54. Keller J, Kafkes A, Basu S, Federico J, Kielhofner G. *The Child Occupational Self Assessment (COSA)* (Version 2.1). Model of Human Occupation Clearinghouse, Department of Occupational Therapy, College of Applied Health Sciences, University of Illinois at Chicago: Chicago, IL; 2005.

55. Iyenger A. A study of the psychometric properties of the OSA [unpublished master's thesis]. University of Illinois at Chicago: Chicago, IL; 2001.

56. Kielhofner G, Forsyth K. Measurement properties of a client self-report for treatment planning and docu-menting therapy outcomes. *Scan J Occup Ther.* 2001;8:131-139.

57. Keller J, Kafke, A, Kielhofner G. Psychometric characteristics of the Child Occupational Self Assessment (COSA) part one: an initial examination of psychometric properties. *Scan J Occup Ther.* 2005;12:118-27.

58. Keller J, Kielhofner G. Psychometric characteristics of the Child Occupational Self Assessment (COSA) part two: refining the psychometric properties. *Scan J Occup Ther.* 2005;12:147-58.

59. Parkinson S, Forsyth K, Kielhofner G. *The Model of Human Occupation Screening Tool* (version 2.0). Model of Human Occupation Clearinghouse, Department of Occupational Therapy, College of Applied Health Sciences, University of Illinois at Chicago: Chicago, IL; 2005.

60. Forsyth K, Parkinson S, Kielhofner G, Keller J, Summerfield-Mann L, Duncan E. The measurement prop-erties of the Model of Human Occupation Screening Tool. [manuscript submitted for publication].

61. Barris R, Kielhofner G, Burch RM, Gelinas I, Klement M, Schultz B. Occupational function and dysfunc-tion in three groups of adolescents. *Occupational Therapy Journal of Research.* 1986;6:301-317.

62. Katz N, Giladi N, Peretz C. Cross-cultural application of occupational therapy assessments: human occupa-tion with psychiatric inpatients and controls in Israel. *Occupational Therapy in Mental Health.* 1988;8:7-30.

63. Olin D. Assessing and assisting the person with dementia: an occupational behavior perspective. *Physical and Occupational Therapy in Geriatrics*. 1985;3:25-32.
64. Neville-Jan A. The relationship of volition to adaptive occupational behavior among individuals with varying degrees of depression. *Occupational Therapy in Mental Health*. 1994;12:1-18.
65. Pizzi MA. Occupational therapy: creating possibilities for adults with human immunodeficiency virus infection, AIDS related complex, and acquired immunodeficiency syndrome. *Occupational Therapy in Health Care*. 1990;7:125-137.

WORK-RELATED ASSESSMENTS: WORKER ROLE INTERVIEW (WRI) AND WORK ENVIRONMENT IMPACT SCALE (WEIS)

Kristjana Fenger, MSc, OT
Brent Braveman, PhD, OTR/L, FAOTA
Gary Kielhofner, DrPH, OTR/L, FAOTA

"Work is the inevitable condition of human life, the true source of human welfare." Tolstoy L. My Religion. *New York: Thomas Y. Crowell and Co; 1885.*

Introduction

The Model of Human Occupation (MOHO)[1] has been widely utilized in work programs and has guided research on injured and disabled workers.[2-7] Two MOHO assessment tools, The Worker Role Interview (WRI)[8,9] and The Work Environment Impact Scale (WEIS),[10] have been developed for work-related contexts and studied internationally.[6,11-14] The WRI assesses psychosocial factors that influence work performance, while the WEIS assesses workplace conditions that impact the worker. Both instruments are used as independent tools, but WEIS and WRI can be administered simultaneously when therapists and patients want to look more closely at environmental factors affecting the worker.[10] The purpose of this chapter is to introduce these instruments, including their development and administration, as well as to demonstrate their application through case examples.

HISTORICAL CONTEXT

In the second half of the 20th century, programs designed for the rehabilitation of injured workers were primarily based on a functional limitations approach. Within this approach, a biomechanical model was widely used in work rehabilitation programs that focused on work capacity or work hardening. These programs simulated the physical demands of a job, building on analyses of work tasks and worksites. Patients engaged in tasks designed to enhance their physical capacity to perform a specific job.[15-17]

With time, research indicated that by focusing only on physical limitations for work, the full range of problems faced by persons with disabilities were not addressed.[18,19] For example, severity of injury in persons with low back pain only partly predicted work disability, while socioeconomic and job-related factors accounted for a larger portion of the variation in outcomes.[19] Interviews at the initiation of work rehabilitation and work prognosis by an experienced team were shown to be better predictors of return to work than biomechanical variables.[18] Consequently, it was recognized that the biomechanical approach overlooked aptitudes, interests, and vocationally relevant skills.[17,19]

The WRI grew out of this context. It was intended to supplement the biomechanical approach by examining psychosocial factors influencing injured or disabled workers. Later, the WEIS was developed to focus more specifically on the work environment of a worker in a specific job.

THE MODEL OF HUMAN OCCUPATION

Both the WRI and the WEIS are designed to reflect key concepts from the MOHO,[1] as well as evidence about factors that influence work outcomes in injured or disabled workers. Braveman[20] reviewed research literature on factors associated with return to work and success at work and organized the factors according to the basic constructs of MOHO. As shown in Table 12-1, most factors that influence return to work can be grouped into the primary theoretical components of MOHO.

MOHO considers both the personal and environmental factors that impact a person with a disability. In the context of work, MOHO directs clinicians to consider workers' motivation vis-à-vis work (volition), how workers pattern their everyday lives (habituation), the capacity for work (performance capacity), and how the environment allows and inhibits participation in work (environmental impact).

Volition includes a worker's: (1) values, or the importance and worth one attaches to work; (2) interests, or the satisfaction and enjoyment experienced while working; and (3) personal causation, which is reflected in thoughts and feelings about capacity for work and effectiveness in the workplace.

Habituation refers to the semi-autonomous patterning of behavior that structures an individual's life. Habituation is the function of: (1) habits, which are tendencies to automatically respond and perform in consistent ways in familiar situations; and (2) roles, which incorporate socially or personally defined status with associated attitudes and expectations for behavior. For the worker, habits regulate how time is spent and how work is done. How a person has internalized the worker role will influence how one engages with others and completes work tasks. Moreover, a person's other life roles can either support or detract from work.

Performance capacity refers to underlying abilities that enable persons to engage in occupation.[1] Performance capacity is not directly assessed in the WRI. Consequently, appropriate work capacity assessments or other functional assessments should be administered along with the WRI when there is any question about work capacity.

MOHO also considers the impact the *environment* has on a worker and worker's performance. Impact refers to whether the environment provides resources to support the worker or obstacles that constrain the worker's ability to meet demands. The physical features of an environment include spaces in which the worker acts and objects the worker comes across at work. The social features of an environment include social groups of which the worker is a part and occupational forms, which refer to the tasks that the worker must perform.

Table 12-1
The Relationship of MOHO Components to Predictive Factors in Return-to-Work Studies

Model Constructs	Model Components	Related Factors Commonly Investigated as Predictive of Return to Work
Volition	Personal causation	Level of perceived disability
		Perceived control over environment
		Educational level
		Perception of fault for injury
		Age
	Values	Gender
		Culture
	Interests	Job satisfaction prior to injury
Habituation	Roles	Work status at time of study (light duty vs. nonworking)
	Habits	Time at job prior to injury
		Attendance record at work prior to injury
Performance capacity	Objective	Nature and severity of injury
		Surgery history
		Diagnosis
	Subjective	Perceived level of pain
Environment	Social groups	Supervisor interaction
		Peer interaction
		Work environment/work stress

MOHO emphasizes that a person's volition and habituation are shaped by culture. This model also emphasizes that the physical and social environments are largely products of culture. Thus, anyone using MOHO should be aware of how cultural factors influence workers and their context. In order to ensure cultural relevance, MOHO assessments are tested across cultures and languages, and this is true of the WRI and WEIS.

The Worker Role Interview

DESCRIPTION

The WRI is a semi-structured interview accompanied by a therapist-administered rating scale where the patient is assessed in relation to return to work in general or to a specific job. Used in the initial rehabilitation assessment process, the WRI is designed to have injured workers or people with longstanding illness or disability discuss various aspects of their past work experience and job settings. The rating of the WRI is based on information collected in an interview. However, therapists are encouraged to assess physical, cognitive, and other functions necessary for work whenever there are questions about work capacity. The outcomes of such assessments are routinely considered when completing the WRI.

A manual is available that describes, in detail, the background of WRI, administration procedures, recommended questions, scoring instructions, rating scale, and case examples.[8] There are 16 items on the 10.0 version of the WRI rating scale form (previously 17 items were included, but one item was deleted because it added little information)[8,9] (Figure 12-1).

The 4-point WRI rating scale includes consideration of how each factor represented in the items influences the patient's likelihood of returning to or succeeding at work. The ratings are: strongly supports (SS), supports (S), interferes (I), and strongly interferes (SI). If there is not enough information to rate the item or the item is not applicable, there is an option to indicate the item is not applicable (N/A). A brief comment supporting each rating is recommended, since it can help when writing a report. When the ratings are completed, they provide a profile of the patient's strengths and weaknesses. This profile is particularly helpful in clarifying multiple factors that influence the patient's potential for achieving rehabilitation success or succeeding in community adaptation. This information can be important in decisions about providing services, placement, necessary supports, discharge planning, and so on.

When completing the ratings for WRI, the therapist can choose one of three different versions of the rating form. The three forms vary in detail and are selected according to the rater's proficiency and knowledge of WRI. The general rating scale is for the expert WRI rater, since it only contains definitions of the 4-point scale. The specific rating scale is generally for an experienced WRI rater, though it can also be used by a novice rater who has studied the manual carefully or who uses the manual as a resource when doing the rating. This scale defines each content area, each item, and has guidelines in the manual on how to score the patient on the items. The criterion rating guide presents the scale in detail, with criteria that serve as a guide to making the rating. This form (see Figure 12-1) is helpful to use when becoming acquainted with the WRI and with therapeutic reasoning based on MOHO in a work rehabilitation context. The descriptive criteria provided on this form can serve as a checklist of areas of occupational functioning that the therapist should consider in assessing the patient and beginning treatment planning.

To guide a WRI interview, there are three different formats of recommended questions. Each is intended for one of three different target groups: (1) injured workers hoping to return to a specific job, (2) patients with longstanding illness or disability who have been out of work for a long time or have limited work history, and (3) patients who may or may not need vocational training. Here, the interview combines the WRI with the Occupational Circumstances Assessment Interview and Rating Scale (OCAIRS).[21] OCAIRS is used to gather general occupational information, and if it emerges that the

Item	Rating	Criteria
3. Takes responsibility	SS	☐ Takes reasonable responsibility for work and/or life situation ☐ Understands aspects of work beyond their control ☑ Is active in seeking to return to or find work
	S	☑ Takes some responsibility for work and/or life situation ☑ Has some understanding of aspects of work beyond their control ☐ Is somewhat active in seeking to return to or find work
	I	☐ Tends to be passive in relation to work and/or life situation ☐ Tends to avoid responsibilities in work and/or life situation ☑ Tends to blame others/circumstances for personal failures ☐ Overly self critical regarding aspects of work beyond their control ☐ Shows little initiative in seeking to return to or find and keep work
	SI	☐ Completely passive in relation to work and/or life situation ☐ Avoids responsibilities ☐ Shows no initiative in seeking to return to or find work ☐ Blames others/circumstances for personal failures
Additional Rater Notes	Is willing and ready to work on improving his chances of finding work. Feels that it is other people's fault that he doesn't have a job e.g. former employer	

Figure 12-1. Example of the Criterion Rating Guide for Item 3.

patient has the possibility of considering work, then the therapist has the opportunity to incorporate necessary WRI questions. If not, then the OCAIRS can be completed alone. This combined format was developed by occupational therapists who were working with patients in a community mental health context and who were charged to identify whether the patient had vocational potential or needs. The OCAIRS is a MOHO-based interview that collects data on 12 major areas: roles, habits, personal causation, values, interests, skills, short-term goals, long-term goals, interpretation of past experiences, physical environment, social environment, and readiness for change.

The questions in all WRI formats are designed to gather information that will provide a holistic picture of the individual's potential as a worker and were developed to broadly represent types of concerns that rehabilitation therapists have about their patients. The content areas of the recommended questions are different for each target group and concern their specific background and experience.

ADMINISTRATION

There are five basic steps in WRI administration procedures:

1. Preparing for the interview, when the therapists collect preliminary data from the patient's record and decide if WRI is appropriate for the patient or not

2. Conducting the interview as a conversation where answers to questions and patient's emotional responses are monitored along with the inquiries made

3. Determining or making reference to underlying work capacity and/or skill, since

the therapist is asked to make a judgment about whether or not the patient's appraisal of his or her own abilities is realistic. This requires the therapist to have some baseline for comparison. This baseline can come from informal observation, but more typically it is from standardized testing or reports of others on the patient's underlying capacities or skills, such as concentration, strength, endurance, and range of motion

4. Preparing evaluation scoring and comments by copying the WRI rating form and rating guidelines or the WRI criterion rating guide from the appendix in the manual

5. Using the WRI for discharge evaluation and to measure change.

DEVELOPMENT AND DEPENDABILITY OF WRI

The WRI was originally developed as a part of a study designed to determine psychosocial variables influencing return to work. It soon became obvious that the tool was very clinically useful, and since then it has been evolving continuously in conjunction with research and practice.

A series of studies of WRI indicate that it is a dependable assessment. Biernacki[22] found it to have high test-retest reliability and high total interrater reliability. Velozo[23] found initial evidence that the 17 WRI items comprised a unidimensional construct of psychosocial capacity for work. In a subsequent study, Velozo[13] found that 15 of 17 items worked together to measure unidimensional construct in a group of 119 workers with low back pain. Two work environment items, boss and work settings, did not work well with the other items. A later study of a refined WRI scale with environmental items that were reworded to emphasize workers' perceptions, showed that all but one item, perception of boss, worked well to constitute a measure of psychosocial capacity for work.[13]

Ekbladh and colleagues[24] investigated the predictive validity of WRI in a 2-year follow-up study of patients attending an insurance medicine investigation center in Sweden. Of the 17 WRI items, five predicted return to work and three were components of the content area "personal causation." These results emphasize the importance of considering the individual's beliefs and expectations of effectiveness at work when assessing patients' work abilities and planning for rehabilitation.

Two studies in Sweden[12] and Iceland[11] examined the psychometric properties of translated versions of WRI utilizing the Multi-Faceted Rasch Measurement (MFRM) approach.[25] The Swedish study examined patients with psychiatric disabilities, while the Icelandic study included patients with various disabilities. Both studies provided evidence that the translated WRI was valid and culturally relevant. Forsyth and colleagues[14] conducted a study of psychometric properties of the WRI rating scale across three countries (Iceland, Sweden, and United States) on 440 participants. The results suggested that 13 items of the scale worked effectively to measure psychosocial capacity for work. The four environmental items appeared to relate more to the environment than to the individual, as might have been expected. The scale validly measured 95% of the participants, who varied by nationality, culture, age, and diagnosis.

CASE STUDY 1: WORKER ROLE INTERVIEW

Thora was a 42-year-old woman who lived in Iceland. She was admitted to a vocational outpatient rehabilitation center after receiving disability pension for over a year because of depression and alcohol abuse. At the time of referral, she had stopped drinking.

Thora was divorced and lived with her two teenagers. She had been a preschool head-master, but stopped working 2 years earlier because she could not cope with the job.

The WRI was administered to Thora to assess her potential for return to a similar kind of work as a preschool teacher. The therapist chose the WRI because she thought psychosocial factors hindered Thora in attending the worker role. Results of the inter-view are shown in Figure 12-2. The following qualitative information was gathered in the interview.

Thora felt as though she hardly managed the home, her children, and taking care of herself. Everything she did was with great effort, and she had no time or energy to work outside the home. When asked, she could only identify two or three tasks that she believed she was able to perform at her former job. She had lost confidence in her own capabilities. Thora could not see any solution to her problems. She was trying to gain more energy by taking short walks once in a while, but she did not attend her yoga les-sons, go swimming, or meet with friends on a regular basis as before. Thora believed she would never work again. She agreed to take part in vocational rehabilitation only to prove to society and herself that she was unable to work.

Thora was proud of the work she had done in the past and found that she had been good at it. When Thora was working, she had many work-oriented goals and found her work very important. Thora felt degraded being on disability pension, but all the same, her enthusiasm for a future career was lost.

Thora's habits were fairly ordered, with reasonably satisfying routines before the divorce. After the divorce, she gave up working, had difficulties managing the home, slept a lot, watched television, and hardly saw friends. She said it was hard to take care of the children but that she had managed and they had helped and were on good terms with her. During hard times Thora got help from psychiatrists and psychologists. Asked about the possibilities of getting a job as a preschool teacher, she said that it would not be a problem. She would get good recommendations and there were always vacant jobs available.

The WRI interview revealed that Thora had both strengths and weaknesses related to work. Her greatest liability was that she had lost control over her situation and confi-dence in herself and her capabilities. She had loved to work and thought she did a great job. Without work, she found herself a less valuable person. Therefore, it was essential to restore her conviction that she could work. The therapist thought her drive for work might be awakened when trying out her abilities and limitations by working for a short time in the beginning and lengthening it as time went by. By starting vocational training, the therapist hoped that Thora would produce more stable habits and routines.

In therapy, Thora needed help to identify resources and barriers within herself and learn new habits. She learned to accept that she needn't do everything 100% and didn't have to finish everything at once. She became good at using feedback to grow and gain respect for herself. She practiced structuring her time and work and learned from coach-ing. Encouragement kept her going. Thora found that the opportunities to perform occu-pations—to succeed or to fail, and if so, start over again, and most often to finish the task in the end—gave her hope. In the closing stages of rehabilitation she had regained belief in her own abilities and experienced joy when working. With much negotiation between Thora and her therapist about future jobs and coaching in every step toward work, she succeeded in getting a job, keeping it, and enjoying it.

As this case illustrates, the WRI provides information on volition, habituation, and perception of environment that influences work success and satisfaction. Using perfor-mance-capacity-oriented assessment alone in this case might have prohibited a revelation of the core problems and a successful intervention focus.

	Rating					Brief comments that support ratings
Personal Causation						
1. Assesses abilities and limitations	SS	S	*	SI	NA	Can only identify few tasks she is able to perform at work. Is not aware of her strengths
2. Expectation of job success	SS	S	I	*	NA	Doesn't think she can work at her former job or any job at all ever
3. Takes responsibility	SS	S	*	SI	NA	She thinks her problem is beyond her control although she makes some effort to get her energy level up
Values						
4. Commitment to work	SS	S	*	SI	NA	Thora took a lot of pride in her work before, had consistent work history, hates being on disability pension
5. Work-related goals	SS	S	I	*	NA	She always had goals in former jobs, now she doesn't
Interests						
6. Enjoys work	SS	*	I	SI	NA	Liked working with people, having the opportunity to work outdoors, having opportunity to go to workshops
7. Pursues interests	SS	S	*	SI	NA	Previously, good match between interests in outdoor activities and people's welfare. Now she only takes walking tours
Roles						
8. Appraises work expectations	*	S	I	SI	NA	Gives examples of job demands and work expectations
9. Influence of other roles	SS	*	I	SI	NA	Salary of a preschool teacher is higher than disability pension. All energy goes to the role of home maintenance, mother, and self care
Habits						
10. Work habits	SS	*	I	SI	NA	Excellent work habits in the past; describes being punctual, accurate, and finishing on time
11. Daily routines	SS	S	*	SI	NA	Previously rather strong, currently weak. Watches TV, makes dinner, and cleans once in a while, with help from children

Figure 12-2. Results of Thora's Worker Role Interview, page 1.

The Work Environment Impact Scale

Workers are most productive and satisfied when their motivation (volition), patterns of work habits (habituation), and capacity for doing and interacting at work fit or match the work environment (physical spaces, objects, social groups, and occupational forms).

12. Adapts routine to minimize difficulties	SS	S	✱	SI	NA	Doesn't adjust exercise routines, has stopped. Tries to do some home activities with frequent breaks
Environment						
13. Perception of work setting	✱	S	I	SI	NA	No problems
14. Perception of family and peers	SS	✱	I	SI	NA	Family and friends encouraged her to start working but have given up, although they are concerned and supportive
15. Perception of boss	SS	✱	I	SI	NA	"My boss liked me and has been asking me to come back, but I would not go to the same position"
16. Perception of coworkers	SS	✱	I	SI	NA	"I liked my coworkers and they liked me. I have never had any difficulties with coworkers"

Figure 12-2. Results of Thora's Worker Role Interview, page 2.

Therefore, the same work environment may affect workers differently. The aim of the WEIS[10] is to determine how a particular work environment impacts a given worker.

DESCRIPTION

The WEIS is a semi-structured interview accompanied by a therapist-administered 4-point rating scale. It was designed to gather information on the worker's perception and experience of work settings from workers with physical or psychosocial disabilities. The interview focuses on the impact of work setting on a worker's performance, satisfaction, and well-being from the point of view of the worker. The target groups are: (1) people presently working and having difficulties at their job, (2) people who are not presently working but intend to go to a specific job or type of work where the work environment is known, and in unique cases, (3) people out of work who can gain from identifying how past work environments impacted their work productivity and satisfaction.

There are 17 items on the WEIS rating scale form,[10] reflecting 17 diverse environmental factors such as physical space, social contacts and supports, temporal demands, objects utilized, and daily job function (Figure 12-3). The rating scale indicates the level of support or interference, provided to the worker. Two ratings imply environmental support: a 4 rating, in exceptional cases, and a 3 rating indicating adequate support. Two ratings suggest that the environment interferes: a 2 rating when there is some interference, and a 1 rating when the interference is perceived to be substantial.

ADMINISTRATION

The WEIS manual introduces and discusses the background of the instrument, the interview process, recommended questions, scoring instructions, and the ratings.[10] There are four basic steps in WEIS's administration procedures:

1. Obtaining appropriate background data, where the therapists collect preliminary data from the patient's record or interdisciplinary staff to determine if the WEIS is appropriate for the patient or not

Time Demands: Time allotted for available/expected amount of work.				
1	✻	3	4	N/A

Comments: When customer volume is high Drew has difficulty accurately completing all tasks to expected levels of performance

Task Demands: The physical, cognitive, and/or emotional demands and opportunities of work tasks.				
1	2	✻	4	N/A

Comments: Aside from problems at high volume times, the task demands match Drew's skills and support work performance

Appeal of Work Tasks: The appeal/enjoyableness or status/value of work tasks.				
1	2	✻	4	N/A

Comments: Drew sees work tasks as less important that his prior type of work but finds the job appealing given its part-time option

Work Schedule: The influence of work hours upon other valued roles, activities, transportation, and basic self-care needs.				
1	2	3	✻	N/A

Comments: Drew enjoys variability of schedule and level of choice over hours he prefers to work

Co-worker Interaction: Interaction/collaboration with co-workers required for job responsibilities.				
✻	2	3	4	N/A

Comments: Drew finds collaborating with others very difficult and prefers to work alone

Work Group Membership: Social involvement with co-workers at work or outside of work.				
✻	2	3	4	N/A

Comments: Drew feels like an outsider and that he does not fit in well with co-workers or his supervisor

Supervisor Interaction: Feedback, guidance, and/or other communication/interaction with supervisor(s).				
1	✻	3	4	N/A

Comments: Drew feels some support and gets feedback but could establish a more effective relationship with his supervisor

Work Role Standards: Overall climate of work setting expressed in expectations for quality, excellence, commitment, achievement, and/or efficiency.				
1	2	✻	4	N/A

Comments: Overall supports work performance with minor problem meeting standards at high volume periods

Work Role Style: Opportunity/expectation for autonomy/-compliance when organizing, making requests, negotiating, and choosing how and what work tasks will be done daily.				
1	✻	3	4	N/A

Comments: Has difficulty following strict work protocols and would

Figure 12-3. Results of Drew's Work Environment Impact Scale, page 1.

prefer more chance to innovate				
Interaction with Others: Interaction/communication with subordinates, customers, clients, audiences, students, or others, excluding supervisor or co-workers.				
1	2	✱	4	N/A
Comments: Mixed: enjoys customers but has difficulty with co-workers				
Rewards: Opportunities for job security, recognition/advancement in position, and/or compensation in salary or benefits.				
1	2	✱	4	N/A
Comments: Drew feels his pay and rewards are adequate for part-time work				
Sensory Qualities: Properties of the work place such as noise, smell, visual or tactile properties, temperature/climate, or air quality and ventilation.				
1	2	3	✱	N/A
Comments: Drew highly enjoys work setting, including music and aromas, etc.				
Architecture/Arrangement: Architecture or physical arrangement of and between work spaces and environments.				
1	2	✱	4	N/A
Comments: Overall supports, although it can be cramped when more than one employee is present				
Ambience/Mood: The feeling/mood associated with the degree of privacy, friendliness, morale, excitement, anxiety, frustration in the work place.				
1	2	✱	4	N/A
Comments: Overall positive except at high volume times when Drew can experience stress				
Properties of Objects: The physical, cognitive, or emotional demands/opportunities of tools, equipment, materials, and supplies.				
1	2	3	✱	N/A
Comments: No problems or difficulties here				
Physical Amenities: Non-work-specific facilities necessary to meet personal needs at work such as restrooms, lunchrooms, or break rooms.				
1	2	3	✱	N/A
Comments: Supports performance, no problems				
Meaning of Objects: What objects signify to a person.				
1	2	✱	4	N/A
Comments: Not highly significant				
General impressions: Overall environment supports performance with exception of difficulties encountered during high volume times and in relations with co-workers and supervisor				

Figure 12-3. Results of Drew's Work Environment Impact Scale, page 2.

2. Conducting the interview, where the therapist carries out the interview like a conversation

3. Completing the rating scale

4. Utilizing the information from the interview to improve the work environment.

DEPENDABILITY

Two studies have been published on the psychometric properties of WEIS. Corner and colleagues,[26] found that the instrument appears to measure a single construct. However, the scale was not as sensitive as preferable in discriminating between individuals. Based on the results of the previous study, Kielhofner and colleagues[27] made revisions of some scale items to clarify their meaning. Then they scrutinized the psychometric properties of the second American English version and the first Swedish versions of WEIS. Results indicated that the WEIS items worked well together to define a single construct, and that the revised instrument had adequate sensitivity and validly measured the subjects.

CASE STUDY 2: WORK ENVIRONMENT IMPACT SCALE

Drew was a 36-year-old man living in Chicago who resided in a supportive living facility for persons with HIV/AIDS. He was referred to occupational therapy for assistance in returning to living independently in his own apartment in the community and for a prevocational assessment. Drew was single but had good support from family and friends. He had completed high school and had a good work history providing secretarial support at a communications company. He had been unemployed for 13 months and was receiving Social Security Disability Insurance (SSDI) when he decided to obtain part-time employment to explore his tolerance for work. He reported having difficulty with fatigue, short-term memory, and often felt "frustrated and short-tempered" because he could not process information as quickly as he used to. At the time of initial assessment, Drew was working three 4-hour shifts a week at a local coffee shop, but was experiencing some problems. His supervisor gave him feedback that his pace of work was too slow, that his coworkers had complained about his attitude, and that he did not consistently follow procedures that were in place to maintain cleanliness and sanitation.

The therapist proposed the administration of the WEIS as part of a larger evaluation plan, and Drew agreed to be interviewed about his work environment. The WEIS was chosen because it would give the therapist and Drew a better understanding of the fit between the work environment of the coffee shop and Drew's current work skills and perceptions of the environment. It was expected that insights gained by administration of the WEIS would help Drew make decisions about what type of work would best meet his needs given his medical condition. Results of the WEIS are presented in Figure 12-3.

Drew reported in the interview that his work tasks had a moderate level of appeal to him. He appreciated being out of his apartment and enjoyed interacting with the customers and his coworkers, although he felt that some of his coworkers "took their jobs too seriously." He noted that the work tasks themselves were not difficult, but that when the coffee shop became busy he was expected to work at a pace that he had difficulty maintaining. He was aware that he sometimes skipped steps such as adequately cleaning items after their use. He also mentioned that he was expected to complete work tasks in a prescribed manner and that there was little room to make decisions on his own, even when he thought his methods of working would be faster. He found this very frustrating.

Through additional discussion, the therapist learned that Drew found the variability of his work schedule appealing and that he had considerable control over which shifts he worked. While Drew typically had more energy in the morning, it was also the busiest and most hectic time to work.

When asked about the physical setting, Drew reacted positively, stating that the coffee shop itself was very pleasant, that he enjoyed working with music in the background, and that he loved the "aromas and constant sensory stimulation" that he encountered. He denied any difficulty utilizing the equipment and objects he came across in his job.

His comments regarding the social environment were notably less positive. Though he stated that he appreciated the diversity he saw in the shop's customers, he did not enjoy the company of his coworkers or of his supervisor. Drew described himself as "feeling out of place" and said that he preferred to work alone. He avoided his coworkers outside of the workplace, felt uncomfortable when his supervisor was present, and complained that the space behind the counter was too small for more than one person to work efficiently. Drew had chosen not to disclose his disability to his coworkers or supervisor, despite noting that he did not think he would encounter any discrimination due to his HIV status.

Through the assessment, Drew and the therapist agreed to explore the following in treatment:

1. Strategies for managing stress and maintaining attention to work tasks, including scheduling fewer morning work shifts

2. The advantages and disadvantages of disclosing his disability to his employer and requesting reasonable accommodations such as priority choice of shifts and more frequent breaks

3. Strategies for developing more positive relationships with his coworkers and his supervisor

4. Strategies for emphasizing Drew's strengths and the parts of the job he found most enjoyable

5. Assessing the long-term impact of part-time employment on Drew's SSDI benefits.

Summary

The Worker Role Interview (WRI) and The Work Environment Impact Scale (WEIS) are two work-related assessments produced within the Model of Human Occupation. The WRI assesses psychosocial factors that influence work performance, while WEIS assesses workplace conditions that impact the worker. Studies indicate the consistency and dependability of both assessments, and they have both been used effectively by occupational therapists around the world and in different languages.

References

1. Kielhofner G. *Model of Human Occupation: Theory and Application.* 3rd. ed. Baltimore, MD: Lippincott Williams & Wilkins; 2002.

2. Barrett L, Beer D, Kielhofner G. The importance of volitional narrative in treatment: an ethnographic case study in a work program. *Work: A Journal of Prevention, Assessment & Rehabilitation.* 1999;12:79-92.

3. Baron K, Littleton MJ. The Model of Human Occupation: a return to work case study. *Work: A Journal of Prevention, Assessment & Rehabilitation.* 1999;12:37-46.

4. Braveman B, Helfrich CA. Occupational identity: exploring the narratives of three men living with AIDS. *Journal of Occupational Science.* 2001;8(2):25-31.

5. Fisher GS. Administration and application of the Worker Role Interview: looking beyond functional capacity. *Work: A Journal of Prevention, Assessment & Rehabilitation.* 1999;12:25-36.

6. Kielhofner G, Braveman B, Finlayson M, Paul-Ward A, Goldbaum L, Goldstein K. Outcomes of a vocational program for persons with AIDS. *Am J Occup Ther.* 2004;58(1):64-72.

7. Mentrup C, Niehaus A, Kielhofner G. Applying the Model of Human Occupation in work-focused rehabilitation: a case illustration. *Work: A Journal of Prevention, Assessment & Rehabilitation.* 1999;12:61-70.

8. Braveman B, Robson M, Velozo C, et al. *The Worker Role Interview* (Version 10.0). Chicago, IL: The Model of Human Occupation Clearinghouse, Department of Occupational Therapy, College of Applied Health Sciences, University of Illinois at Chicago; 2005.

9. Velozo C, Kielhofner G, Fisher G. *A User's Manual for the Worker Role Interview (WRI)* (Version 9.0). Chicago, IL: The Model of Human Occupation Clearinghouse, Department of Occupational Therapy, College of Applied Health Sciences, University of Illinois at Chicago; 1998.

10. Moore-Corner RA, Kielhofner G, Olson L. *A User's Guide to Work Environment Impact Scale (WEIS)* (Version 2.0). Chicago, IL: The Model of Human Occupation Clearinghouse, Department of Occupational Therapy, College of Applied Health Sciences, University of Illinois at Chicago; 1998.

11. Fenger K, Keller J. Worker Role Interview: testing the psychometric properties of the Icelandic versions. *Scand J Occup Ther.* 2007;14(3):160-172.

12. Haglund L, Karlsson G, Kielhofner G, Lai JS. Validity of the Swedish version of the Worker Role Interview. *Scand J Occup Ther.* 1997;4:23-29.

13. Velozo C, Kielhofner G, Gern A, et al. Worker Role Interview: toward validation of a psychosocial work-related measure. *J Occup Rehabil.* 1999;9(3):153-168.

14. Forsyth K, Braveman B, Kielhofner G, et al. Psychometric properties of the Worker Role Interview. *Work. A Journal of Prevention, Assessment and Rehabilitation.* 2006;27:313-318.

15. Bettencourt CM, Carstrom P, Brown SH, Lindau K, Long CM. Using work simulation to treat adults with back injuries. *Am J Occup Ther.* 1986;40:12-18.

16. Caruso LA, Chan DE, Chan A. The management of work-related back pain. *Am J Occup Ther.* 1987;41:112-117.

17. Matheson LN, Ogden LD, Vilette K, Schultz K. Work hardening: occupational therapy in industrial rehabilitation. *Am J Occup Ther.* 1985;39:314-321.

18. Frederickson BE, Trief PM, Van Beveren P, Yan HA, Baum S. Rehabilitation of the patient with chronic back pain: a search for outcome predictors. *Spine.* 1988;13:351-353.

19. Waddell G. A new clinical model for the treatment of low back pain. *Spine.* 1987;12:632-644.

20. Braveman B. The Model of Human Occupation and prediction of return to work: a review of related empirical research. *Work: A Journal of Prevention, Assessment & Rehabilitation.* 1999;12:13-23.

21. Forsyth K, Deshpande S, Kielhofner G, et al. *A User's Manual for The Occupational Circumstances Assessment Interview and Rating Scale* (Version 3.0). Chicago, IL: The Model of Human Occupation Clearinghouse, Department of Occupational Therapy, College of Applied Health Sciences, University of Illinois at Chicago; 2005.

22. Biernacki SD. Reliability of the Worker Role Interview. *Am J Occup Ther.* 1993;46(9):797-803.

23. Velozo C. *Final report: Demographic and Intervention Factors in Return to Work: A Database Approach.* NIDRR grant H133C901. 1991.

24. Ekbladh E, Haglund L, Thorell L-H. The Worker Role Interview-Preliminary data on the predictive validity of return to work of clients after an insurance medicine investigation. *J Occup Rehabil.* 2004;14(2):131-141.

25. Linacre JM. *Many-Facet Rasch Measurement.* Chicago, IL: MESA Press; 1989.

26. Corner RA, Kielhofner G, Lin F-L. Construct validity of a work environment impact scale. *Work: A Journal of Prevention, Assessment & Rehabilitation.* 1997;9:21-34.

27. Kielhofner G, Lai J, Olson L, Haglund L, Ekbadh E, Hedlund M. Psychometric properties of the Work Environment Impact Scale: a cross-cultural study. *Work: A Journal of Prevention, Assessment & Rehabilitation.* 1999;12:71-77.

ROLE ASSESSMENTS USED IN MENTAL HEALTH

Victoria P. Schindler, PhD, OTR, BCMH, FAOTA

"The concept, role, is primarily a dramatic one, deriving centuries ago from the wooden scroll on which the early actor's lines were written. In its present form...it is that which holds two realities, the everyday and the imaginative, in a paradoxical relationship to one another." Landy RJ. The dramatic basis of role theory. The Arts in Psychotherapy. *1991;18(1):29.*

Introduction

This chapter will introduce an evaluation and treatment intervention designed to assist individuals diagnosed with schizophrenia to develop social roles and their underlying task and interpersonal skills. This evaluation and treatment intervention is entitled Role Development. It is a frame of reference or a set of guidelines for clinical practice. It is designed to give practitioners the theoretical background and concrete steps to implement this intervention.

Roles are patterns of behavior and the foundation of all social behavior, and they are commonly referred to as social roles. *Social roles* are life roles that are the foundation of our relationships with our families, friends, work, and community. Some social roles are spouse, community member, student, and friend. Enacting roles that are important and meaningful to us produces contentment, joy, and satisfaction.[1-4]

Roles can be learned in a functional or dysfunctional manner. An individual can be highly adept at performing many aspects of a role or can be lacking in skills or motivation to perform a role successfully and consistently. To enact a role effectively, individuals need a repertoire of task and interpersonal skills, and these skills are the foundation of roles.[2,5]

The development of roles can be disrupted in individuals diagnosed with a mental illness. The more disabling the mental illness, the more it affects the learning of and ability to sustain social roles.[4,6] One of the most severe types of mental illness is schizophrenia.[7] Individuals diagnosed with schizophrenia often have deficits in learning and/or maintaining the task and interpersonal skills necessary to enact positive, socially acceptable roles.[5,8-10]

For individuals diagnosed with schizophrenia, commonly available treatments such as medication and activity programs alleviate symptoms and promote involvement in activity and social interactions. However, activity programs may not address the development of social roles or the specific skills that are nested in these roles. Additional treatment methods with demonstrated effectiveness are required to develop these skills and roles.[11,12] One such method is treatment based on a set of guidelines for clinical practice. Sets of guidelines for practice describe the assessment and intervention methods necessary to promote change within a specific theoretical foundation. Staff trained in the use of a set of guidelines for practice are then able to use their skills and knowledge to facilitate positive growth and change in their patients.[13]

Role Development,[14] a set of guidelines for clinical practice, has been developed to provide direction for health care practitioners to assist individuals diagnosed with schizophrenia to learn social roles and their underlying task and interpersonal skills. Role Development is operationally defined as an intervention based on a theoretical set of guidelines for practice that address the development of meaningful social roles and the skills that are the foundation of these roles. Role Development is a theory-based, individualized intervention in which staff and patient work collaboratively to identify and develop the patient's social roles and the skills associated with these roles. When Role Development is implemented by rehabilitation staff, it provides a common link and theoretical foundation on which to base intervention.[2,14,15]

As with all sets of guidelines for practice, the Role Development Guidelines link theory to practice and consist of four parts: (1) theoretical base, (2) function-dysfunction continuums, (3) behaviors indicative of function and dysfunction, and (4) methods to promote positive change. The theoretical base of Role Development provides a description of an individual's need to learn and feel competent and successful in social roles. It describes how learning takes place, the learning of typical and atypical roles, and the therapeutic tools that assist in the process of developing roles. The continuums and the behaviors indicative of function and dysfunction provide a means to evaluate an individual's skills (task and interpersonal) and roles (eg, worker, student, group member, friend). The postulates to promote positive change describe specific methods to assist an individual to develop skills and roles.[1,2,14]

Role Development: A Set of Guidelines for Clinical Practice

THEORETICAL BASE

The theoretical information for the Role Development set of guidelines for practice was derived primarily from the Role Acquisition frame of reference.[2] A primary source for the theoretical base of the Role Acquisition frame of reference is social learning theory.[16] The theoretical base of Role Development addresses five principles: (1) the nature of the individual, (2) what needs to be learned, (3) how learning takes place, (4) typical and atypical development, and (5) appropriate tools.

The Nature of the Individual

All individuals have an inherent need to explore their environment and to experience a sense of competency and mastery in various aspects of daily living. This is especially true in aspects of the environment that are of interest to the individual. These interests develop from exploration and from the amount of worth placed on them by the individual's family and cultural group.[2,15,17]

What Needs to be Learned

An individual's societal group and cultural orientation specify what one learns and categorizes into social roles.[18,19] An individual's interests and goals also influence roles. Skill competence also has been viewed as an integral part of role satisfaction and manifestation.[5,20,21] The foundation of all roles is task skills and interpersonal skills. To enact a role effectively, individuals need a repertoire of task and interpersonal skills. *Task skills* are those skills that address one's sensorimotor, cognitive, and psychological functions as they relate to the completion of tasks. Task skills that are basic to roles include paying attention, following directions, and solving problems related to a task. *Interpersonal skills* are those skills that address one's cognitive, psychological, and social functions as they relate to interactions with others. Interpersonal skills basic to roles include initiating and sustaining a conversation, and expressing one's ideas and feelings. Task and interpersonal skills are learned and refined as one participates in social roles. The social roles one may learn in this set of guidelines for practice include worker, student, friend, and group member.[5,22,23]

How Learning Takes Place

Learning of task and interpersonal skills and social roles occurs according to two processes: (1) the socialization process, and (2) the application of the principles of learning. The socialization process describes the agent and the setting that facilitate the learning of a role. The agent is the individual responsible for collaborating with the patient regarding what is to be learned, providing feedback, and rewarding positive growth. An agent can be a positive role model who consistently and clearly defines expectations, provides constructive feedback, and rewards positive growth, or a negative role model who neglects this process or engages in this process in a destructive or harmful manner. For example, a parent who gently and consistently teaches a child appropriate moral and societal values would be viewed as a positive agent. To the contrary, a parent who ignores or neglects these teachings or teaches them in a way that is contrary to society's norms (eg, teaching a child that the use of illegal drugs is acceptable) would be viewed as a negative agent. The ideal settings for the learning of adequate socialization are settings in which relevant behavior is "elicited, evoked, required, and permitted."[2,3,16,21]

In the Role Development Guidelines, the agent is clearly a facilitator. As a facilitator, the agent adheres to several principles. First, the agent assumes that the individual has knowledge of needs regarding roles and skills. The individual, in collaboration with the agent, sets the agenda for therapy. Secondly, the agent accepts the individual's report as relevant information. Hence, it is of the utmost importance to develop a plan that incorporates the individual's stated desires, goals, and feedback. The final assumption is that the agent does not promote change, but creates an environment to facilitate change.[24]

Settings in the socialization process should provide enough stimulation to generate interest, and practice of skills should be encouraged. For example, an ideal setting is one that is safe and has enough activities and interactions to stimulate exploration, competency, and mastery. A setting that is deprived, unsanitary, or harmful is not conducive to learning.[2,25]

Learning also occurs through the use of the *Principles of Learning*. These principles are psychological tenets that serve as a foundation to learning. A summation of these principles is as follows:

1. Learning is influenced by an individual's inherent capacities, age, sex, interests, culture, and motivation.

2. Learning is more likely to occur when learning goals are set by the individual and when the individual understands what is to be learned and the rationale for learning.

3. Learning is increased when the individual is an active participant in learning and when learning begins at the individual's current level and proceeds at a comfortable rate.

4. Frequent repetition, trial and error, reinforcement and feedback, and a supportive environment are important aspects of the learning process.

5. Anxiety affects learning differently, and conflicts and frustrations must be recognized and addressed.[2]

Typical and Atypical Development

Typical development occurs when an individual interacts in an environment that promotes exploration, competency, and mastery. There are an adequate number of agents, and the agents are positive role models. The settings have an appropriate amount of stimulation and incentives to encourage the learning of social roles. The individual is motivated to explore and develop new roles in a satisfying manner. In *atypical development*, the number of agents may be inadequate, and/or some of the agents may be unable or unwilling to encourage appropriate learning. Settings may be deprived or harmful. Atypical development could also occur due to a major life disruption such as illness or the loss of a role partner.[2,25]

Typically, the learning of roles follows a normal developmental progression.[22,26,27] This typical development of roles can become severely hindered by a diagnosis of mental illness. The more disabling the mental illness, the more it impacts on the learning of social roles. One of the most severe types of mental illness is one that encompasses schizophrenic disorders.[6,28-30] Instead of progressing through the typical development of roles and skills, many individuals diagnosed with schizophrenic disorders learn roles that are deviant or passive in nature and do not promote independent functioning in the community.[23,28,29,31-35]

Appropriate Tools

The tools used to evaluate performance and promote change in this set of guidelines for practice include the nonhuman environment (ie, everything in an environment other than the individuals), conscious use of self (ie, therapeutic use of self), the teaching-learning process (teaching activities required for independent living), purposeful activities, activity analysis and synthesis (the process of developing, examining, and selecting suitable activities), group dynamics, therapeutic groups, and activity groups. Within this set of guidelines for practice, tools should emphasize active participation in activities as opposed to passive participation or random activity. Activities should be real and tangible as opposed to abstract. In order to be successful in a variety of roles, one must be involved in "doing" the skills or components of these roles.[2,5,6,23,36-40]

FUNCTION/DYSFUNCTION CONTINUUMS

This set of guidelines for practice describes two categories of function/dysfunction continuums: skills and social roles. *Skills* include: 1) task skills and 2) interpersonal skills. The skills involve coordination among an individual's motor, sensory/perception, process, psychological, communication/interaction, and social functions. *Social roles* are: (1) worker, (2) student, (3) group member, (4) friend, (5) family member, (6) parent, (7) community member, (8) health maintainer, and (9) home maintainer. The task skills and interpersonal skills are necessary components for participation in social roles.[2]

BEHAVIORS INDICATIVE OF FUNCTION/DYSFUNCTION

The continuums are described in relation to behaviors indicative of dysfunction. The absence of these behaviors indicates function. The categories and continuums are adapted from Mosey[2] and Rogers, Sciarappa, and Anthony[41] and are as follows:

The behaviors indicative of function and dysfunction are the assessments used to evaluate the specific roles and skills. There is an assessment for each role within the function/dysfunction continuums (eg, worker, student, group member, friend, family member, community member, health maintainer, home maintainer) and for the task skills and interpersonal skills.

POSTULATES TO PROMOTE POSITIVE CHANGE

The postulates to promote positive change are the specific methods (eg, activities and interactions) to engage the individual in the development of roles. The postulates describe the way in which the therapist selects and adapts activities, arranges and modifies the therapeutic environment, and uses the self as a therapeutic tool to promote change in the patient.[1,2,13] The postulates can be found in an article written by the author for *Occupational Therapy in Mental Health*.[42]

IMPLEMENTATION OF ROLE DEVELOPMENT

To implement the Role Development Guidelines, the therapist follows a set of instructions that are summarized briefly. First, the therapist conducts an initial interview with the patient to determine the roles and skills the patient would like to address. The therapist and the patient discuss the types of activities and interactions in which the patient could participate in order to develop the task and interpersonal skills that compose the desired role. Then, the therapist observes the patient in groups and completes the appropriate assessments for skills and roles based on the observation and interview. Next, the therapist develops a treatment plan in collaboration with the patient. At least weekly, and more often if necessary, the therapist and the patient meet for approximately 15 to 30 minutes to discuss the patient's progress with the treatment intervention and develop a plan for the following week. The therapist documents a weekly progress report based on this meeting. Modifications to the treatment plan are made accordingly. Details regarding implementation of Role Development can be found in an article written by the author in *Occupational Therapy in Mental Health*.[42]

Literature Review

THE DEVELOPMENT OF ROLE DEVELOPMENT GUIDELINES

The primary source for the Role Development Guidelines is Role Acquisition, a frame of reference developed by Mosey.[2] The Role Acquisition frame of reference was modified for this study, resulting in Role Development. The theoretical base of Role Acquisition consisted primarily of Mosey's original work. This was expanded upon in the Role Development Guidelines to include some of the seminal literature on role theory,[3,18,19,21,43] social learning theory,[16] and skill development.[5,6,36]

An historical review of role theory begins in the 1930s and continues to evolve today. The concept of *role* originated in drama in the form of a wooden scroll on which the actor's lines were written.[44] The evolution of role theory focused on two schools of thought: structural functionalism and symbolic interactionism. *Structural functionalism* views roles as the expected behaviors of an individual's status or position in a social structure.[3,18,43] *Symbolic interactionism*, to the contrary, states that human behavior is attributable more to an individual's unique characteristics and perceptions than to an overlying social structure.[19,45,46] Social learning theory[16] also had an impact on the development of role theory. Central concepts such as modeling, reinforcement, punishment, and consequences can be applied to the way in which one learns a role. Current thinking is that a variety of roles can have a positive influence on an individual's ability to function in society. Multiple roles equip a person to deal with a wide variety of situations and to compensate for disappointment in one role by succeeding in other roles.[47] Unfortunately, multiple roles can also cause role strain. Also, for individuals diagnosed with schizophrenia, multiple roles may be impractical. Recently, Wolfensberger[4] developed Social Role Valorization, a theory that addresses how society devalues individuals such as the mentally ill, the poor, and prisoners—individuals who have few roles, or negative roles such as criminal.

The Documented Use of Role Development Guidelines

Three research studies have been conducted on Role Development to date. A larger-scale study was conducted at a maximum-security psychiatric facility.[14,43,48] Two studies incorporating multiple single-subject case studies were conducted at a community mental health center.[49] These studies will be briefly summarized.

Study A: Research Conducted at a Maximum-Security Psychiatric Facility

The purpose of this study[14,42,48] was to examine if adults diagnosed with schizophrenia who resided in a forensic setting demonstrated improved task and interpersonal skills and social roles when involved in an individualized intervention based on Role Development, compared to an intervention based on a multidepartmental activity program (MAP).

METHOD

Participants

Patient participants were adult males, 18 to 55 years of age, who were diagnosed with schizophrenia and were receiving antipsychotic medication. A total of 84 patients were admitted to the study, with 42 participants each in the experimental and comparison groups. All patients completed written informed consent forms. No participants withdrew from the study. Eighteen rehabilitation department staff participated in the Role Development training and implementation, including two art therapists. Training occurred over 10 weeks for a total of 15.5 hours. All staff completed written informed consent forms.

Procedures

The study used a repeated measures pretest-posttest design with an experimental group (Role Development program) and a comparison group (MAP). Quantitative and qualitative measures were used to collect data. Participants in both groups were assessed with four instruments upon admission to the study and at 4, 8, and 12 weeks of participation in the study. The instruments were the Role Functioning Scale,[50] the Task Skills Scale, the Interpersonal Skills Scale,[2,41] and the Role Checklist.[51] Inter-rater reliability, test-retest reliability, and Cronbach's alpha measure of internal consistency were established for three of the four instruments prior to the study.[42] Reliability studies were not conducted for the Role Checklist, as this is a self-report checklist. Independent raters, blind to the purpose of the study, conducted the initial and repeated measures of functioning. Qualitative measures included patient interviews and staff focus groups.

The comparison group participated in the existing MAP routinely offered by the facility. The MAP is a nonindividualized therapeutic intervention designed to encourage the productive use of time and socialization in a group setting.[52] The experimental intervention, Role Development, was a new treatment and an enhancement of the existing MAP. Once the experimental group began, staff were monitored biweekly for fidelity to the intervention via completion of fidelity checklists by the staff and the principal investigator.

Results

Data analysis included quantitative and qualitative results. There were no demographic differences between participants in the experimental and comparison groups. Within-group tests, between-group tests, ANCOVA, MANCOVA, and repeated measures ANOVA were conducted. Data analysis indicated that participants in the Role Development program showed statistically significant improvement ($p < .05$) in the development of task skills, interpersonal skills, and role functioning, especially at 4 weeks of treatment, in comparison to participants in the MAP. Qualitative data from staff focus groups and patient interviews supported the findings. A complete description of this study can be found in Schindler.[42]

Study B: Research Conducted at a Community Mental Health Center

PURPOSE OF THE STUDY

Two studies were conducted to examine if adults diagnosed with severe and persistent mental illness who attended a community mental health center demonstrated improved task and interpersonal skills and social roles when involved in Role Development. The first study was a pilot study as a precursor to the second study. Both studies used a single-subject case study design with pretest and posttest follow-up at 8 weeks.[53,54] Qualitative interview questions at pretest and posttest were used to supplement quantitative findings. This design was selected to continue the assessment of Role Development in a different setting (ie, outpatient setting) and with a more focused view on the process involved in role and skill development. Master's level students conducted the treatment intervention and participated in weekly supervision to maintain fidelity to the treatment intervention.

Participants

The first study (ie, the pilot study)[49] included two participants. The second study consisted of six men and four women.[55] All participants were diagnosed with a severe and persistent mental illness. The same assessments used in Study A were used as pretest and posttest measures in these studies. The pilot study documented findings as two case studies. Both patients demonstrated improvement in the majority of scores from pretest to posttest. However, their improvement was primarily documented in a case study format. Results of the second study used the Wilcoxon Signed Ranks Test which demonstrated a statistically significant improvement in role functioning ($p = .02$), interpersonal skills ($p = .029$), and task skills ($p = .05$).

Description of Assessment Tools

- Task Skills Scale: The Task Skills Scale was developed by Schindler[42] based on the Role Acquisition frame of reference authored by Mosey.[2] The Task Skills Scale assesses areas of functioning required to complete basic daily tasks. Eight areas are assessed and outlined on the scale, located in Appendix F. Individuals are observed and then rated on a scale of 1 to 5, with 1 being the lowest level of functioning and 5 being the highest level of functioning.

- Interpersonal Skills Scale: Like the Task Skills Scale, the Interpersonal Skills Scale was developed by Schindler[42] based on the Role Acquisition frame of reference authored by Mosey.[2] The Interpersonal Skills Scale assesses the skills related to cognitive, psychological, and social functioning within interpersonal interactions. Like the Task Skills Scale, eight areas are assessed and outlined on the scale, located in Appendix G. Individuals are observed and then rated on a scale of 1 to 5, with 1 being the lowest level of functioning and 5 being the highest level of functioning.

- Role Scales: Individual scales were developed for nine roles (worker, student, friend, group member, parent, family member, community member, health maintainer, and home maintainer). Each of these scales describes behavior within the specific role and uses the same 1 to 5 rating scale as the Task Skills Scale and the Interpersonal Skills Scale. These role scales can be found in Appendices H through P.

RELIABILITY AND VALIDITY OF THE ASSESSMENT TOOLS

A study was conducted to establish inter-rater reliability, internal consistency, and test-retest reliability on the Task Skills Scale and Interpersonal Skills Scale.[2,41]

Four raters were recruited for the reliability studies. All raters had clinical backgrounds. Training in the administration of the scales was conducted. A schedule was developed in which each staff rater was paired with every other rater (ie, R1/R2, R1/R3, R1/R4, R2/R3, etc.).

A total of 12 individuals were observed and interviewed by four raters, and the rating scales were completed. This was a group of convenience. Twelve individuals participated because this was conducted within a pilot study and 12 individuals is common practice for a pilot study. The age of the patients ranged from 18 to 49; the mean age was 37 years with a standard deviation of 8.4. Eight of the patients were Caucasian (66%), and four of the patients were African American (33%). Eleven of the patients were never married (92%), and one patient was divorced (8%). Length of stay varied from less than 1 month to greater than 1 year; the mean was 2.5 months with a standard deviation of 2.1.

Inter-rater reliability and internal consistency were obtained for the scales (Table 13-1).

Alpha coefficients were conducted. Alpha coefficient for the Task Skills Scale was .99 (N = 32); for the Interpersonal Skills Scale it was .99 (N = 32).

To assess inter-rater reliability, bivariate correlations were conducted on every item in every scale for all four raters (Task Skills Scale—eight items, Interpersonal Skills Scale —eight items).

The Interpersonal Skills Scale had correlations ranging from .70 to .88: interacts comfortably with peers (.70); interacts comfortably with staff (.73); communicates accurately and expresses self clearly (.75); controls impulsive, offensive, and/or annoying behavior (.75); keeps all statements appropriate to context (.79); ability to initiate, respond to, and sustain verbal interactions (.80); uses appropriate nonverbal behavior and tone of voice (.83); cooperates as a member of a group (.88).

The Task Skills Scale had correlations ranging from .81 to .93: tolerates frustration (.81); ability to organize task in a logical manner (.86); willingness to engage in doing tasks (.87); rate of performance (.88); attention to detail (.88); ability to follow directions (.90); ability to maintain concentration on task (.90); and physical capacity (.93).

Once inter-rater reliability and internal consistency were established, a pilot study to determine test-retest reliability was conducted.

A total of 12 individuals were observed and interviewed by three raters, and the rating scales were completed. These patients were observed and interviewed on two consecutive Tuesday afternoons, at the same time of day, in the same rehabilitation group, and by the same raters. Demographics and correlations described pertain to 11 patients because one of the patients severely decompensated in the span of 1 week. The age of the patients ranged from 26 to 54; the mean age was 41 years with a standard deviation of 8.9. Nine of the patients were Caucasian (82%), and two of the patients were African American (18%). Ten of the patients were never married (91%), and one patient was widowed (9%). Length of stay varied from less than 1 month to greater than 1 year; the mean was 2.5 months with a standard deviation of 1.7. Test-retest reliability was obtained for the Role Functioning Scale, the Task Skills Scale, and the Interpersonal Skills Scale.

To assess test-retest reliability, bivariate correlations were conducted on every item in every scale (Role Functioning Scale—four items, Task Skills Scale—eight items, Interpersonal Skills Scale—eight items).

The Interpersonal Skills Scale had correlations ranging from .82 to 1.0: interacts comfortably with peers (.82); interacts comfortably with staff (.84); communicates accurately and expresses self clearly (.89); controls impulsive, offensive, and/or annoying behavior (.90); keeps all statements appropriate to context (.85); ability to initiate, respond to, and sustain verbal interactions (1.0); uses appropriate nonverbal behavior and tone of voice (.86); cooperates as a member of a group (.89).

The Task Skills Scale had correlations ranging from .81 to .93: tolerates frustration (.93); ability to organize task in a logical manner (.81); willingness to engage in doing tasks (.87); rate of performance (.82); attention to detail (.87); ability to follow directions (.82); ability to maintain concentration on task (.93); and physical capacity (.93).

CONVERGENT VALIDITY

The purpose of this study was to determine if convergent validity exists between the Task Skills Scale (TSS) and the Occupational Therapy Task Observation Scale (OTTOS), and the Interpersonal Skills Scale (ISS) and the Specific Level of Functioning Assessment Scale (SLOF). This study incorporated a quantitative methodological design. The hypothesis was that convergent validity exists between the TSS and the OTTOS, and the ISS and the SLOF.[56]

Table 13-1

Alpha Coefficients, Inter-rater Reliability, and Test-Retest Reliability: Pilot Study

n = 12

Scale	Alpha Coefficient	Inter-rater Reliability	Test-Retest Reliability
Role Functioning	.98	.84 to .97	.81 to .92
Interpersonal Skills	.99	.70 to .88	.82 to 1.0
Task Skills Scale	.99	.81 to .93	.81 to .93

Sample

There were 30 participants in the study: 50% were male and 50% were female; 50% were Caucasian and 50% were African American. All of the participants were attendees of the day treatment center program and had a diagnosis of a severe and persistent mental illness.

Instruments

- The Task Skills Scale: The OTTOS assesses the task and general behaviors of individuals diagnosed with mental illness. This scale has 10 descriptors of task performance (Part 1) and 5 descriptors of general behaviors (Part 2). Each item is scored on a range of 0 (maximal dysfunction) to 10 (no evidence of dysfunction). Interrater reliability and convergent validity were established. Convergent validity was established with the Comprehensive Occupational Therapy Evaluation Scale (COTE) and the Milwaukee Evaluation of Daily Living Skills.[57]

- The Interpersonal Skills Scale: The SLOF[56] is a behavioral rating instrument developed by the New Jersey Division of Mental Health and Hospitals in order to assist staff at the state hospitals in developing goal-oriented treatment plans. The SLOF consists of 43 behavioral items grouped into six subscales. These areas include physical functioning, personal care skills, interpersonal relationships, social acceptability, activities of community living, and work skills. For the purpose of this study, two of the subscales of the SLOF were used (interpersonal relationships and social acceptability). The SLOF uses a rating of 1 to 5, with 1 being highly atypical and 5 being highly typical.

Several measures of reliability and validity have been established on this assessment tool. Inter-rater reliability, internal consistency, construct validity, and convergent validity were established. Convergent validity was established with the Global Assessment of Functioning Scale.[58]

Results

The Spearman Rho correlation test was used to determine nonparametric correlations between the TSS and the OTTOS. The correlation between the total mean score for the TSS and the total mean score for the OTTOS was statistically significant (r = .709; p = .01). The correlation between the total mean score for the TSS and the total mean score for the Task Behavior subscale of the OTTOS was statistically significant (r = .813; p = .01). The correlation between the total mean score for the TSS and the total mean score for the General Behavior subscale of the OTTOS was statistically significant (r = .370; p = .05).

The Spearman Rho correlation test was used to determine nonparametric correlations between the ISS and the SLOF. The correlation between the total mean score for the ISS and the total mean score for the SLOF was significant (p = .761; p. = .01). The correlation between the total mean score for the Interpersonal Relationships subscale of the SLOF and the total mean score for the ISS was significant (r = .749; p = .01). The correlation between the total mean score for the Social Acceptability subscale of the SLOF and the total mean score for the ISS was significant (r = .44; p = .01).

Administration of the Assessment Tools

GUIDELINES FOR OBSERVATION

Individuals should be observed in an activity that elicits the behavior outlined on the particular scale. Observation should be conducted for one half hour or for the length of time necessary to observe all of the behaviors outlined on the scale. The rater should be as inconspicuous as possible, and the environment should be comfortable for the individual being rated. The rater should observe all behaviors prior to rating the scale.

GUIDELINES FOR SCORING EACH OF THE INSTRUMENTS

Each scale is provided with a 1 to 5 rating scale. A rating of 1 indicates the individual is performing significantly below essential performance standards, and a rating of 5 indicates the individual is performing significantly above essential performance standards. A rating of 3 indicates the individual is meeting essential performance standards. If an individual is doing what is required for adequate performance in the behavior or interaction, a rating of 3 is assigned. If the individual is performing somewhat below standards, a rating of 2 is assigned. If the behavior is significantly below standards, a rating of 1 is assigned. In contrast, if the individual is performing somewhat above standards, a rating of 4 is assigned. If the individual is performing significantly above standards, a rating of 5 is assigned.

Summary

This chapter described the assessment tools used with the Role Development set of guidelines for practice. Role Development was described, including the theoretical base, the function/dysfunction continuums, the behaviors indicative of function/dysfunction, and the postulates to promote positive change. Implementation of Role Development was described. A literature review was provided, including the development of and documented use of Role Development. Two research studies were described. The assessment tools, including the TSS, the ISS, and the Role Scales were described. Research studies establishing reliability and convergent validity of the scales were described. Finally, the methods to administer the scales were outlined. The scales are located in Appendices F through P.

References

1. Kielhofner G. *Model of Human Occupation.* 3rd ed. Baltimore, MD: Lippincott Williams and Wilkins; 2002.
2. Mosey AC. *Psychosocial Components of Occupational Therapy.* New York, NY: Raven Press; 1986.
3. Parsons T. *The Social System.* Glencoe, IL: The Free Press; 1951.
4. Wolfensberger W. A brief overview of social role valorization. *Mental Retard.* 2000;38:105-123.
5. Liberman RP, Wallace CJ, Blackwell G, Eckman TA, Vaccaro JV, Kuehnel TG. Innovations in skills training for people with serious mental illness: the UCLA social and independent living skills modules. *Innovations & Research.* 1993;2(2):46-59.
6. Anthony WA. Recovery from mental illness: the guiding vision of the mental health system in the 1990's. *Innovations & Research.* 1993;2(3):17-24.
7. American Psychiatric Association. *Diagnostic and Statistical Manual of Mental Disorders IV-R.* 4th ed. Washington, DC: Author; 2000.
8. Anzai N, Yoneda S, Kumagai N. Training persons with schizophrenia in illness self- management: a randomized controlled trial in Japan. *Psychiatr Serv.* 2002;53:545-547.
9. Mann NA, Tandon R, Butler J, Boyd M, Eisner WH, Lewis M. Psychosocial rehabilitation in schizophrenia: beginnings in acute hospitalization. *Arch Psychiatr Nurs.* 1993;7:154-162.
10. Torres A, Mendez LP, Merino H. Improving social functioning in schizophrenia by playing the train game. *Psychiatr Serv.* 2002;53:799-801.
11. Lehman AF, Steinwachs DM. At issue: translating research into practice: the Schizophrenia Patient Outcomes Research Team (PORT) treatment recommendations. *Schizophr Bull.* 1998;24(1):1-10.
12. Roy-Byrne PP, Sherbourne CD, Craske MG. Moving treatment research from clinical trials to the real world. *Psychiatr Serv.* 2003;54:327-332.
13. Mosey AC. *Applied Scientific Inquiry in the Health Professions: An Epistemological Orientation.* 2nd ed. Bethesda, MD: American Occupational Therapy Association; 1996.
14. Schindler VP. A role development intervention for persons with schizophrenia. *Psychiatr Serv.* 2004;55(1):88-89.
15. Kielhofner G. *A Model of Human Occupation.* Baltimore, MD: Williams and Wilkins; 1985.
16. Bandura A. *Social Learning Theory.* Englewood Cliffs, NJ: Prentice-Hall; 1977.
17. Kielhofner G. *A Model of Human Occupation.* 2nd ed. Baltimore, MD: Williams and Wilkins; 1995.
18. Durkheim E. *The Rules of Sociological Method.* Chicago, IL: The University of Chicago Press; 1938.
19. Mead GH. *On Social Psychology.* Chicago, IL: The University of Chicago Press; 1964.
20. Kipper DA. The dynamics of role satisfaction: a theoretical model. *J Group Psychother Psychodrama Sociometry.* 1991;44(2):71-86.
21. Sarbin TR. Role theory. In: Lindzey G, ed. *Handbook of Social Psychology.* Cambridge, MA: Addison-Wesley; 1954:223-258.
22. Black MM. The occupational career. *Am J Occup Ther.* 1976;30:225-228.
23. Versluys HP. The remediation of role disorders through focused group work. *Am J Occup Ther.* 1980;34:609-614.
24. Pollock N, McColl M. Assessment in client-centred occupational therapy. In: Law M, ed. *Client-Centered Occupational Therapy.* Thorofare, NJ: SLACK Incorporated; 1998:89-105.
25. Parsons T. Illness and the role of the physician: a sociological perspective. *Am J Orthopsychiatr.* 1951;21:452-460.
26. Matsutsuyu J. Occupational behavior—a perspective on work and play. *Am J Occup Ther.* 1971;25:291-294.
27. Thoits PA. Multiple identities and psychological well being: a reformulation and test of the social isolation hypothesis. *Am Soc Rev.* 1983:48;174-187.

28. Pearlin LI. Role strains and personal stress. In: Kaplan HB, ed. *Psychosocial Stress: Trends in Theory and Research.* New York, NY: Academic Press; 1983:3-33.
29. Shannon PD. Work-play theory and the occupational therapy process. *Am J Occup Ther.* 1972;26:169-172.
30. Wessen AF. The apparatus of rehabilitation: an organizational analysis. In: Sussman MB, ed. Sociol and Rehab. Washington, DC: American Sociological Association and the Vocational Rehabilitation Administration, US Department of Health, Education and Welfare; 1965:148-179.
31. Dickerson A, Oakley F. Comparing the roles of community-living persons and patient populations. *Am J Occup Ther.* 1995;49:221-228.
32. Gove W, Lubach JE. An intensive treatment program for psychiatric inpatients: a description and evaluation. *J Health Soc Behav.* 1968;9(4):225-236.
33. Heard C. Occupational role acquisition: a perspective on the chronically disabled. *Am J Occup Ther.* 1976;31:243-247.
34. Karmel M. The internalization of social roles in institutionalized chronic mental patients. *J Health Soc Behav.* 1970;11(9):231-235.
35. Susser MW, Stein Z, Mountey GH, Freeman, HL. Chronic disability following mental illness in an English city. Part I: total prevalence in and out of mental hospital. *Soc Psych.* 1970;5:64-76.
36. Fidler GS. The task-oriented group as a context for treatment. *Am J Occup Ther.* 1969;32:305-310.
37. Jodrell RD, Sanson-Fisher R. Basic concepts of behavior therapy: an experiment involving disturbed adolescent girls. *Am J Occup Ther.* 1975;29:620-624.
38. Mosey AC. *Activities Therapy.* New York, NY: Raven Press; 1973.
39. Smith AR, Tempone VJ. Psychiatric occupational therapy within a learning theory context. *Am J Occup Ther.* 1968;22:415-425.
40. Wanderer ZW. Therapy as learning: behavior therapy. *Am J Occup Ther.* 1974;28:207-208.
41. Rogers ES, Sciarappa K, Anthony WA. Development and evaluation of situational assessment instruments and procedures for persons with psychiatric disabilities. *Vocational Evaluation and Work Adjustment Bulletin.* 1991;Summer:61-67.
42. Schindler VP. Occupational therapy in forensic psychiatry: role development and schizophrenia. *Occup Ther Ment Health.* 2004;20:3-4.
43. Merton RK. *Social Theory and Social Structure.* Chicago, IL: The Free Press of Glencoe; 1957.
44. Landy RJ. The dramatic basis of role theory. *Arts in Psychother.* 1991;18:29-41.
45. Blumer H. *Symbolic Interactionism: Perspective and Method.* Englewood Cliffs, NJ: Prentice-Hall; 1969.
46. DeMarrias KD, LeCompte MD. *The Way Schools Work.* 2nd ed. White Plains, NY: Longman; 1995:34-38.
47. Stephan CW, Stephan WG. *Two Social Psychologies.* 2nd ed. Belmont, CA: Wadsworth Publishing; 1990.
48. Schindler V. Role development: an evidenced-based intervention for individuals diagnosed with schizophrenia. *Psychiatr Rehab J.* 2005;28(4):391-394.
49. Schindler VP, Baldwin SA. Role Development: application to community based clients. *Israeli J Occup Ther.* 2005;14(1):E3-E8.
50. Goodman SH, Sewell DR, Cooley EL, Leavitt N. Assessing levels of adaptive functioning: the role functioning scale. *Comm Ment Health J.* 1993;29:119-131.
51. Oakley F. *The Role Checklist.* Bethesda, MD: US Department of Health and Human Services–National Institutes of Health; 1981.
52. Clark F, Azen SP, Zemke R, Jackson J, Carlson M, Mandel D, et al. Occupational therapy for independent-living older adults. *J Am Med Assoc.* 1997; 278:1321-1326.
53. Campbell DT, Stanley JC. *Experimental and Quasi-experimental Designs for Research.* Chicago, IL: Rand McNally College Publishing; 1963.
54. Portnoy LG, Watkins MP. *Foundations of Clinical Research: Applications to Practice.* 2nd ed. Upper Saddle River, NJ: Prentice-Hall; 2000.
55. Schindler V. Developing roles and skills in community-based adults with severe and persistent mental illness. *Occupational Therapy in Mental Health*: In press.
56. Goldman D, Rodriguez C, Saunders D, Shiman A, Solomon A. *Convergent validity between the Interpersonal Skills Scale and the Specific Level of Functioning Scale (SLOF) and the Task Skills Scale and the Occupational Therapy Tasks Observation Scale (OTTOS)* [Unpublished masters thesis]. Pomona, NJ: Richard Stockton College of New Jersey.
57. Margolis RL, Harrison SA, Robinson HJ, Jayaram G. Occupational Therapy Task Observation Scale (OTTOS): a rapid method for rating task group psychiatric patients. *Am J Occup Ther.* 1996;50(5):380-385.
58. Schneider LC, Struening EL. SLOF: a behavioral rating scale for assessing the mentally ill. *Soc Work Research Abs.* 1983;19:9-21.

14

THE BAY AREA FUNCTIONAL PERFORMANCE EVALUATION

James P. Klyczek, PhD, OTR
Elizabeth Stanton, PhD, OTR/L

"The occupational therapist's skilled observation, use of specific assessments, and interpretation of results leads to a clear delineation of problems and probable causes." American Occupational Therapy Association. Occupational therapy practice framework: domain and process. Am J Occup Ther. 2002;56:609-639.

Introduction

The purpose of this chapter is to describe the historical development of the original and revised Bay Area Functional Performance Evaluation (BaFPE); the administration and scoring of the two BaFPE components—the Task Oriented Assessment (TOA) and the Social Interaction Scale (SIS); and standardization of the BaFPE, including numerous studies examining the validity and reliability of the TOA and SIS. Samples on which current norms have been developed for the TOA are described, as well as research testing the influence of various factors, such as age, education, gender, and culture, on the development of norms. Clinical application of the BaFPE to psychiatric inpatients, patients with eating disorders, and skilled nursing residents is reviewed, and a description of how the TOA and SIS have been used to evaluate patient progress in research studies is provided. Finally, suggestions for further research on the BaFPE are provided with an invitation to therapists to take part in the continued development of this standardized occupational therapy functional performance evaluation.

Theoretical Basis

While the theoretical foundation of the BaFPE shares some features characteristic of psychoanalytic, developmental, and biopsychosocial models, Bloomer and Williams[1] based the BaFPE primarily on the acquisitional,[2] occupational behavior, adaptational, and functional restoration frames of reference. The underlying principles of the BaFPE, "like those of the acquisitional frame of reference, imply that functional performance can be measured...[and that patients] may be helped to become more functional through exposure to situations in which more adaptive behavior can essentially be practiced."[1]

The necessity of maintaining a balance among the daily life tasks of work, play, rest, and sleep is emphasized in the occupational behavior frame of reference, as is the focus on occupational role and acquisition of skills and habits necessary to facilitate the development and performance of occupational behavior.[3,4] Occupational behavior is the result of dynamic interactions between persons and the environments in which they function.[5]

Bloomer and Williams viewed adaptation as critical to an individual's overall functional performance, and adaptation was an important consideration in developing the BaFPE.[1] They viewed dysfunction as "the lack or loss of skill acquisition...[and that] functional behavior [should] be considered a prerequisite to the acquisition of occupational behavior."[1] In arguing for a renewed focus on occupational performance, Fisher stated, "our uniqueness has been in the use of occupation as a curative or restorative force as well as in the view that enhanced occupational performance is the desired goal of therapy."[6]

The BaFPE is also viewed by its developers as consistent with the Model of Human Occupation (MOHO) developed by Kielhofner and others.[6-12] The model is used to describe how occupational behavior is motivated, organized, and performed in various contexts. While previous versions of the MOHO addressed performance as drawing on functional capacities such as communication/interaction skills, process skills, and perceptual-motor skills, the most current conceptualization recognizes the importance of the underlying components of performance, but emphasizes the subjective experience of the lived body.[12]

The *Occupational Therapy Practice Framework* offers concepts consistent with those on which the BaFPE is based, particularly the domains related to performance skills and contexts.[13] Underlying the ability to perform occupational behavior are motor skills (eg, mobility, coordination, and strength); process skills such as attending to and organizing various aspects of a task; and communication/interaction skills, which entail verbal and nonverbal methods of exchanging information and relating to others in the context of occupation. According to the *Framework*, the social context represents one of seven that influence patient performance.

Bloomer and Williams stated that there are two skills necessary for general function in the environment—the ability to engage in goal-directed and task-oriented activities with objects in the environment, and the ability to interact with other people in the environment in a socially acceptable way.[14] Their goal was to develop a valid and reliable tool that would appropriately assess general components of functioning needed to perform activities of daily living (ADL).[15]

HISTORICAL DEVELOPMENT

The BaFPE was developed by Judith Bloomer and Susan Williams in 1977 and 1978 at Langley Porter Psychiatric Institute at the University of California Medical Center in San Francisco to meet the need for a standardized assessment of functional performance.[16] Williams and Bloomer defined functioning as "employing useful activity to achieve an active mode of adaptation to the environment."[16] This process or activity would include the ability to satisfy physiological and psychological needs through interaction with both people and objects in the environment. The term *functional* "...pertains to this definition of functioning, and is a descriptive adjective connoting purposeful activity and active adaptation to the environment."[15]

Williams and Bloomer also stated that activity can be classified into the functional areas of self-care, work, and leisure, and that functional skill is the foundation of everyday performance that integrates the motoric, social, cognitive, psychological, and sensory-integrative performance components. They use the term *functional* to pertain to "an individual who is able to perform, synthesizing these components."[15]

The present BaFPE is composed of the TOA and SIS.[15] The TOA assesses one's ability to act on the environment in goal-directed ways and contains five tasks used to provide information about the patient's cognitive, performance, and affective areas of functioning. The SIS assesses social behaviors observed in five different settings.

Originally conceptualized as a single evaluation, with the TOA and SIS as two subtests from which an overall BaFPE score was derived, the BaFPE was later revised with the TOA and SIS used together or separately, but with no overall BaFPE score. The authors cautioned that information from either the TOA or SIS alone is not a measure of functional performance. *Functional performance*, as defined by the test authors, requires evaluation of the patient's ability to interact with both objects and people in the environment.

The BaFPE was revised based on feedback from clinicians and the results of data analysis, and was published in a second edition in 1987.[15,17] The purposes of revision were to reduce ambiguity of some of the functional parameters, clarify administration instructions, and provide additional guidance in score interpretation and reporting. According to Williams and Bloomer,[15] the main revisions were as follows:

1. Separate use and scoring of the TOA and SIS.

2. The TOA Bank Deposit Slip task was changed to the Money and Marketing task, because the former task may have been biased against patients without checking accounts. The revised task is more common and retains the processes of the former task.

3. The TOA House Floor Plan task was changed to the Home Drawing task, because it was difficult to score and may have been subject to local house design. A more common list of room names and more carefully defined residence are provided in the revised task.

4. One of the original 10 TOA parameters was dropped (decision making), three were revised (paraphrase, thought disorder, task completion), and three new parameters were defined (errors, efficiency, general affective impression), resulting in 12 functional parameters.

5. The functional parameters were newly organized into cognitive, performance, and affective components to facilitate scoring and interpretation of results.

6. Timing was formalized as part of the performance component.

7. The Qualitative Signs and Referral Indicators section was added to the TOA rating sheets to screen for organicity.

8. Rather than using one single overall rating for the SIS, five settings are now specified for evaluating social behavior.

9. A Self-Report of Social Interaction, similar to the SIS, was developed for patients as a means for assessing perceptions and insights related to their own social functioning.

10. The TOA and SIS rating sheet formats were revised, and summary score sheets were developed to facilitate reporting results.

Since publication of the second edition of the BaFPE, numerous studies have been conducted to examine the validity and reliability of the TOA, and norms on psychiatric inpatients and patients with eating disorders have been developed.

Administration and Scoring

TOA

Description

The TOA is designed to gather information about an individual's functioning in a one-to-one setting through five task-oriented activities. The TOA was originally developed for use in inpatient or outpatient psychiatric settings, but, as discussed later, has been used with other populations and is appropriate in any situation in which information about an individual's task-oriented functioning is desired.

TOA Tasks

The TOA is composed of five tasks that include a range of difficulty and structure:

1. *Sorting Shells*: 10 categories of shells are sorted by size, shape, and color.

2. *Money and Marketing*: The amount of money needed to purchase specific items is calculated, the ability to purchase the items with available money and a mock check is determined, and the amount of change from the transaction is calculated.

3. *Home Drawing*: A floor plan for a home is drawn, with the patient following specific instructions about what should be included.

4. *Block Design*: A block design is duplicated from memory or with the use of a cue card if needed.

5. *Kinetic Person Drawing*: A person doing something is drawn.

The TOA begins with a preassessment interview to elicit information about the patient's current or past functioning, and to develop rapport and explain what the patient will be doing during the assessment. The patient is tested at a table or desk in a room with as few distractions as possible. Testing materials for the five tasks are prepared by the examiner prior to the test.

Scoring the Functional Parameters

The individual is rated on 12 functional parameters during each task. Ratings range from (1) markedly dysfunctional or inappropriate to (4) almost always functional or appropriate. Behavioral guidelines are provided on rating sheets for evaluating the 12 parameters for each task. The parameters are organized into three components:

1. Cognitive Component

   - Memory for written and oral instructions
   - Organization of time and materials
   - Attention span
   - Evidence of thought disorder
   - Ability to abstract

2. Performance Component
   •   Task completion
   •   Errors
   •   Efficiency
3. Affective Component
   •   Motivation and compliance
   •   Frustration tolerance
   •   Self-confidence
   •   General affective and behavioral impression

At the beginning of each task, the therapist reads instructions to the patient, which the patient is asked to restate. If the patient cannot restate the general idea of the task after one repetition of instructions, the task is not completed. The patient's performance is scored during the task, using the rating sheet provided for each task. A stopwatch is used to time each task, and the patient is asked to stop if the maximum allowable time has been used. Some areas on the task rating sheets may be scored after the task has been completed, but, with experience, the therapist should be able to complete all ratings during testing.

Qualitative Signs and Referral Indicators

Following completion of each task, the therapist completes the Qualitative Signs and Referral Indicators (QSRI) section of the rating forms by checking off any of the observations noted during testing. The QSRI contains general and task-specific observations that indicate possible organic factors, suggesting the need for referral for further evaluation.

Summary Score Sheet

Scores on the five task rating sheets are then transferred to the TOA Summary Score Sheet, and the scores are then summed up to derive parameter, component, task, and total TOA scores. Check marks recorded on the QSRI section of the task rating sheets are summed up and transferred to the TOA Summary Score Sheet. Although the QSRI scoring is not included in the formal TOA score, if more than 20 of the 141 symptoms are checked, or if any starred QSRI items are checked, consultation or further testing is considered.

Interpretation

TOA scores may be interpreted in three ways. They may be interpreted first by examination of parameter and component scores, which provide information about the patient's strengths and needs in various area of functioning. For example, a patient may score well in the performance areas, but poorly in the affective areas. The second way is by examination of task scores. Because the tasks range in difficulty and structure, performance trends may become evident, eg, when the patient performs better in more structured tasks. The third way of interpreting TOA scores is by comparison to norms, which allows the therapist to compare the patient's performance to an appropriate reference group. This avenue of interpretation will become more useful when more extensive norms are developed for the TOA.

SOCIAL INTERACTION SCALE

Description

The SIS is used to assess seven categories of verbal and nonverbal social interaction behaviors considered important to overall functioning. It is intended to be completed within 24 hours of the TOA to obtain a valid assessment of the two types of functioning. Behavior is assessed in five social setting situations:

1. *One-to-One Interview*: During an interview or administration of the TOA.

2. *Mealtime*: A group setting in which group interaction must be possible, such as several individuals eating together at the same table.

3. *Unstructured Group Situation*: A group setting in which there is no expectation regarding the patient's performance (such as a common-living or group-gathering area) and no stimuli (such as a TV being played) that precludes the opportunity for social interaction.

4. *Structured Activity Group*: A planned group activity or recreational game setting in which social interaction is expected by the leader.

5. *Structured Oral Group*: Any group that focuses on discussion among members, ranging from oral group therapy to any type of discussion group, such as a community meeting or current events group. Williams and Bloomer cite research indicating that multiple observations across situations are necessary for accurate assessment of social skills.[18-22] They suggest that the SIS is best completed with frequent observations in multiple situations by the therapist, as well as other staff working with the patient.[15]

Scoring the Functional Parameters

An individual is rated on a 5-point scale on seven functional parameters across five social situations. Behavioral guidelines for the ratings are provided on the rating forms. Ratings range from 1 to 5, with 1 indicating that assessment was not possible due to the degree of dysfunction. The ratings of 2 through 5 are used to reflect a continuum of performance from (2) markedly dysfunctional or inappropriate to (5) almost always functional or appropriate.

The seven parameters of social interaction rated on the SIS scoring form include:

1. *Verbal Communication*: Quantity and quality of verbal interaction

2. *Psychomotor Behavior*: Motor effect of psychological processes, reflected in hypo- or hyperactivity

3. *Socially Appropriate Behavior*: Quality of behavior in relation to cultural and social expectations

4. *Response to Authority Figures*: Quality of interaction with and response to people who influence power or control over the individual

5. *Independence/Dependence*: Appropriateness of self-reliance and self-direction

6. *Ability to Work With Others*: Quantity and quality of peer interactions in work- or task-oriented settings

7. *Participation in Groups or Program Activities*: Ability to take part in activities that require social interaction

Not all seven parameters are scored in each situation. The SIS is completed through direct observation by the examiner, although corroboration by other team members is desirable. A minimum of 10 minutes of observation in each social setting is recommended, with the SIS completed within a 1- to 2-day period.

SIS Scoring Sheet

Parameter scores are derived by summing up the ratings for each situation and dividing this number by the number of rated observations. For example, scores of 4, 2, 2, 3, and 2 for the verbal communication parameter across the five situations yield a parameter score of 13/5 or 2.6. The situation scores are derived by summing up all parameter scores for that situation. The total SIS score is derived by totaling the five situation scores. For interpretation of situation scores, the sum of the parameter scores for a situation is divided by the number of parameters scored.

Interpretation

Methods for interpreting SIS scores are similar to those of the TOA. Parameter and situation scores may be examined to identify a patient's strengths and needs in relation to the seven categories of verbal and nonverbal interaction, and in relation to structured versus unstructured and group versus one-to-one situations. SIS normative data on two reference groups are provided in the BaFPE manual,[15] but the small number of subjects (n = 20, n = 35) makes comparison of patient scores difficult. As with the TOA, this avenue of interpretation will become more useful when more extensive norms are developed.

Standardization

Test standardization is a long and complex process that involves developing a consistent protocol for administration and scoring, testing of the tools' validity and reliability, and definition of norms. The administration and scoring of the BaFPE are clearly described in the manual provided with the test kit. The focus of this section is to describe a number of studies that have been conducted to examine the validity and reliability of the original and revised BaFPE. First, a brief overview defining the various types of validity and reliability testing conducted on the TOA and SIS is provided.

Validity and Reliability

Validity of a tool, in a general sense, refers to whether the tool is measuring what it was intended to measure. *Concurrent validity* refers to the correlation between scores on the tool under study and scores for the same individual on another tool, with established or accepted validity measuring the same construct concurrently. The correlation should be high enough to indicate that the new tool is valid, but not so high as to suggest that the new tool is identical to the existing tool. New tools may be developed because they are less expensive, easier or quicker to administer and score, and more reliable than existing tools.[23] *Discriminant validity* is a measure of the ability of a tool to differentiate between various groups. For example, can a functional assessment distinguish differences in ability between functionally disabled individuals and nonimpaired individuals? Is the tool useful for determining which individuals are in need of intervention? *Predictive validity* is the extent to which the scores on one measure successfully predict a particular outcome. For example, how well do lower scores on a discharge ADL evaluation relate to the need for increased caregiver support postdischarge? *Construct validity* is a measure of whether a tool tests the construct for which it was intended, such as functional performance in the case of the BaFPE.

The *reliability* of a tool refers to whether the measurements obtained are consistent and predictable. *Inter-rater reliability*, or inter-rater agreement, refers to the consistency of measurements obtained by different raters.[24] *Intra-rater reliability*, or test-retest reliability, refers to the consistency of measurements by the same rater.[23] Refer to Chapter 23 for a thorough review of validity and reliability.

Validity on the Original Version of the TOA

CONCURRENT

Bloomer and Williams[1] conducted a concurrent validity study on the original TOA with the Functional Life Scale (FLS)[25] and the Global Assessment Scale (GAS).[26] Correlations between the TOA and the FLS and GAS were .43 and .45, respectively. Correlations between the composite BaFPE (TOA and SIS) and the FLS and GAS were .52 and .57 at P < .001, respectively. Bortone also found a positive, but not statistically significant, correlation between the BaFPE and GAS scores of 23 schizophrenic and borderline patients.[27]

Cheeseman[28] tested 20 patients diagnosed with brain vascular disease with the TOA, FLS, and Jebsen Hand Function Test.[29] The correlation between the composite BaFPE and the FLS was .62, which was consistent with Bloomer and Williams' original field study results (r = .52).[1] Cheeseman reported a statistically significant correlation (P < .0005) between BaFPE scores and the Jebsen for the nonaffected hand that suggested that "adequate motor skills are necessary to successfully perform tasks on the TOA."[17]

Kaufman[30] studied the concurrent validity of the TOA by comparing TOA scores of 16 psychiatric inpatients with their scores on the Kohlman Evaluation of Living Skills (KELS)[31] and reported that the composite BaFPE and TOA correlations to both were .84 at P < .001. The highest correlation between the KELS and TOA tasks was with the House Floor Plan task with r = .82.

DISCRIMINANT

Several studies lend support to the discriminant validity of the original TOA. In initial field testing, it was found that patients exhibiting higher degrees of psychotic behavior scored lower on the BaFPE.[1] Bortone found that patients diagnosed with borderline personality disorder scored higher on the BaFPE than patients with schizophrenic disorders.[27] Also, patients with borderline personality disorder scored lower on the TOA than the SIS, but the reverse was true for patients with schizophrenia.

Wener-Altman, Wolfe, and Staley examined the use of the BaFPE with adolescents.[32] They tested 19 male and 29 female psychiatric inpatients ranging in age from 13 to 17 years with a mean of 15.45 years. Primary diagnoses of subjects were conduct disorders (48%), adjustment disorders (21%), schizophrenia or affective disorders (18%), and character disorders (13%). They found a significant correlation between diagnosis and TOA, but those with more severe impairments, such as schizophrenia, scored less well.

Other researchers report different findings. Olson and Jamal completed the most extensive published study on the original BaFPE with 211 inpatients.[33] They found no statistically significant differences in TOA or composite BaFPE scores by diagnosis among patients diagnosed with schizophrenia, depression, or manic depression.

Brockett examined the discriminant validity of the BaFPE and reported significant differences in scores of 50 patients tested at a Canadian general hospital from scores of patients tested in San Francisco.[34] They suggested that the differences might have been due to cultural differences and, therefore, questioned the validity of the BaFPE.

PREDICTIVE

The relationship between the TOA, the Nurse's Observation Scale for Inpatient Evaluation (NOSIE-30),[35] and an adaptation of the Comprehensive Evaluation of Basic Living Skills (CEBLS)[36] was studied by Accardi.[37] His sample of 7 males and 12 females, primarily White, ranged in age from 21 to 72, with a mean age of 40.5 years. Correlations between the TOA and NOSIE-30 were .66 (P < .001); and .63 (P < .005) between the TOA and the adapted CEBLS. Houston, Williams, Bloomer, and Mann stated that "Accardi's findings support the use of the BaFPE as a predictor of functional performance, as determined by two other functional assessments given concurrently."[17]

In addition to their research on the BaFPE discriminant validity, Olson and Jamal reported that TOA scores correlated significantly with aftercare residential placement.[33] Also, BaFPE-based recommendations regarding legal conservatorship correlated significantly with actual treatment-team decisions regarding conservatorship.

CONSTRUCT

Bloomer and Williams established the initial construct validity of the BaFPE via their findings that patients' BaFPE discharge scores were significantly higher than admission scores. They also found high correlations between the TOA tasks and parameters, with most in the .70 to .89 range.[1] Wener-Altman et al reported positive correlations between the TOA parameters and total TOA score ranging from .25 to .88.[32] Olson and Jamal also found high internal correlations for the TOA, SIS, and composite BaFPE.[33] Finally, Mason found that most of the TOA parameters did not correlate significantly with the SIS parameters, which suggests that the TOA and SIS are measuring different aspects of functional performance.[38]

Francis and Cermak's study with 20 patients with schizophrenia and 20 nondiagnosed subjects supported the validity of the Sorting Shells and House Floor Plan tasks on the original TOA.[39] They randomly divided subjects into original and modified task groups, each composed of 10 diagnosed and 10 nondiagnosed subjects. Subjects in the original group performed the original tasks, while subjects in the modified task group used buttons instead of shells for the sorting task and were given a simplified 5-room square house instead of the 10-room L-shaped house in the original TOA. It was hypothesized that subjects would perform better on the modified tasks because they were more relevant and familiar than the existing tasks. Diagnosed subjects performed more poorly than nondiagnosed subjects on both tasks as expected, but "the use of a different medium did not differentially affect the performance of the patients with schizophrenia,"[39] thus lending support to the validity of the existing tasks.

Validity on the Revised Version of the TOA

CONCURRENT

The concurrent validity of the TOA has been tested with the revised Allen Cognitive Levels Test (ACL), the Global Assessment Scale (GAS), three subtests of the Wechsler

Adult Intelligence Scale (WAIS), Part 1 of the American Association on Mental Deficiency Adaptive Behavior Scale (AAMD-ABS), and the Scorable Self-Care Evaluation (SSCE).

Newman[40] studied the relationship between TOA scores and cognitive level, as assessed with the revised ACL Test[41] with 21 inpatients. All TOA tasks, except sorting shells, correlated significantly with the ACL at P <.05. Newman also reported that the TOA and ACL correlated significantly with the GAS.

Testing the hypothesis that intelligence influences functional performance, Thibeault and Blackmer[42] examined the relationship between scores on the TOA and three subtests of the WAIS[43] with 26 male and 34 female subjects ranging in age from 21 to 75 years. Subjects were diagnosed with either schizophrenia (n = 31) or depression (n = 29). Correlations between the total TOA score and the Digit Symbol, Block Design, and Picture Completion subtests were .60, .67, and .58 (P < .05), respectively. The authors stated that these positive correlations are evidence of the TOA validity, "but the correlations are not so high as to suggest that the two tests assess the same dimensions of human functioning."[42]

Klyczek and Mann[44] tested the concurrent validity of the TOA with Part I of the AAMD-ABS.[45,46] The sample included 67 psychiatric inpatients with a mean age of 30.8 years, 73% of whom were male. The correlation between the TOA and the total ABS Part I score was .32 at P < .05. Correlations ranged from -.19 between the eating subdomain of the ABS and the Kinetic Person Drawing (KPD) task of the TOA, to .58 between the socialization domain of the ABS and the Sorting Shells task of the TOA. The authors suggested that the ABS' fair reliability may have resulted in the low correlation between the two tests.

Mercer Castilla and Klyczek[47] examined the relationship between parameter, component, and total task scores on the KPD task of the TOA and the personal care, housekeeping chores, work and leisure, and financial management subscales of the SSCE[48] to determine the extent to which scores on a projective drawing task (TOA-KPD) correlate with measures of functional performance (SSCE). Correlations between the tests ranged from .10 to -.42 (inverse scoring) and were not statistically significant. The correlation between the total TOA and total SSCE scores was -.28 and was not statistically significant. The authors concluded that the KPD is not a valid measure of functional performance when used alone.

DISCRIMINANT

The discriminant validity of the TOA has been tested with a number of samples, including psychiatric inpatients versus outpatients, patients with eating disorders versus nondiagnosed patients, adult psychiatric patients versus nondiagnosed adults, and elderly psychiatric patients versus nondiagnosed elderly.

Curtin and Klyczek published the first study examining differences in TOA scores for inpatient and outpatient samples.[49] Subjects included 31 psychiatric outpatients in an adult day-training program and 29 psychiatric inpatients matched by age and years of education. Outpatient subjects had an average age of 58.6 years and 9.5 years of education. Inpatient subjects had an average age of 53.6 years and 10.8 years of education. The majority of subjects were White females in both groups. The inpatient group scored significantly higher on the Sorting Shells task and on all cognitive and performance parameters, except attention span and evidence of thought disorder. The inpatient group scored significantly lower on all affective component parameters, except self-confidence. The total TOA score was 6.8 points higher for the inpatient group, but this difference was not statistically significant.

The authors noted that the inpatient group had almost twice as many subjects with a diagnosis of mood disorder than with schizophrenia, while the outpatient group had almost four times as many subjects with a diagnosis of schizophrenia than mood disorder. Longer psychiatric histories were also noted for subjects in the outpatient sample. The authors concluded that differences between inpatient and outpatient TOA scores do exist, but suggest that these differences may be due to diagnosis and chronicity.

Konieczny reported very good discriminant validity of the TOA with 63 patients diagnosed with eating disorders and a sample of 64 nondiagnosed subjects.[50] The samples were matched on age, race, gender, occupation, education in years, educational degree, and marital status. The age range of subjects was 14 to 58 years in the diagnosed group, and 14 to 54 years in the nondiagnosed group. The mean age was 24.4 years in both groups. There were no significant differences between groups on any of the matching variables. Diagnosed subjects scored significantly lower on the total TOA score, all five task scores, all three component scores, and all parameter scores, except evidence of thought disorder. The largest differences were observed in the affective component and parameters, and the smallest differences were observed in the performance component and parameters.

Lissner examined the discriminant validity of the TOA with 60 individuals with a diagnosis of mental illness and 60 nondiagnosed subjects.[51] The samples were matched on gender, age, ethnicity, education level, years of education, and marital status. Each sample included 18 male and 42 female subjects. Subjects' ages ranged from 19 to 59 (M = 27.7) in the diagnosed sample and from 19 to 66 (M = 27.4) in the nondiagnosed sample.

Based on discriminant analysis, Lissner concluded that 18 of the 21 ratings analyzed (12 parameter, 3 component, 5 task, total) have sufficient discriminant validity. Three parameters, including memory for written/oral instructions, evidence of thought disorder, and motivation and compliance, do not possess discriminant validity.

Stoffel matched 20 nondiagnosed subjects over 60 years old with 20 subjects with a DSM-III-R diagnosis receiving treatment in an adult psychiatric day treatment program.[52] Subjects in the diagnosed sample had diagnoses of schizophrenia (55%), mood disorder (30%), psychoactive substance-use disorder, organic mental disorder, or other psychotic disorders (15%). Subjects' ages ranged from 61 to 85, with a mean of 71.65 years in the diagnosed sample and 72.75 years in the nondiagnosed sample. There were no significant differences between samples on age, gender, ethnicity, or years of education. The results showed that the diagnosed subjects scored lower on all TOA ratings, except the motivation/compliance parameter. Differences between the groups were statistically significant for the total TOA score and cognitive and performance component scores, as well as for 6 of the 12 parameter scores. Stoffel stated that her findings indicate that discriminant validity does exist on the TOA for the cognitive component, performance component, and total TOA scores, but that further research, with a larger sample, is necessary to validate the lack of difference between the samples on the affective component score.

The TOA as the Standard

Interestingly and indicative of growing support for the validity of the TOA, two studies have been conducted testing the concurrent validity of other tools with the TOA.

Tardif[53] examined the concurrent validity of the Functional Needs Assessment (FNA)[54] with the TOA with 10 male and 17 female patients ranging in age from 33 to 85 years, with a mean age of 58.9 years. Subjects were diagnosed with schizophrenia (63%), organic mental disorders (22%), or mood disorders (15%). Tardif found that the Sorting Shells and Home Drawing tasks significantly correlated with four of the six clinical program scores on the FNA. The TOA cognitive component scores significantly correlated with all six FNA clinical program scores, and the total TOA and total FNA scores correlated with r = .54 at P < .01.

As a "show-me" assessment, the FNA is used to evaluate actual functional performance. The premise that the TOA is useful for evaluating the functional parameters underlying component skills was supported by the largest correlation (r = .59, P < .001), which was found between the total TOA score and the preplacement clinical program of the FNA, composed of the following skills: care of living quarters, laundry skills, social etiquette, planning and decision making, and leisure skills.

Rogers[55] failed to establish the concurrent validity of the Milwaukee Evaluation of Daily Living Skills (MEDLS)[56] with the TOA with seven male and eight female psychiatric outpatients. Ages of subjects ranged from 17 to 66, with a mean age of 40. The majority of correlations were low and nonsignificant. Scores on only 4 of the 20 MEDLS subtests correlated significantly with the total TOA. These included use of transportation (r = .80), medication management (r = .70), use of money (r = .61), and brushing teeth (r = .50), all at P < .05. Rogers stated that her findings are limited by a small, nonrandomly selected sample.

Reliability of the TOA

ORIGINAL VERSION

Bloomer and Williams tested the inter-rater reliability of the TOA with 62 diagnosed and 20 nondiagnosed subjects.[1] Correlations for the TOA total and BaFPE total were .99. A field study conducted in 1981 with 51 diagnosed and 50 nondiagnosed subjects showed correlations ranging from .86 to .99 for the total TOA score, and .82 to .97 for the BaFPE total.

REVISED VERSION

Williams and Bloomer reported that the inter-rater reliability of the revised TOA is higher than the original.[15] They evaluated interrater reliability with four pairs of occupational therapists. Each team evaluated 25 patients with a DSM-III diagnosis. Complete data on 91 subjects were evaluated with Pearson's Product-Moment Correlation Coefficients. Approximately 80% of the correlations equaled or exceeded .80. The average correlations for the total TOA and the cognitive, performance, and affective components were .96, .93, .96, and .85, respectively. According to Williams and Bloomer, "correlation coefficients for 10 of the original 16 scales on the TOA improved...three were lower, and three remained about the same. The items added to the revised instrument showed high correlations."[15]

Evaluation of the internal consistency of the revised TOA showed the overall range of correlations to be .29 to .84, with an average of .60. The intercorrelations for the parameters and component areas were higher than for the tasks, but not "high enough to suggest that any item or task should be eliminated from the TOA format."[15]

Conducting further analysis on the TOA data collected on 266 psychiatric patients from which the 1991 standard scores for the TOA were developed,[57] Mann and Huselid reported that the internal reliability of the TOA "is excellent (alpha coefficient = .93),"[58] which indicates high intercorrelation among the items on the test.

It should be noted that little research has been conducted with the SIS in comparison to the numerous studies that have examined the TOA. As will be discussed later in the Further Research section of this chapter, few therapists have reported using the SIS.[59]

Validity on the Original Version of the SIS

CONCURRENT

Bloomer and Williams examined the concurrent validity of the SIS with the FLS and GAS, and reported correlations of .46 and .53, respectively.[1] The correlation between the SIS and the socialization component of the FLS was .42 at $P < .001$. Accardi found that correlations between SIS scores and NOSIE-30 and adapted CEBLS scores ranged from .46 to .69 at $P < .05$.[37] Kaufman reported a correlation of .74 between the SIS and the KELS.[30]

PREDICTIVE

Olson and Jamal found positive correlations between TOA scores and aftercare placement; however, SIS scores did not correlate with those placements.[33] Wener-Altman, Wolfe, and Staley found a significant negative correlation ($r = -.39$, $P < .01$) between length of stay and total SIS score in a study with 48 adolescent psychiatric inpatients.[32]

Reliability of the SIS

ORIGINAL VERSION

The mean inter-rater reliability correlations on the original SIS ranged from .54 to .72 for the seven parameters and was .86 for the total SIS score.[1] Bortone reported moderate to perfect agreement among raters on all SIS parameters in an "inter-rater agreement analysis" of SIS scores for 30 schizophrenic and borderline patients.[27]

REVISED VERSION

According to Williams and Bloomer, the inter-rater reliability for the revised SIS improved substantially from the original version, although the SIS correlations were lower than those for the TOA.[15] The inter-rater reliability on the original SIS ranged from .54 to .72, while the correlations ranged from .56 to .94 ($P < .001$) on the revised SIS. Inter-rater reliability on the five observation situations ranged from .74 to .94 ($P < .001$). Internal reliability of the SIS was also examined. The overall range of correlations was .35 to .87 ($P < .001$).

NORMS

While tests of validity are used to establish that an instrument actually measures what it was intended to measure, and tests of reliability are used to determine the consistency or predictability of scores, norms enable the therapist to compare a particular patient's score with the scores of a larger group of individuals similar to the patient tested. Normed scores are often presented in the form of standard scores. According to Mann, Klyczek, and Fiedler, "results of testing are more easily understood when presented in some form of standard deviation units and, thus, are more appropriate for clinical documentation."[60]

General Psychiatry

Mann et al published the first norms on the revised TOA, using data on 144 psychiatric inpatients.[60] These norms were later expanded to include data on 266 psychiatric patients.[57] The sample was composed of 118 male and 148 female subjects ranging in age from 14 to 70 years old, with a mean age of 30.7 years and a mean of 11.5 years of education. Standard scores were presented for each of the component task summary scores, component summary scores, parameter total scores, total task summary scores, and the total TOA score.

EATING DISORDERS

Stanton, Mann, and Klyczek presented percentile scores for anorexic (n = 37) and bulimic (n = 28) patient samples for TOA component total scores and total TOA scores, as well as mean scores and standard deviations for the three components and their respective parameters.[61] The anorexic sample was composed of 1 male and 36 females ranging in age from 14 to 49 years, with a mean of 22.8 years. The bulimic sample was composed of 28 females ranging in age from 16 to 58 years, with a mean of 27.4 years. The authors provide examples for reporting test results. They stated that their findings are limited in generalization due to a small sample composed of patients from only one private psychiatric hospital, but further stated that the TOA can be used to identify patient problems in cognitive processing and with actual performance.

Factors Affecting Norms

GENERAL

Thibeault and Blackmer's study with 60 psychiatric patients showed no significant differences in TOA scores that were based on type or dosage of medication.[42] However, in evaluating the effect of electroconvulsive therapy (ECT), they found that non-ECT patients (n = 41) scored significantly higher than ECT patients (n = 19) on the memory, organization, and attention span parameters; the cognitive component total; the Block Design Task total; and the total TOA. They also found differences in TOA scores by education, with more highly educated patients scoring significantly higher than less-educated patients.

AGE

Thibeault and Blackmer found that younger adult patients scored significantly higher on the TOA than older patients.[42] In contrast, Wener-Altman et al found that older adolescent patients scored significantly higher on the TOA and SIS than younger adolescent patients.[32] In a study with 30 adolescents receiving psychiatric services at a residential placement center, Peterson found that older adolescents scored higher on the TOA than younger adolescents, but the differences were not statistically significant.[62]

LENGTH OF STAY

Thibeault and Blackmer reported no difference in TOA scores based on number of hospital admissions or total time in a hospital for adult psychiatric patients.[42] However, Wener-Altman et al found a significant negative correlation: $r = -.39$, $P < .01$ between length of stay and total SIS scores for adolescent psychiatric inpatients.[32]

GENDER

Most studies have not identified differences in TOA scores by gender. Crouch tested gender differences on the TOA with 33 male and 33 female psychiatric patients matched on diagnosis, age, years of education, highest educational degree achieved, ethnicity, and marital status.[63] Both male and female groups were composed of 28 White and 5 African American subjects. Males ranged in age from 15 to 68 years, with a mean age of 37.15 years and a mean of 9.88 years of education. Females ranged in age from 15 to 69 years, with a mean age of 37.61 years and a mean of 10.58 years of education. There were no significant differences between the male and female groups on any of the matching variables. Crouch reported no significant differences on any of the TOA parameter, component, task, or total scores between groups. These findings are similar to those found with adult psychiatric patients[42] and with adolescent psychiatric inpatients in which no gender differences were found on the revised TOA, original TOA, or SIS, respectively.[32]

Tornabene used a nondiagnosed sample of 25 male and 25 female subjects to test gender differences on the TOA.[64] The two groups were matched on age, race, years of education, and marital status. There were no significant differences between groups on the matching variables. In contrast to previous research,[32,42,63] Tornabene found significant differences on four parameter and two component scores on the TOA, with females scoring significantly higher than males on the memory for written/oral instructions parameter and the cognitive component total, and males scoring significantly higher than females on the task completion, errors, efficiency parameters, and performance component total. There were no significant differences between groups on the total TOA score. Peterson also found that females scored significantly higher than males ($P = .01$) on the cognitive parameters in a study with adolescents at a residential placement center.[62]

CULTURE

Cultural factors were cited as a possible reason scores on the original BaFPE for 50 patients tested in a Canadian general hospital differed significantly from patients tested in San Francisco.[34] No further research into cultural differences was located in a recent search of the literature.

Clinical Application

Based on results of face-to-face, in-depth interviews with 30 occupational therapists from 4 cities who use the BaFPE, Managh and Cook identified seven primary reasons that occupational therapists use the BaFPE.[59] These reasons include:

1. Implicit departmental policy requires use of the BaFPE.

2. The BaFPE can be administered and scored more quickly than alternate assessments.

3. The BaFPE is used as a screening, either to determine if occupational therapy intervention is necessary for a patient or to place a patient in a particular occupational therapy group.

4. The BaFPE is used in response to the preference of multidisciplinary treatment teams for standardized rather than nonstandardized assessments.

5. The BaFPE supports clinical observations and complements other life skills assessments.

6. The BaFPE is a therapeutic medium by which patient self-esteem and self-confidence can be enhanced.

7. The BaFPE emphasizes the performance of action, rather than patient self-report.

Bruce and Borg find utility in being able to rate the impact of psychological states on performance.[65] However, these authors offer a critique of the tasks used to assess function. "With the exception of money management and grocery market tasks, the nature of these assessment tasks are not likely to be tasks that are necessary for the patient to function in his or her everyday environment."[65]

Other researchers have reported that the TOA and SIS are useful in evaluating patients with eating disorders or bipolar disorder, some skilled nursing home residents, and patient progress in research studies.

EATING DISORDERS

In their research to develop TOA norms for the eating disorder population, Stanton, Mann, and Klyczek state that the TOA "results can be useful in confronting defense mechanisms, particularly patient denial that eating patterns have had any significant negative effects [and that] the House Floor Plan and Kinetic Person Drawing may be used by the skillful clinician as projectives, although this is not part of the standardized scoring system."[61]

Wozniak hypothesized that the sense of ineffectiveness experienced by patients with eating disorders, as measured by the ineffectiveness subscale of the Eating Disorders Inventory (EDI),[66] would be reflected in their scores on the self-confidence and general affective impression parameters of the TOA.[67] BaFPE-TOA and EDI scores for 63 patients diagnosed with eating disorders were analyzed. Low and nonsignificant correlations resulted in rejection of the hypothesis. However, these results are consistent with Stanton et al, who stated that "feelings of ineffectiveness, often verbalized by anorexic patients, are not always related to poor performance."[61] Interestingly, Wozniak reported a low to moderate but nonsignificant correlation between the total TOA score and the EDI perfectionism subscale score. Konieczny later found that the smallest difference in TOA scores between subjects with an eating disorder and nondiagnosed subjects was on the performance component total and the task completion, errors, and efficiency parameters.[50]

BIPOLAR DISORDER

Tse, Yeats, and Walsh[68] used the TOA, along with other measures of function and affect, to evaluate a 51-year-old male who had difficulty sustaining meaningful work. The authors found that TOA scores supported other findings suggesting that the subject of this single case study was highly functional when he was euthymic, and that he did not seem to have any residual areas of dysfunction despite a long history of bipolar disorder.

Concerned with mathematical difficulties in adolescents with remitted bipolar disorder, Lagace, Kutcher, and Robertson[69] administered the Money and Marketing subtest of the TOA to three groups of adolescents (bipolar disorder, major depressive disorder, and no history of psychiatric disorder), along with a variety of achievement and intelligence tests. The researchers found no differences among groups for task accuracy; however, the group with bipolar disorder took significantly ($p < 0.001$) more time to complete the task than the other two groups. This and other study results suggest to the authors that a specific pattern of cognitive processing dysfunction may be present in adolescents with bipolar disorder that warrants further research and programs for remediation in mathematics.

SKILLED NURSING RESIDENTS

Applicability of the TOA with skilled nursing residents was studied by Mann and Small Russ.[70] They analyzed TOA data on 13 male and 29 female residents aged 47 to 93 years old (M = 75.4). Approximately 25% (range = 17% to 29%) of the residents were rated at the lowest possible score on the five TOA tasks, suggesting that the "TOA is appropriate for nursing home patients at the middle and higher end of cognitive and physical abilities, but for some patients...it is not practical."[70] The authors offer a number of examples to illustrate how lack of stimulation in the nursing home environment influences resident behavior, which is reflected in poor performance on the TOA and interpretation of drawings completed in the Kinetic Person Drawing task.

The authors suggest various opportunities that should be afforded nursing home residents to improve quality of care. Although they suggest that the TOA may not be appropriate for up to 25% of this population, the use of such tools as the TOA possibly could help therapists develop appropriate treatment programs for residents.

Evaluation of Patient Progress in Research Studies

The TOA was reported useful for evaluating patient progress to compare the effectiveness of a cognitive rehabilitation treatment modality to a traditional one-to-one task-oriented approach for attention disorder in 29 patients with chronic schizophrenia. Although study results indicated no significant difference between the two treatment methods, patients showed significant improvement on scores in the TOA Sorting Shells task and on the self-confidence and motivation parameters across four of the five tasks and on the efficiency parameter across all five TOA tasks.[71]

The SIS was used by Staron to evaluate changes in patients' interpersonal communication skills in a study in which the effectiveness of verbally-oriented versus activities-oriented group treatment approaches in a psychiatric day treatment program were compared.[72] The SIS was administered prior to and at the completion of a 12-week treatment protocol. Eighteen patients received the oral therapy approach in 45-minute/once-per-week treatment groups, while 17 patients received the same amount of an activities-oriented approach. All patients continued to receive the same treatment services regularly provided in the program. Results indicated that there were no significant differences between the two treatment methods, but patients in both groups showed significant improvement in SIS scores.

Further Research

VARIATIONS IN BaFPE ADMINISTRATION

Results of the survey conducted by Managh and Cook, described earlier, showed variations in occupational therapists' use of the BaFPE. Common variations included not using the QSRI, not using the SIS, modifying the administration and scoring of the TOA, and infrequent reference to the available normative data.[59]

Approximately 20% of therapists reported they never used the QSRI. Almost 50% of therapists who did use the QSRI only used it if the patient previously exhibited organic signs. Some therapists indicated they could identify signs of organic involvement in other situations without the QSRI. Lack of use of the SIS was attributed to lack of time to rate the SIS and because social interaction was already routinely assessed in therapy groups.

Common modifications to the TOA protocol involved altering task timing by allowing patients to finish tasks, even if allowable time had expired; altering the TOA verbatim instructions because they were viewed by some therapists as demeaning or because they wanted to ensure patient success on the task; and not following the scoring protocol due to lack of time. Few therapists used the TOA norms because of concern about the small sample size or lack of comparative reference for patients they were evaluating.

When variations such as these are made to test protocol, therapists are no longer administering a standardized test. Although lack of use of the SIS is apparently common, as demonstrated by Managh and Cook's survey results and the lack of published studies on the SIS (compared to the TOA), therapists are only assessing task-oriented behavior and not functional performance as intended by the test authors.

DEVELOPMENT OF A SHORTER TOA

Development of a shortened version of the TOA, containing only 24 rather than 60 ratings, has been explored.[58] Using multiple regression and factor analyses on data originally used to formulate the 1991 TOA standard scores,[57] four parameter ratings were eliminated (attention span, evidence of thought disorder, efficiency, and motivation/compliance), as well as two tasks (Home Drawing and Block Design). The correlation of total TOA scores between the full and shortened versions of the TOA was high (r = .94).

Summary

Research on the use of the BaFPE continues. Therapists are invited and encouraged by the test authors to participate in the ongoing testing and refinement of the BaFPE and in the development of national norms for the TOA and SIS. Therapists who do not see themselves as researchers or who cannot find the time to conduct research in their own clinics may become involved in BaFPE research by developing relationships with academics or other researchers currently working on the BaFPE. The therapist can serve an important role in the research process by securing approval from the clinic or hospital administration to collect research data in the therapist's department. It is important to note that graduate occupational therapy students have made useful contributions to the current research on the BaFPE. Developing relationships with graduate occupational therapy students, who may be studying the BaFPE, is another possible avenue for therapists to become involved in clinical research.

References

1. Bloomer J, Williams S. *The Bay Area Functional Performance Evaluation*. Research ed. Palo Alto, CA: Consulting Psychologists Press; 1979:12,15.
2. Mosey A. *Three Frames of Reference for Mental Health*. Thorofare, NJ: SLACK Incorporated; 1970.
3. Reilly M. A psychiatric OT program as a teaching model. *Am J Occup Ther*. 1966;20:61-67.5.
4. Reilly M. The educational process. *Am J Occup Ther*. 1969;23:299-307.
5. Barret L, Kielhofner G. Theories derived from occupational behavior perspectives. In: Crepeau E, Cohn E, Boyt Schell B. *Willard & Spackman's Occupational Therapy*. 10th ed. Philadelphia, PA: Lippincott Williams & Wilkins; 2003: 209-233.
6. Fisher A. Uniting practice and theory in an occupational framework. *Am J Occup Ther*. 1998;52:509-521.
7. Kielhofner G. A model of human occupation, part 2. Ontogenesis from the perspective of temporal adaptation. *Am J Occup Ther*. 1980;34:657-663.
8. Kielhofner G. A model of human occupation, part 3. Benign and vicious cycles. *Am J Occup Ther*. 1980;34:731-737.
9. Kielhofner G. The model of human occupation. In: Kielhofner G. *Conceptual Foundations of Occupational Therapy*. Philadelphia, PA: F.A. Davis; 1992:154-169.
10. Kielhofner G, Burke J. A model of human occupation, part 1. Conceptual framework and content. *Am J Occup Ther*. 1980;34:572-581.
11. Kielhofner G, Burke J, Igi C. A model of human occupation, part 4. Assessment and intervention. *Am J Occup Ther*. 1980;34:777-788.
12. Kielhofner G. *Model of Human Occupation*. 4th ed. Philadelphia, PA: Lippincott Williams & Wilkins; 2007.
13. American Occupational Therapy Association. Occupational therapy practice framework: Domain and process. *Am J Occup Ther*. 2002; 56: 609-639.
14. Bloomer J, Williams S. The Bay Area Functional Performance Evaluation. In: Hemphill B, ed. *The Evaluative Process in Psychiatric Occupational Therapy*. Thorofare, NJ: SLACK Incorporated; 1982:255-308.
15. Williams S, Bloomer J. *Bay Area Functional Performance Evaluation*. 2nd ed. Palo Alto, CA: Consulting Psychologists Press; 1987:1-2,11.
16. Bloomer J, Williams S, Houston D. In progress—short reports on psychosocial assessment, The Bay Area Functional Performance Evaluation. *OTMH*. 1980;1(2):41-42.
17. Houston D, Williams S, Bloomer J, Mann W. The Bay Area Functional Performance Evaluation: Development and standardization. *Am J Occup Ther*. 1989;43:170-183.
18. Bellack A. Recurrent problems in the behavioral assessment of social skills. *Behavior Research and Therapy*. 1983;21(1):29-41.
19. Carlsmith J, Ellsworth P, Aronson E. *Methods of Research in Social Psychology*. Reading, MA: Addison-Wesley; 1976.
20. Kazdin A. *Behavior Modification in Applied Settings*. Homewood, IL: The Dorsey Press; 1975:67-82.
21. Murphy K, Martin C, Garcia M. Do behavior observation scales measure observation? *J Appl Psychol*. 1982;67(5):562-567.
22. Paul G, Lentz R. *Psychosocial Treatment of Chronic Mental Patients: Milieu Versus Social Learning Program*. Cambridge, MA: Harvard University Press; 1977:111-126.
23. Stein F. Research analysis of occupational therapy assessments used in mental health. In: Hemphill B, ed. *Mental Health Assessment in Occupational Therapy, An Integrative Approach To the Evaluative Process*. Thorofare, NJ: SLACK Incorporated; 1988:223-247.
24. Ottenbacher K. *Evaluating Clinical Change*. Baltimore, MD: Williams & Wilkins; 1986:84-87.
25. Sarno J, Sarno M, Levita E. The Functional Life Scale. *Arch Phys Med Rehabil*. 1973;54:214-220.
26. Endicott J, Spitzer R, Fleiss J, Cohen J. The Global Assessment Scale. *Arch Gen Psychiatry*. 1976;33:766-771.
27. Bortone J. *Functional Component Skills Associated With DSM-III Diagnoses of Schizophrenia and Borderline Personality Disorders Thesis*. New York, NY: New York University; 1984:51.
28. Cheeseman J. *An Investigation of the Concurrent Validity of the Bay Area Functional Performance Evaluation for Patients With Brain Vascular Disease* [thesis]. Richmond, VA: Virginia Commonwealth University; 1980.
29. Jebsen R, Taylor N, Trieschmann R, Trotter M, Howard L. An objective and standardized test of hand function. *Arch Phys Med Rehabil*. 1969;50:311-319.
30. Kaufman L. *A Comparison of Performance on the Bay Area Functional Performance Evaluation and the Kohlman Evaluation of Living Skills by Adult Psychiatric Patients* [thesis]. Boston, MA: Sargent College of Allied Health Professions, Boston University; 1982.
31. McGourty L. *Kohlman Evaluation of Living Skills*. Seattle, WA: KELS Research, Box 33201; 1979.

32. Wener-Altman P, Wolfe A, Staley D. Utilization of the Bay Area Functional Performance Evaluation with an adolescent psychiatric population. *Can J Occup Ther.* 1991;58:129-136.

33. Olson B, Jamal J. *The BaFPE: Standardization and Clinical Application in Acute Adult Psychiatry.* Irvine, CA: University of California Irvine Medical Center; 1987.

34. Brockett M. Cultural variations in Bay Area Functional Performance Evaluation scores—considerations for occupational therapy. *Can J Occup Ther.* 1987;54:195-199.

35. Honigfeld G, Gillis R, Klett, C. NOSIE-30: a treatment sensitive ward behavior scale. *Psychological Reports.* 1966;19:180-182.

36. Casanova J, Ferber J. Comprehensive Evaluation of Basic Living Skills. *Am J Occup Ther.* 1976;30:101-105.

37. Accardi M. *The Bay Area Functional Performance Evaluation: A Validity Study* [thesis]. Boston, MA: Boston School of Occupational Therapy, Tufts University; 1985.

38. Mason J. *Observer Ratings Versus Self-report of Social Interaction As Assessed by the Bay Area Functional Performance Evaluation.* Halifax, Nova Scotia: Dalhousie University; 1985.

39. Francis E, Cermak S. Comparison of two subtests of the Bay Area Functional Performance Evaluation. *OTMH.* 1987;7:99-114.

40. Newman M. *Cognitive Disability and Functional Performance in Individuals With Chronic Schizophrenic Disorders* [thesis]. Los Angeles, CA: University of Southern California; 1987. Thesis.

41. Allen C. *Occupational Therapy for Psychiatric Diseases: Measurement and Management of Cognitive Disabilities.* Boston, MA: Little, Brown; 1985.

42. Thibeault R, Blackmer E. Validating a test of functional performance with psychiatric patients. *Am J Occup Ther.* 1987;41:515-521.

43. Wechsler D. *WAIS Manual: Wechsler Adult Intelligence Scale.* New York, NY: The Psychological Corporation; 1955.

44. Klyczek J, Mann W. Concurrent validity of the Task-Oriented Assessment component of the Bay Area Functional Performance Evaluation with the American Association on Mental Deficiency Adaptive Behavior Scale. *Am J Occup Ther.* 1990;44:907-912.

45. Nihira K, Foster R, Shellhaas M, Leland H. *AAMD Adaptive Behavior Scale.* Washington, DC: American Association on Mental Deficiency; 1969.

46. Nihira K, Foster R, Shellhaas M, Leland H. *AAMD Adaptive Behavior Scale, 1974 Revision.* Washington, DC: American Association on Mental Deficiency; 1974.

47. Mercer Castilla L, Klyczek J. Comparison of the Kinetic Person Drawing Task of the Bay Area Functional Performance Evaluation with measures of functional performance. *OTMH.* 1993;12(2):27-38.

48. Clark EN, Peters M. *The Scorable Self-Care Evaluation.* Thorofare, NJ: SLACK Incorporated; 1984.

49. Curtin M, Klyczek J. Comparison of BaFPE-TOA scores for inpatients and outpatients. *OTMH.* 1992;12(1):61-75.

50. Konieczny T. *Discriminant Validity of the BaFPE TOA as an Evaluation Tool for Patients With Eating Disorders* [thesis]. Buffalo, NY: D'Youville College; 1996.

51. Lissner J. *Discriminant Validity of the Bay Area Functional Performance Evaluation Task Oriented Assessment* [thesis]. Buffalo, NY: D'Youville College; 1996.

52. Stoffel E. *Discriminant Validity of the Revised Bay Area Functional Performance Evaluation—Task Oriented Assessment for An Elderly Population* [thesis]. Buffalo, NY: D'Youville College; 1994.

53. Tardif M. *Concurrent Validity of the Functional Needs Assessment With the Task Oriented Assessment Component of the Bay Area Functional Performance Evaluation* [thesis]. Buffalo, NY: D'Youville College; 1993.

54. Dombrowski L. *Functional Needs Assessment Program for Chronic Psychiatric Patients.* Tucson, AZ: Therapy Skill Builders; 1990.

55. Rogers E. *A Study of the Concurrent Validity of the Milwaukee Evaluation of Daily Living Skills with the Bay Area Functional Performance Evaluation* [thesis]. Buffalo, NY: D'Youville College; 1992.

56. Leonardelli C. *The Milwaukee Evaluation of Daily Living Skills: Evaluation in Long-Term Psychiatric Care.* Thorofare, NJ: SLACK Incorporated; 1988.

57. Mann W, Klyczek J. Standard scores for the Bay Area Functional Performance Evaluation Task Oriented Assessment. *OTMH.* 1991;11(1):13-24.

58. Mann W, Huselid R. An abbreviated Task Oriented Assessment (Bay Area Functional Performance Evaluation). *Am J Occup Ther.* 1993;47:111-118.

59. Managh M, Cook J. The use of standardized assessment in occupational therapy: The BaFPE-R as an example. *Am J Occup Ther.* 1993;47:877-884.

60. Mann W, Klyczek J, Fiedler R. Bay Area Functional Performance Evaluation (BaFPE): standard scores. *OTMH.* 1989;9:1-7.

61. Stanton E, Mann W, Klyczek J. Use of the Bay Area Functional Performance Evaluation with eating disordered patients. *OTJR.* 1991;11(4):227-237.

62. Peterson B. *A Preliminary Examination of BaFPE-TOA Scores for Adolescents With Psychiatric Disorders* [thesis]. Buffalo, NY: D'Youville College; 1996.

63. Crouch A. *Gender Bias in the Bay Area Functional Performance Evaluation—Task Oriented Assessment* [thesis]. Buffalo, NY: D'Youville College; 1994.

64. Tornabene P. *Gender Differences of a Nonpatient Population on the Bay Area Functional Performance Evaluation* [thesis]. Buffalo, NY: D'Youville College; 1995.

65. Bruce MA, Borg B. *Psychosocial Frames of Reference: Core for Occupation-Based Practice*. 3rd ed. Thorofare, NJ: SLACK Incorporated; 2002.

66. Garner D, Olmsted M, Polivy J. Development and validation of a multidimensional eating disorder inventory for anorexia nervosa and bulimia. *Int J Eat Disord*. 1983;2:15-35.

67. Wozniak L. *The BaFPE-TOA and the EDI in Relation to Individuals With a Diagnosis of Eating Disorders* [thesis]. Buffalo, NY: D'Youville College; 1991:128.

68. Tse S, Yeats M, Walsh A. A single case study: striving for stability and work—"it's a real bastard of a disease." *Work*. 1999;12(2):151-157.

69. Lagace D, Kutcher S, Robertson H. Mathematics deficits in adolescents with Bipolar I Disorder. *Am J Psychiatry*. 2003;160(1):100-104.

70. Mann W, Small Russ L. Measuring the functional performance of nursing home patients with the Bay Area Functional Performance Evaluation. *Physical and Occupational Therapy in Geriatrics*. 1991;9(3):113-129.

71. Brown C, Harwood K, Hays C, Heckman J, Short J. Effectiveness of cognitive rehabilitation for improving attention inpatients with schizophrenia. *OTJR*. 1993;13(2):71-86.

72. Staron R. *The Effectiveness of Activity Versus Verbal Therapy in Improving Interpersonal Communication Skills* [thesis]. Buffalo, NY: D'Youville College; 1992.

THE ASSESSMENT OF OCCUPATIONAL FUNCTIONING—COLLABORATIVE VERSION

Janet H. Watts, PhD, OTR/L
Sandra M. Newman, MS, OTR/L

"Whoever knows himself is truly wise!" Chaucer G. The Canterbury Tales. *New York, NY: Oxford University Press;1998:178-200.*

Introduction

The Assessment of Occupational Functioning—Collaborative Version (AOF-CV) is a theory- and research-based, semi-structured screening tool appropriate for use in a variety of contexts. It is designed to: (1) efficiently collect a broad range of complex, inter-related qualitative information on key components of the Model of Human Occupation (MOHO) that supports or hinders occupational performance, and (2) identify areas needing more in-depth evaluation. The AOF-CV incorporates research-based changes and is formatted for either therapist administration or self-administration with therapist follow-up. Watts and Madigan[1] developed the current collaborative version after using the original AOF with varied groups, experimenting with a self-administered format, and further instrument development research. The original AOF[2] was based directly on the original MOHO, and while this model has been revised, the AOF-CV continues to be compatible with the current model's theory and practice.[3] This chapter will present an overview of the AOF-CV, a discussion of its relationship to MOHO and the *Occupational Therapy Practice Framework (Framework)*, a summary of instrument development and clinical utility research, and a case study.

Overview

DESCRIPTION AND FORM

The AOF-CV is a semi-structured, self-report screening instrument based on MOHO that collects information about patients' perceptions of their strengths and limitations in the areas of values, personal causation, interests, roles, habits, and skills. It does not directly address underlying performance capacities (eg, musculoskeletal constituents) or environmental variables. It yields an Occupational Profile, numerical ratings, information for the Occupational Analysis, and it is recommended as an initial screening tool. It consists of a one-page administration protocol, a one-page cover sheet that asks about recent employment history and reasons for job changes, a 22-question interview schedule coded to model components, and a 5-point rating scale.

PURPOSE

The AOF-CV offers a theory-based, self-report assessment with established psychometric properties. It was developed as an initial screening tool to be supplemented with other history-taking assessments and direct observation. Thus, it was designed to be as efficient as possible, while yielding clinically useful information.

ADMINISTRATION

The AOF-CV can be used either as a paper-and-pencil self-report with therapist follow up or as a semi-structured interview. It should be used only with patients who are capable of responding thoughtfully to an interview. The interviewer should have good interview skills and knowledge of MOHO.

For patient administration with therapist follow-up, the therapist simply asks the patient to complete the interview form. The therapist then reviews the responses, probing or clarifying as needed, and rates the items. Probing and clarification are indicated if the specified questions elicit:

1. No reply
2. A request for clarification
3. An answer suggesting the interviewee misunderstood the question
4. A superficial response
5. Any other indications of miscommunication, whether by the interviewer or patient

Using the interview form as a self-assessment tool with therapist follow-up may not only enhance accuracy over either an interview or self-assessment used alone, but it also: (1) permits more time for the patient's unpressured, uninhibited self-reflection; (2) integrally involves the patient in the therapy planning process; and (3) saves time. The self-assessment with therapist follow-up has the potential to improve both assessment effectiveness and efficiency.

For therapist administration, the therapist follows the interview format, using parenthetical probes or clarifications as needed. Responses are noted on the interview schedule and provide information needed to mark the rating form.

Ratings of interpersonal and communication skills are based on either the therapist's experience conducting the entire interview or on the therapist's review and use of follow-up questions to interview the patient.

Theoretical Base

RELATIONSHIP OF THE AOF-CV TO THE MODEL OF HUMAN OCCUPATION

MOHO[3] provides the conceptual framework for this evaluation. This model conceptualizes human occupation as being composed of volition, habituation, and performance capacities, with these capacities being interrelated aspects of the whole person. Volition is made up of personal causation, values, and interests. Habituation is made up of roles and habits. Performance capacities incorporate both objective physical and mental components and subjective experiences. Occupational performance capacity is the demonstrated ability to perform motor, process, and communication and interaction skills in the context of occupational performances.

MOHO uses systems thinking to describe humans' occupational functioning as flexibly assembled in such a way that the person, the task, and the environment all contribute to behavior. Thus, the human system continually creates its structure through the ongoing interaction of the person, task, and environment. At any point in time, any of these can become the lead contributing factor toward creating behavior, depending on their relative importance. The parts of the system are related "heterarchically," that is:

> [The parts] will interact with each other in ways that depend on the situation. In a heterarchy, each component contributes something to the total dynamic...Heterarchy is manifest through human occupation. When we consider any thought, emotion, or action, the parts of the human being and the environment cooperate together according to local conditions created by what each element brings to the total dynamic.[3(p35)]

While MOHO incorporates much more complexity, these core concepts serve as a basis for discussing the AOF-CV.

The AOF-CV relates to MOHO in these ways:

1. It deals with a group of core concepts (ie, aspects of the volitional, habituation, and performance capacities), not the entire model in its complexity.

2. It focuses on the person more than the task or environment.

3. It addresses structure more than process.

4. It provides screening-level information, not detailed data about all model elements.

5. It was developed to systematically ask questions about the person's volition, habituation, and occupational performance skills.

The AOF-CV assesses the structure of the volition subsystem by asking questions about a person's: (1) beliefs about their abilities and sense of control (ie, personal causation), (2) convictions about occupations, beliefs about how time should be used, and related goals (ie, values), and (3) favorable dispositions toward certain occupations (ie, interests). Structure of the habituation subsystem is assessed in the AOF-CV by examining aspects of roles and habits.

Occupational performance skills questions are general and yield information about how persons perceive their performances of movement, dealing with processes, and social communication and interaction. These were originally conceptualized as part of a performance subsystem; however, in the current model these are addressed as performance capacities.

RELATIONSHIP OF THE AOF-CV TO THE *OCCUPATIONAL THERAPY PRACTICE FRAMEWORK*

The AOF-CV most directly addresses *Framework* items in the following areas: Performance in Areas of Occupation, Performance Skills, Performance Patterns, Activity Demands, and Patient Factors. It does not specifically address context. Table 15-1 correlates the most directly related concepts; however, many other domain areas are diffusely addressed by the AOF-CV.

The AOF-CV initiates a patient-centered approach to the evaluation stage of the OT Process. It contributes critical information toward development of the Occupational Profile and the Analysis of Occupational Performance. It also stimulates a collaborative patient/therapist dialogue and patient self-reflection. The process of completing the AOF-CV yields a broad picture of patient needs, concerns, and problems, while focusing on issues related to the domain of occupational therapy.

Instrument Development Research

The AOF-CV is the current, refined version of the original Assessment of Occupational Functioning (AOF). Reliability and validity estimates for the AOF-CV have been developed through systematic study.[2,4-13] The original AOF was developed as a semi-structured interview and rating scale for a therapist who needed a brief, comprehensive, theory-based evaluation that could help establish treatment priorities for physically disabled or aged residents. Research on the original AOF with 83 community-based and institutionalized elderly persons provided initial support for dimensionality, with AOF items corresponding consistently with MOHO components. It also provided preliminary support for reliability and validity, as well as guidance for revisions. Test-retest and inter-rater reliabilities for total scores were generally acceptable, with a few low item scores. Concurrent validity was supported by correlations with the Life Satisfaction Index-Z[14] and by the demonstrated ability to distinguish between institutionalized and community-based subjects. However, Geriatric Rating Scale[15] correlations were mixed. Such research findings informed the first revision of the AOF.[6]

Watts, Brollier, Bauer, and Schmidt[12] compared the AOF (first revision) to the revised Occupational Case Analysis Interview and Rating Scale (OCAIRS)[16] in a study with 41 patients with schizophrenia and five occupational therapists who had used both instruments. The occupational therapists found the instruments to be clinically valuable and provided suggestions for refinements. Concurrent validity was supported[5] by correlations with the Global Assessment Scale.[17] Quantitative and qualitative data from 11 experts supported AOF (1st revision) content validity,[6] and this study's findings informed the second AOF revision.[13]

Validity of the AOF-CV (second revision) has been examined in various studies. Morgan[10] studied the ability of the AOF (second revision) to distinguish between 25 healthy elderly persons in a retirement home and 25 intermediate care facility residents. The total score and component scores for personal causation, roles, habits, and skills differed significantly, whereas value and interest scores did not, adding further support for validity and utility of the AOF with elderly persons. Baber's[4] research supported concur-

Table 15-1
OTPF and Related AOF-CV Concepts

OTPF Category	AOF-CV Related Components
Areas of Occupation: ADL, IADL, education, work, play, leisure, social participation	Interest discrimination, range Values: enacted through selection of meaningful activities
Performance Skills: motor, process, communication/interaction	Motor and communication/interpersonal skill performance
Performance Patterns: habits, routines, roles	Habit pattern organization, social-acceptability, flexibility Occupational role balance, comfort, security
Activity Demands: eg, social demands (relates to social and cultural contexts)	Occupational role: understanding role demands and obligations Values: social appropriateness/personal standards
Patient factors reside within the patient and may affect occupational performance	
Body Functions/Global Mental Functions: energy and drive → motivation, interests, values	Personal causation: belief in internal control, confidence in a range of skills and competence at personally relevant tasks, hopeful anticipation for success Interest pursuit Values: demonstrated through personal goals; enacted through selection of meaningful activities
Body Functions/Specific Mental Functions: higher level cognitive functions → time management; problem solving	Values—temporal orientation expressed as awareness of past, present, and future events and beliefs about how time should be used Problem-solving skill performance
Body Functions/Specific Mental Functions: language → receptive and expressive spoken language	Communication skills

rent validity of the AOF (second revision) in relation to the Quality of Life Index (QLI)[18] in a study with 30 physically disabled persons recently out of rehabilitation. The AOF (second revision) personal causation, interests, roles, and skills components correlated moderately to strongly with conceptually similar QLI items, but there were no conceptually similar QLI habit items, and the values correlation was not statistically significant. Additionally, Viik, Watts, Madigan, and Bauer[11] established preliminary validity for use of the AOF (second revision) with an alcoholic population using the Alcohol Dependence Scale[19] in a study with 48 persons.

In 1991, the AOF-CV (research version) was created to:

1. Clarify communication among diverse English-speaking cultures (ie, Australian Aboriginal and non-Aboriginal populations)

2. Simplify items

3. Reformat the rating sheet

4. Add administration guidelines

5. Combine related questions

6. Reword items to be compatible with optional self-administration.

Research on the AOF-CV (research version) has examined: (1) content validity, (2) appropriateness of terminology across cultures, and (3) which patients could effectively use it in the self-administration format.[7,9] McGuigan examined content validity[9] by surveying experts from several English-speaking countries (ie, Australia, Canada, New Zealand, and the United States), asking them to match AOF-CV items to the model components from which they were derived. This yielded a similar pattern to that established in previous research.[6] Qualitative findings suggested that, while the language of the instrument seemed to pose no problems, there was a need to interpret items relative to cultural values. For example, one person commented on the cross-cultural difficulties of the item "Do you feel in control of your life?" because, with Maori and Pacific Islanders, the good of the group takes precedence over the good of the individual.

Elliott and Newman[7] explored the utility and effectiveness of AOF-CV (research version) self-administration with 27 psychiatric patients. The study found that higher Mini-Mental Status[20] scores (≥ 27), educational level, and verbal ability indicate which patients may complete it independently with limited follow-up. Overall, 89% of the questions were effectively answered independently, and therapist follow-up required an average of 12 minutes. Therapists noted that patients gained useful insights from the process. Thus, the study supported AOF-CV (research version) utility when used as a self-assessment with therapist follow-up. The instrument was refined in 1993 based on findings from McGuigan and Elliott and Newman's research to produce the current AOF-CV.[1] Finally, 20 anonymous online surveys electronically submitted between June 2004 and July 2005 indicated that the AOF-CV was uniformly useful; overall usefulness and ease of use were rated superior by all.

Case Example: Tom

Tom is a 35-year-old man who sustained a right hand crush injury at work; his right hand is dominant. He fractured his ring finger and dislocated his middle finger. The tips of his small finger and ring finger were amputated. He began outpatient hand therapy when the temporary pins were removed from his fingers 2 months after the accident. Tom has a history of substance abuse.

Tom has lived with his significant other, Debbie, for 7 years and they have two young children. They had been living on the west coast, but Debbie wanted to move east to be closer to Tom's family. Tom was not eager to be located near his family, but felt that the west coast was not the best place to raise his children. Tom believed that the west coast lifestyle did not provide a healthy environment for children. He had been employed installing/finishing floors prior to the move and took great pride in his detailed work in some luxurious homes. After the move, he performed temporary work until he found a similar job just 1 month prior to his injury. His significant other works in an office and his sister provides day care for the children.

QUALITATIVE INFORMATION/OCCUPATIONAL PROFILE

Tom completed the AOF-CV as self-administered with therapist follow-up.

Values

Tom reported deriving meaning from spending time with his children. His short-term goals involved finding activities for the children and himself that also included his significant other. He felt that he could make better use of his time and that he was not as attentive to the children as he could be. His long-term goal was to be self-employed so he could spend more time with his family.

Personal Causation

Tom felt that he had limited control over his life. His family is very opinionated about how he should run his life and raise his children. He believes that his significant other is immature and spoiled. Since they have moved east, Debbie sides with his family when conflicts arise. The hand injury has compounded the friction between them because he is unable to work full-time and has to rely on his family more. In the past, he has taken great pride in his woodworking skills and now has doubts about his ability to return to that line of work.

Interests

Tom likes to read, fish, hike, and ride his bike. He also expressed an interest in learning how to play the guitar or violin. Due to his hand injury, he is unable to pursue many of his interests, so he spends most of his time reading about various topics on-line. He also feels that taking care of the problems in his relationship with his significant other is a priority.

Roles

Tom's current roles are father, partner, and homemaker. Since he injured his hand, he no longer fulfills the role of a worker. Since he has been out of work, he enjoys spending more time with his children and performing domestic tasks such as cooking. Although he wants to return to work, he is taking advantage of this time off to decrease the stress of daily responsibilities on Debbie and to work on their relationship.

Habits

Prior to the injury, Tom's daily routine involved getting up, fixing breakfast for his family, and then going to work. After work, he would spend time with his children and help out with any housework. Although his children still go to his sister's home for day care, he is able to spend more time with them since the injury. Because Debbie works, he does most of the housework and has dinner ready when she comes home. He doesn't understand why Debbie doesn't appreciate his efforts or why his family is critical of how he spends his time.

Skills

Although his injury is to his dominant hand, Tom has the ability to use his right thumb and index finger to perform light self-care and homemaking. He is able to lift or hold only light objects. He is concerned about how much use he will regain in his hand in order to return to his previous line of work, which involved lifting tools like hammers and power saws and operating them with precision.

AOF-CV RATINGS

The following ratings were made by his therapist after completion of the AOF-CV, with 1 meaning "very little" and 5 meaning "very likely". Thus, higher ratings indicate more commitment to or engagement in the specified concept. Scores of 1-3 suggest possible areas for more detailed evaluation.

1. Values:

   meaningfulness – 3

   occupational goals – 4

   personal standards – 4

   temporal orientation – 4

2. Personal Causation:

   belief in control – 3

   belief in skill – 3

   belief in efficacy – 3

   expectancy of success – 4

3. Interests:

   discrimination – 4

   pattern – 5

   potency – 2

4. Roles:

   balance – 2

   internalized expectations – 2

   perceived incumbency – 2

5. Habits:

   degree of organization – 2

   social appropriateness – 3

   rigidity/flexibility – 3

6. Skills:

   motor skills – 3

   process skills – 2

   communication/interpersonal skills – 2

OCCUPATIONAL ANALYSIS

Tom is a young man with many interests and goals. Prior to his hand injury, he already felt limited by the lack of control over his life. His limitations were exacerbated by the injury, which left him with range of motion and strength deficits in his dominant hand. He lost his role as a worker, which previously gave him much pride and satisfaction. He no longer pursued his interests and did not spend his time in goal-related activities. Thus, education in time management was planned to facilitate a balance of his interests, values, and roles. Identifying short-term goals and providing the means to successfully achieve them may enhance his confidence in his abilities and give him a sense of accomplishment. During the rehabilitative process, it is anticipated that he will feel that he has regained control over his life. His ultimate goal is to return to work and pursue his long-term goal of being self-employed.

TREATMENT IMPLICATIONS

Values

Assist Tom with identifying and prioritizing his short- and long-term goals, and set realistic timeframes for each.

Personal Causation

Provide hand therapy to increase the functional use of his right hand. Successful engagement in work-related activities should increase Tom's sense of efficacy. He needs to rely less on his family in order to gain control of his life. He expressed an interest in moving out of state to be away from his family, but he needs to regain adequate use of his hand and return to work first.

Interests

Explore his many interests and pursue the ones that are compatible with his values, his limited use of his right hand, and his financial constraints.

Roles

Identify the sources of conflict in his relationship with his significant other and work on resolving the issues. Explore constructive ways to increase the attention he gives to his children. Identify the skills required to return to work and provide opportunities to practice those skills.

Habits

Identify ways that his time could be better spent. Provide a daily schedule to reduce wasted time and increase time spent in goal-oriented tasks.

Skills

Provide graded activities that are related to returning to work in order for Tom to regain confidence in his abilities and realize his limitations.

RESPONSE TO TREATMENT

During therapy, Tom participated in graded activities to experience both success and the appropriate challenge. Whenever possible, he was given choices to enhance his sense of personal control. One of his short-term goals that involved his values and interests was to go on a camping trip with his family. He planned a successful outing, which improved his confidence in his parent and partner roles. He took great pride in his ability to set up the tent despite the limited use of his right hand. In another activity, he used his wood working skills to construct a model wooden car for his son. He especially enjoyed mixing paints to achieve the exact desired colors for the model. It reminded him of his expertise in mixing stains when he previously finished hardwood floors. He gained a sense of competency and improved self-esteem by completing the activity. During therapy, he developed a sense of hope that he had the potential to achieve his goals, including returning to work.

Summary

This chapter presented an overview of the AOF-CV, demonstrated its basis in research and compatibility with occupation-based theory and practice, and illustrated its use. The AOF-CV arose from a clinical need, and its development has been informed by both instrument development research and therapist feedback regarding its clinical value. Its strength lies in how it efficiently generates a breadth of critical information for treatment and discharge planning, its applicability to varied settings, the reflection it stimulates within patients, its ability to identify salient psychosocial issues regardless of the diagnosis or patient situation, and the collaborative relationship it stimulates between patient and therapist.

References

1. Watts JH, Madigan MJ. Assessment of Occupational Functioning—Collaborative Version. 1993. Available at the Virginia Commonwealth University Department of Occupational Therapy website: http://www.sahp.vcu.edu/occu/
2. Watts JH, Kielhofner G, Bauer DF, Gregory MD, Valentine DB. The Assessment of Occupational Functioning: a screening tool for use in long-term care. *Am J Occup Ther.* 1986; 40:231-240.
3. Kielhofner G. *Model of Human Occupation: Theory and Application.* 3rd ed. Baltimore, MD: Lippincott Williams & Wilkins; 2002.
4. Baber KP. Construct validity inferences about the Assessment of Occupational Functioning for persons with physical disabilities. 1988. (Unpublished master's degree research project. Information available from the Department of Occupational Therapy, Virginia Commonwealth University/Medical College of Virginia, MCV Box 980008, Richmond, VA 23298-0008.)
5. Brollier C, Watts JH, Bauer D, Schmidt W. A concurrent validity study of two occupational therapy evaluation instruments: the AOF & OCAIRS. *Occupational Therapy in Mental Health.* 1988;8(4):49-59.
6. Brollier C, Watts JH, Bauer D, Schmidt W. A content validity study of the Assessment of Occupational Functioning. *Occupational Therapy in Mental Health.* 1988;8(4):29-47.
7. Elliott KR, Newman SM. A concurrent validity study of the 1991 Research Version of the Assessment of Occupational Functioning. 1993. (Unpublished master's degree research project. Information available from the Department of Occupational Therapy, Virginia Commonwealth University/Medical College of Virginia, MCV Box 980008, Richmond, VA 23298-0008.)
8. Hopkins SE, Schmidt WC. A comparison and concurrent validity examination of two evaluation instruments used with psychiatric patients. 1986. (Unpublished master's degree research project. Information available from the Department of Occupational Therapy, Virginia Commonwealth University/Medical College of Virginia, MCV Box 980008, Richmond, VA 23298-0008.)
9. McGuigan PM. Content validity of the 1991 Research Version of the Assessment of Occupational Functioning. 1993. (Unpublished master's degree research project. Information available from the Department of Occupational Therapy, Virginia Commonwealth University/Medical College of Virginia, MCV Box 980008, Richmond, VA 23298-0008.)

10. Morgan R. The Assessment of Occupational Functioning: use as an elderly screening tool. 1988. Unpublished master's degree research project. Information available from the Department of Occupational Therapy, University of Indianapolis, 1400 E. Hanna Ave., Indianapolis, IN 46227.
11. Viik MK, Watts JH, Madigan MJ, Bauer D. Preliminary validation of the Assessment of Occupational Functioning with an alcoholic population. *Occupational Therapy in Mental Health*. 1990;10:19-33.
12. Watts JH, Brollier C, Bauer D, Schmidt W. A comparison of two evaluation instruments used with psychiatric patients in occupational therapy. *Occupational Therapy in Mental Health*. 1988;8(4):7-27.
13. Watts JH, Brollier C, Bauer D, Schmidt W. The Assessment of Occupational Functioning: the second revision. *Occupational Therapy in Mental Health*. 1988;8(4):61-88.
14. Wood V, Wylie ML, Sheafor B. An analysis of a short self-report measure of life satisfaction: correlation with rater judgments. *J Gerontol*. 1969;24:465-469.
15. Plutchik R, Conte MA, Lieberman M, Bakur M, Grossman J, Lehrman N. Reliability and validity of a scale for assessing the functioning of geriatric patients. *J Am Geriatrics Society*. 1970;18:491-500.
16. Kaplan K, Kielhofner G. *Occupational Case Analysis Interview and Rating Scale*. Thorofare, NJ: SLACK Incorporated; 1989.
17. Endicott J, Spitzer R, Fleiss J, Cohen J. The Global Assessment Scale: a procedure for measuring overall severity of psychiatric disturbance. *Arch Gen Psychiatry*. 1976;33:766-771.
18. Ferrans C, Powers M. Quality of Life Index: development and psychometric properties. *Advances in Nursing Science*. 1985;8(1):15-21.
19. Skinner HA, Horn JL. *Alcohol Dependence Scale (ADS) User's Guide*. Toronto: Addiction Research Foundation; 1984.
20. Folstein MF, Folstein SE, McHugh PR. Mini-Mental State, a practical method for grading the cognitive state of patients for the clinician. *J Psychiatr Res*. 1975;12:189-198.

THE ROLE CHECKLIST

Anne E. Dickerson, PhD, OTR/L, FAOTA

"If we confine ourselves to one life role, no matter how pleasant it seems at first, we starve emotionally and psychologically. We need a change and balance in our daily lives. We need sometimes to dress up and sometimes to lie around in torn jeans." Crosby FJ. Juggling: The Unexpected Advantages of Balancing Career and Home for Women and Their Families. *New York, NY: The Free Press; 1991.*

Introduction

The Role Checklist is a clinical assessment tool used by occupational therapists to help identify the occupational performance of patients through the identification of roles and the values of those roles. It was originally developed by Frances Oakley[1] as a means to describe and evaluate the construct of "roles" within the Model of Human Occupation (MOHO).[2-5] While the idea behind the Role Checklist has evolved significantly in the MOHO, it remains a viable assessment for determining participation in roles and the value of enacted roles. This chapter presents the current understanding of roles in the MOHO, a description of the Role Checklist, its clinical usage, the results of research studies on the Role Checklist, and a case study.

Occupational Therapy and Roles

Occupational therapy's overall goal is to assist individuals in the engagement of daily life activities that are meaningful and purposeful. This includes enabling the individual to participate in valued occupational roles. In fact, roles have been identified as part of the domain of occupational therapy within the performance patterns of the *Occupational Therapy Practice Framework*.[6] Brånholm and Fugl-Meyer[7] found a link between fulfillment of occupational roles and life satisfaction in both young and old individuals, while others have described role loss in the elderly and its link to life dissatisfaction.[8-10]

Addressing role dysfunction has long been recognized as an appropriate task for occupational therapists.[8,11-16] Disruption to role performance and life satisfaction is likely when individuals incur disabilities that necessitate unwanted changes in their lifestyles, particularly individuals who experience a sudden, traumatic injury or illness. Not only must he or she deal with an immediate change in performance capacities, but the abrupt loss of one or more roles that constitute an important component of his or her self-image must also be dealt with. For example, the young male skateboarder who becomes a quadriplegic in an accident must deal not only with losing his ability to perform the activities of daily living (ADL), but also with losing his ability to participate in a major life role through which he often defined himself to others. Caregivers are also at risk of role dysfunction due to the often overwhelming demands of caring for individuals with disabilities[17] or aging parents.

Individuals may lose their sense of self when they experience role loss because the loss can undermine confidence, lead to depression and lack of motivation, degrade self-image, and ultimately block the rehabilitation process.[16] As part of the domain of occupational therapy, therapists can assist individuals in maximizing their abilities by teaching them new habits and skills so they can resume old roles or assume new ones.

Model of Human Occupation

The MOHO offers an explanation of "how occupation is motivated, patterned, and performed,"[5(p13)] which elucidates occupation in terms of volition, habituation, and performance capacity. Roles are identified as part of the phenomena of *habituation* (pattern), the term used to convey the idea of how routine, automatic behaviors are organized to flow within each individual's environments or habitats.

Kielhofner[5] identifies habits and roles as the two processes that "preserve" the strategies of action underlying the established patterns of behavior referred to as habituation. Within MOHO, habits and roles are theorized to shape much of what we do in the contexts of our social and physical environments.

Through interaction within the social environment, an individual acquires and learns the identity and behaviors associated with any number of roles. That is, the individual *internalizes a role*.[5] Specifically, Kielhofner[5] refers to the internalized role as "the incorporation of a socially and/or personally defined status and a related cluster of attitudes and actions."[5(p72)] This internalization is the development of a sense of relationship between an individual and others within the context of their environment. As an individual interacts with other people, the ease and structure of those interactions are assisted by the fact that one interacts within roles. People respond in a predictable and appropriate manner when they share a common idea of what behaviors roles prescribe. Roles facilitate appropriate action and interaction. Such role behavior patterns are identified by MOHO as *role scripts*, which provide guidelines of how to behave in specific situations within a social environment without much conscious awareness.[5] For example, when I am in a public place with my children, I will intervene immediately to stop any misconduct with either child in my role as a mother. Role scripts do not prescribe exactly what I am going to say or do, but they facilitate a swift, intuitive reaction since the role as mother has been internalized and can be enacted automatically, thereby allowing my energy and concentration to be directed at whatever else I might be doing. Others who observe my actions generally accept them as appropriate because, as members of my cultural group, they are familiar with what behaviors are expected within the role of mother. They may indicate this acceptance with some acknowledgement such as a nod or smile that further reinforces my understanding and enactment in my role as a mother. Thus, an important function of roles is to direct and/or constrain behavior. Since society depends on its members to function within roles, certain role behaviors are expected and serve to maintain social order and the cohesiveness of groups.

MOHO has identified three ways in which roles influence occupation.[5] First, roles influence the manner and style of our interactions, as well as the content. For example, in my role as mother to my son, my manner likely would be authoritative when telling him to not use his fingers while eating. While in the role of spouse, I may be more appealing or humorous when suggesting to my husband not to use his fingers. Second, roles shape the kinds of actions we do to carry out a particular role. Within a public place, it would be appropriate to verbally tell my son to quiet down if he was speaking too loudly. My action would be expected by others within a similar cultural group. Third, roles partition daily and weekly cycles into times when we ordinarily inhabit certain roles. My mother role typically is enacted in the late afternoon when assisting my children with homework, after moving in and out of worker, friend, and teacher roles during the day. Roles are tied to cyclical time, or recurrences, and by occupying parts of our daily routine they give regularity to our occupational behavior.

Finally, any given social role may have occupational, personal-sexual, or familial-social dimensions.[18] The role of mother has occupational, personal, and familial dimensions. Typically, it is the occupational dimension that is of primary concern to the occupational therapist. The occupational nature of a role is recognized when the role facilitates play, leisure, or productive behavior. The Role Checklist was developed to delineate occupational roles and to evaluate an individual's participation in and value of their particular roles.

Role Checklist

DESCRIPTION

The purpose of the Role Checklist is to assess an individual's occupational role performance, indicating an individual's role identification as well as the value that an individual attaches to his or her roles. It is a written inventory that is appropriate for adolescents, adults, and older adults with physical or psychosocial dysfunction.

Since it was designed to identify the occupational behavior of patients, the roles identified on the checklist are roles that provide opportunities to fulfill behavior within an occupational performance dimension. The 10 roles included in the checklist are student, worker, volunteer, caregiver, home maintainer, friend, family member, religious participant, hobbyist/amateur, and participant in organizations. Each of these roles is briefly described, with a reference to the frequency with which the role is enacted. These frequencies are included in the definition, since fulfilling the role should include *doing* something within the role rather than merely stating a relationship to that role. For example, being a friend establishes a relationship and, based on the feelings while doing something with a friend at least once a week, shows enactment of occupational behavior. There is also an "other" category on the checklist for the individual to identify enacted occupational roles that are not listed.

The assessment is based on self-report. Usually, it is completed as the therapist interviews a patient; however, the assessment can be completed independently by the patient. The instrument takes approximately 15 minutes to complete and consists of two parts.

In addition, a summary sheet has been developed for viewing and interpreting results more easily.

Part One asks the patient to consider each of the 10 roles listed on the Checklist as to whether they have performed each role in the past, are presently fulfilling the role, or anticipate fulfilling that role in the future. The "past" refers to any time up until the preceding week. The "present" refers to the past week (7 days), including the day of the administration of the Checklist. The "future" refers to tomorrow or any day thereafter.

Part Two asks the patient to indicate the value of each of the roles delineated in the Checklist, regardless of whether they have fulfilled the role or not. The degree to which the individual values each role is indicated by three choices: "not at all valuable," "somewhat valuable," or "very valuable."

Appendix Q is a copy of the Role Checklist as well as the directions that have been developed to standardize the administration of the Checklist.

RESEARCH AND CLINICAL USE OF THE ROLE CHECKLIST

If roles are deemed a component in the domain of occupational therapy, as they are in the *Framework*[6] under Performance Patterns, it should be addressed by occupational therapists in our diverse settings. The Role Checklist is a convenient and easy assessment tool to gather initial information about role performance. It can be utilized with individuals from adolescence to older adulthood and is not specific to any diagnostic category. The Role Checklist can be used to identify problems with continuity of role performance, specifically whether or not the patient is fulfilling the same roles in the present as he or she has in the past and plans to fulfill in the future. Other problems can also be identified. For example, the Role Checklist can illustrate visually to an individual that he or she is attempting to fulfill too many roles and is stressed by the demands of each of the roles. Additionally, since the assessment addresses the value of roles, it can be used to identify role loss that could be associated with problems of self-identity and self-esteem. With the assessment of role value, the Checklist can compare an individual's role participation and role value. Individuals who participate in roles that are not highly valued or do not participate in roles they do value may demonstrate frustration and/or lack of motivation. Contradictions between goals and current life situations or functional status may lead to occupational dysfunction. Most importantly, the completion of the Role Checklist can provide a mechanism for dialogue between therapist and patient about issues that are often difficult to articulate and define.

As a useful assessment tool for occupational therapists, the Role Checklist can be used in a variety of settings and should be presented as an important tool for the profession. It has been translated into several languages (eg, Spanish, Portuguese, French, Arabic, German, and Swedish), and although it has been developed with the MOHO, it can be used independently of the model or with other models that include role performance. Since its development, the Role Checklist has been used in research studies as a tool or methodological instrument for examining role performance. Appendix R is an annotated bibliography of many of these studies. Appendix S is an annotated bibliography of studies that specifically support the reliability and/or validity of the Role Checklist. Appendix T offers examples of papers that use the Role Checklist as an occupational therapy intervention tool.

Case Study

Doris is a 78-year-old White female who has been widowed for 4 years from her second husband. Doris has lived in a rural community for most of her adult years, moving from a three-story family home to a mobile home when she and her first husband wanted to stop climbing stairs. Doris has five grown children—two living within 10 miles, one living within a 2-hour drive, and two living in different states. All of them but her oldest son are in regular contact; the rest have maintained good relations with their mother and siblings. Doris was married to her first husband Frank for almost 50 years when he died from a sudden heart attack. Within a year of his death, Doris married George, a good friend of both Doris and Frank. That was a happy marriage until his death 4 years ago.

Doris's background is German; she is 5 feet, 11 inches tall, and has been overweight most of her adult life. She never had diabetes, but she has had high blood pressure since her early 40s and osteoarthritis since her 50s. Over the past 25 years, she has had three hip replacements, one being replaced when it wore out a few years ago. She has also had a knee replacement. Recovery from all these surgeries has been difficult due to her size. Additionally, during the knee replacement Doris suffered a minor stroke and had severe "sun-downing" effects. The doctor reported to her daughter that "we almost lost her on the table." Doris also has a frozen right shoulder that significantly impacts her ability to reach, but she has refused surgery to replace the joint due to the slow recovery from prior surgeries. Doris needs canes and/or a walker to walk. Unfortunately, due to stomach ailments, Doris is very limited in choices of arthritis medications and therefore has chronic pain in her joints, limiting her mobility.

Over the past 3 years, Doris recognized that she needed to consider moving from the country to some form of retirement community. With only a small pension and Social Security income, she put herself on the list of a church run retirement home in a nearby city that has independent apartments as well as a skilled nursing facility. The waiting list was 2 years. In the meantime, Doris sold her mobile home and moved to an apartment in the country until her apartment at the home was available.

Doris continues to drive, although she limits herself to only back roads or city blocks with which she is familiar. She has short-term memory deficits from the stroke, which she recognizes and becomes frustrated with when she cannot remember something. She likes to paint, read, scrapbook, do crossword puzzles, and watch television. She used to knit, but now finds that too hard on her vision and arthritic fingers. Doris has always liked to travel, but due to her decreased mobility, she limits her travels to shopping trips, church, and visits to friends or family. However, even this is limited because steps have become more difficult for her to negotiate and both her children who live nearby have significant steps to their homes.

Doris recently moved into the retirement apartment. She misses having a porch to sit on in the country and is not used to so many neighbors. Doris is very involved with her church, but it is at least 15 miles away in the country, not close to her new location. Doris has been depressed, frustrated with her limitations, and has decreased use of her right arm since her move. She was referred to an occupational therapist by her general physician, to be seen at the skilled nursing facility within her retirement community as an outpatient. One of the assessments was the Role Checklist. Table 16-1 is a summary of the results.

Table 16-1
Role Checklist Summary Sheet

DATE: June 2005

NAME: Doris Ross   AGE: 78

Sex: ☐ Male   ☑ Female   Retired: ☑ Yes   ☐ No

Martial Status: ☐ Single ☐ Married ☐ Separated ☐ Divorced ☑ Widowed

Overview	Perceived Incumbency			Value Designation		
Role	Past	Present	Future	Not At All	Somewhat	Very
Student	✓			✓		
Worker	✓			✓		
Volunteer	✓		✓		✓	
Caregiver	✓		✓		✓	
Home maintainer	✓	✓	✓		✓	
Friend	✓		✓			✓
Family member	✓	✓	✓			✓
Religious partici-pant	✓		✓			✓
Hobbyist/Amateur	✓		✓			✓
Participant in organizations	✓			✓		
Other _____						

COMMENTS

The occupational therapist collaborated with Doris on activities and exercises to increase the functional abilities of her right arm. Additionally, the therapist evaluated Doris within her living space to ensure that Doris was able to complete her ADLs independently. Doris needed assistance with some of her dressing because she cannot reach back to pull up zippers or attach a bra in the back. Together, the therapist and Doris devised methods to get a bra with a front attachment. The occupational therapist also helped Doris organize her small kitchen to accommodate the items she would need on the shelves she could reach. Doris already had a raised toilet seat, arm rails and hand grips in the bathroom, and was independent in bathing and toileting.

The Role Checklist showed that Doris highly valued the roles of friend, family member, religious participant, and hobbyist. She had all these roles in the past; however, she only continued to participate as a family member, as her children continued to check in on her in the new setting. It was clear that her participation in the occupations of friendship, religious participant, and hobbyist had been disrupted by either the move to the new apartment or her decreasing abilities. The occupational therapist talked to Doris about her hobbies. Doris was a painter but had not been able to paint in her new apartment as there was no area to set up her materials. Together, the therapist and Doris found a spot that could be cleared in her bedroom and organized the area so that Doris would be able to leave her paints out so she could participate in this occupation on a daily basis. Doris had been overwhelmed with the move and had decided she could no longer visit friends or go to her church. The therapist worked with Doris in determining how she could maintain contact with her friends at both her church and from her prior living environment. In contacting the church members, there was support from members who would come to pick up Doris if she would no longer be able to drive. Just the knowledge of this support assisted Doris in adjusting to the move and understanding that she would be able to continue to participate in the roles of friend and religious participant. The therapist also helped Doris review the activity schedule of the retirement center. Doris was delighted to find out there was a church service every Thursday night as well as a community meal that was offered once a week.

In this case, the occupational therapist used a bottom-up approach to address mobility issues with Doris's right arm, but used a top-down approach in determining what occupations were important to her. This ensured that she was able to participate in her chosen occupations and showed her how she could maintain or improve her quality of life after moving to a totally new environment. The Role Checklist was used to facilitate the conversation between patient and therapist.

Summary

This chapter summarizes the concept of roles in occupational therapy, specifically within the MOHO. The Role Checklist, a clinical assessment developed under the model, is described. The Role Checklist was designed as a response to the need to assess the roles of occupational therapy patients efficiently and effectively. The written inventory identifies a respondent's perceived role participation and the degree to which each role is valued along a temporal continuum that includes 10 predefined roles. Information gathered from the instrument can be used to help in patient assessment in terms of role participation, valuation of roles, role balance, and future orientation.

Appendices R, S, and T illustrate reliability and validity studies of the Role Checklist, research that have used the Role Checklist in their methodology, and papers describing how the Role Checklist is used clinically. Although the numbers of these studies and descriptions are numerous, further research is needed. Reliability studies with patient populations are needed, as well as other concurrent validity studies with other role assessment tools or occupational performance instruments. Studies demonstrating the usefulness of the instrument with other groups of patients, including minority groups, would be valuable. Finally, long-term studies would be useful to determine whether using the Checklist in occupational therapy treatment does indeed predict future role performance or the preparation to enter new roles.

References

1. Oakley F. The Model of Human Occupation in Psychiatry [unpublished master's degree project]. Richmond, VA: Department of Occupational Therapy, Medical College of Virginia, Virginia Commonwealth University; 1982.
2. Kielhofner G, Burke J. Conceptual framework and content, part 1. A model of human occupation. *Am J Occup Ther.* 1980;34:572-581.
3. Kielhofner G, Burke J. Components and determinants of human occupation. In: Kielhofner G, ed. *A Model of Human Occupation.* Baltimore, MD: Williams & Wilkins; 1985:12-36.
4. Kielhofner G. *A Model of Human Occupation: Theory and Application.* 2nd ed. Baltimore, MD: Williams & Wilkins; 1995:71-72.
5. Kielhofner G. *A Model of Human Occupation: Theory and Application.* 3rd ed. Baltimore, MD: Williams & Wilkins; 1995:63-80.
6. American Occupational Therapy Association. Occupational therapy practice framework: domain and process. *Am J Occup Ther.* 2002:609-639.
7. Brånholm I, Fugl-Meyer AR. Occupational role preference and life satisfaction. OTJR. 1992;2:159-171.
8. Duellman MK, Barris R, Kielhofner G. Organized activity and the adaptive status of nursing home residents. *Am J Occup Ther.* 1986;40:618-622.
9. Gregory MD. Occupational behavior and life satisfaction among retirees. *Am J Occup Ther.* 1983;37:548-553.
10. Smith NR, Kielhofner G, Watts JH. The relationship between the volition, activity pattern & life satisfaction in the elderly. *Am J Occup Ther.* 1986;40:278-283.
11. Heard C. Occupational role acquisition. *Am J Occup Ther.* 1977;31:243-247.
12. Hallett JD, Zasler ND, Maurer P, Cash S. Role change after traumatic brain injury in adults. *Am J Occup Ther.* 1994;48:241-246.
13. Kielhofner G, Harlan B, Bauer D, Maurer P. The reliability of historical interview with physically disabled respondents. *Am J Occup Ther.* 1986;40:551-556.
14. Matsutsuyu J. Occupational behavior—a perspective on work and play. *Am J Occup Ther.* 1971;25:291-294.
15. Rogers JC, Holm MB. Occupational therapy diagnostic reason: a component of clinical reasoning. *Am J Occup Ther.* 1991;45:1045-1053.
16. Versluys H. Remediation of role disorders through focused group work. *Am J Occup Ther.* 1980;34:609-614.
17. Frosch S, Gruber A, Jones C, et al. The long term effects of traumatic brain injury on the roles of caregivers. *Brain Injury.* 1997;11:891-906.
18. Oakley F, Kielhofner G, Barris R, Reichler RK. The Role Checklist: development and empirical assessment of reliability. *OTJR.* 1986;6:157-170.

PART VI:
BIOLOGICAL AND SPIRITUAL
ASSESSMENTS

OT-QUEST ASSESSMENT

Emily Schulz, PhD, OTR/L, CFLE

"…theory is all-important in helping a therapist decide what to do…when therapists use theory, they must establish a link between the general concepts and postulates made by the theory and the specific client or client group to whom they are providing services. This process…is aided by a technology for application. This technology aids therapists to make the link between theory and practice by providing specific tools, procedures, and examples." Koenig HG, McCullough ME, Larson DB. Handbook of Religion and Health. *New York, NY: Oxford University Press; 2001.*

Introduction

This chapter will first offer a definition of spirituality for occupational therapy and explore the role of spirituality in occupational therapy intervention. A spirituality assessment tool for occupational therapy practice—The OT-QUEST—will be presented, including the history of its development, reliability and validity, rationale, administration, and scoring; along with a case study illustrating its use. Finally, a discussion of the tool's strengths and limitations, and suggestions for future research will be provided.

Literature Review

General interest in spirituality and its use in health care has been on the rise.[1-5] Studies have been conducted demonstrating the positive impact of spirituality, faith, and religion on the physical, mental, and emotional health issues of persons with a variety of conditions.[6-10] In the occupational therapy literature addressing spirituality, the focus has primarily been on exploring the term as it relates to occupation[11-21] or investigating its role in practice.[2,22-27] The next section of this chapter will first offer a definition of spirituality for occupational therapy along with a three-dimensional model, followed by a discussion of the role of spirituality in occupational therapy.

DEFINITION OF SPIRITUALITY

Through a review of the literature, it becomes apparent that spirituality is a multi-dimensional construct.[4,28] First, to clarify an issue that is often raised, spirituality and religion are not the same thing, although they can overlap for some people.[29] Koenig, McCollough, and Larson, who have researched religion and health extensively,[30] differentiate between spirituality and religion. They explain that *spirituality*, when compared to religion, is "individualistic, less visible and measurable, less formal, less orthodox, less systematic, emotionally oriented, inward directed, not authoritarian, [as having] little accountability, and ... [being] unifying, not doctrine oriented."[30(p18)] They describe *religion*, in contrast, as "community focused, observable, measurable, objective, formal, orthodox, organized, behavior oriented, [having] outward practices, [being] authoritarian in terms of behaviors, and [having] a doctrine separating good from evil."[30(p18)] In summary, religion, when compared to spirituality, appears to be more concerned with rules and rituals, while spirituality focuses more on personal meaning and the experience of unity.[29,30]

When describing spirituality in the literature, most health care professions seem to focus on the quality of unity or connectedness as a main characteristic of the term.[4,31-41] Connectedness, according to the literature, can be to the self,[31] others,[31,33,35,38,41] the world,[33,35,41] and the divine as well.[33,38,41]

Occupational therapy literature, because of the profession's unique attention to meaningful occupation, seems to concentrate on the expressive aspect of spirituality when discussing its nature.[11-21,42,43] According to the occupational therapy literature, the expression of one's of spirituality can manifest through a person's reflections,[17,18,21,43] narratives,[16,20] and actions.[12-15,19]

Finally, because human beings are embodied on a physical plane of existence (rather than on some ethereal realm, for instance), the natural laws of physics apply to us, including those of linear time.[44] While there are some theories in quantum physics[45,46] and metaphysics[47] in which time and physical matter are viewed as illusions—for those rare individuals in an enlightened state, for example—most humans beings, including most occupational therapy patients, have not achieved such a state and therefore are still subject to the laws of physics and linear time.

The definition offered in this chapter is for the majority of human beings rather than those who are enlightened, as the enlightened most likely will not require occupational therapy services. For the majority of humanity, it is through the act of existing on the physical plane, with its confines of linear and historical/cultural time and physical/societal barriers and facilitators,[48] that a demand for mastery[49,50] and an opportunity for the human spirit to shine forth and evolve[51] are created.

Indeed, Adolf Meyer stated that it is humankind's ability to remember the past, recognize and use the present moment, and realize that there is a future to plan for that separates us as a species from the rest of the animal kingdom.[52] In fact, it is during the present moment that a state of flow can occur for a person engaged in a meaningful creative occupation.[53,54]

Therefore, taking into consideration the literature, a definition of spirituality for occupational therapy is: *experiencing a meaningful connection to our core selves, other beings, the world, and/or a greater power, as expressed through our reflections, narratives, and actions, within the context of space and time.* This definition is illustrated in Figure 17-1.

In the model depicted in Figure 17-1, spirituality as a whole is viewed as a mystery. The model can be used to portray a person's spirituality in a moment in time or a person's spiritual evolutionary process across linear time. The three dimensions of spirituality

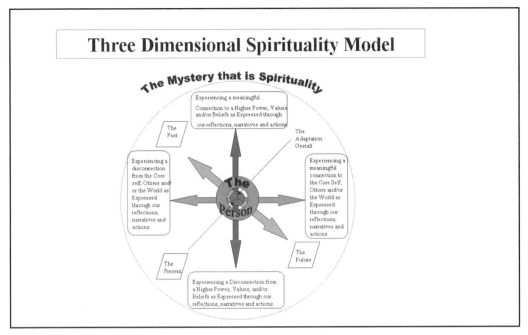

Figure 17-1. Three Dimensional Spirituality Model.

illuminated in the model are the vertical element (on a continuum from connectedness to disconnectedness to a greater power, which includes the divine, values, and beliefs); the horizontal element (on a continuum from connectedness to disconnectedness to self, others, and the world); and the temporal element (past, present, and future). The individual person is in the center of the model and holistically adapts to challenges in life[49-50] across linear time, and as this occurs, may change in levels of connectedness/disconnectedness to the vertical and horizontal aspects of spirituality. The model is fluid and dynamic.[51]

Figures 17-2 through 17-5 illustrate examples of types of people at the extremes of the four quadrants of the model in a snapshot of time for the purpose of clarifying how the model works: high connectedness to both vertical and horizontal elements (Figure 17-2), high connectedness to the horizontal element with high disconnectedness to the vertical element (Figure 17-3), high disconnectedness to both the vertical and horizontal elements (Figure 17-4), and high disconnectedness to the horizontal element with high connectedness to the vertical element (Figure 17-5). These are merely examples, as most likely the majority of humans do not fall into the extremes, nor do people necessarily stay in one quadrant, due to the dynamic nature of the model across linear time as previously mentioned.

THE ROLE OF SPIRITUALITY IN OCCUPATIONAL THERAPY

Many occupational therapy scholars have questioned the role of spirituality in the profession.[4,22,23,25,27] After all, occupational therapists are not clergy, nor are they trained to be clergy. In fact, even though most occupational therapists value highly their own spirituality, many have not been trained on how to address spirituality in practice.[22] It is definitely not the role of the occupational therapist to proselytize, attempt to convert, or

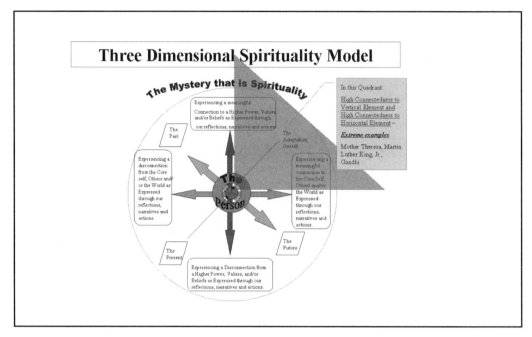

Figure 17-2. Quadrant 1—High Connectedness to Vertical Element and High Connectedness to Horizontal Element.

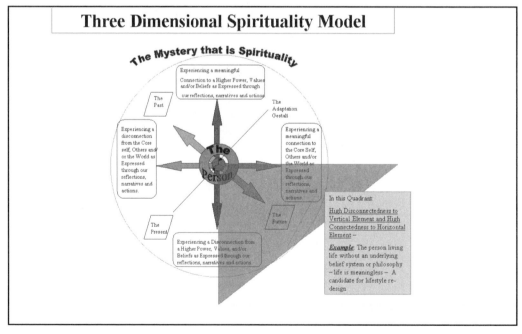

Figure 17-3. Quadrant 2—High Disconnectedness to Vertical Element and High Connectedness to Horizontal Element.

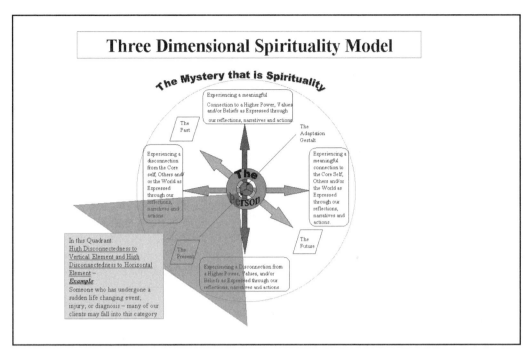

Figure 17-4. Quadrant 3—High Disconnectedness to Vertical Element and High Disconnectedness to Horizontal Element.

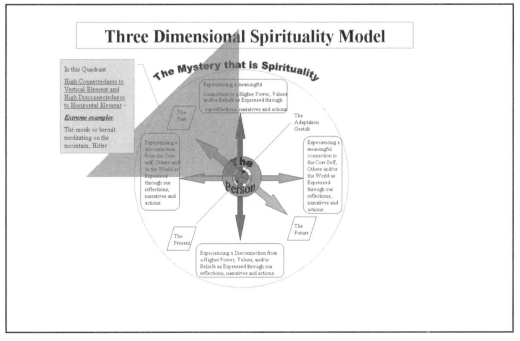

Figure 17-5. Quadrant 4—High Connectedness to Vertical Element and High Disconnectedness to Horizontal Element.

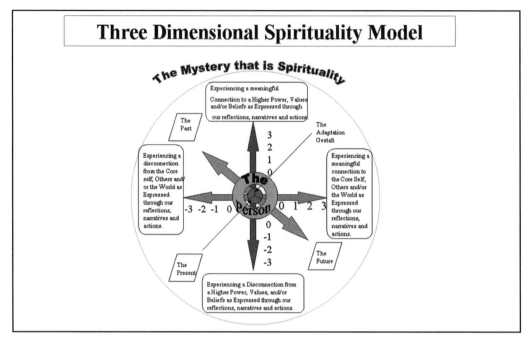

Figure 17-6. Three Dimensional Spirituality Model with Numbers Included to Quantify Levels of Connectedness to Vertical and Horizontal Elements.

otherwise coerce a patient into embracing the therapist's own spiritual or religious beliefs. And for patients who are in a spiritual crisis or need spiritual counseling, after actively listening to him or her, it is appropriate for the occupational therapist to refer the patient to a chaplain or clergy member of that patient's faith, rather than trying to counsel the patient.[51] That being said, what are suitable boundaries to adhere to when approaching the issue of spirituality in practice? This is a legitimate question, and is best addressed by remembering our profession's domain of concern: facilitating the engagement of people in their meaningful occupations for optimum participation in their environments.[48]

According to the *Occupational Therapy Practice Framework*, spirituality is, at its most basic level, about the essential underlying foundation that provides meaning in life for human beings.[48] Therefore, if we tap into our patients' spirituality, we can discover what is meaningful to them, and thus collaboratively create treatment goals, plans, and interventions that are client-centered and have the potential to be truly powerful, healing, and transformative.[51,55] By facilitating the engagement of patients in the occupations or outward manifestations of their spirituality or faith (or their values or beliefs, for nonreligious people), occupational therapists can address spirituality in a way that is ethically sound and within the domain of the profession.

USING THE DEFINITION OF SPIRITUALITY AND SPIRITUALITY MODEL TO GUIDE CLINICAL REASONING

Perhaps the above point can best be illustrated by Figure 17-6 and Table 17-1. Figure 17-6 is the now-familiar three-dimensional model of spirituality with the addition of numbers on a continuum from -3 to +3 for both the vertical elements and the horizontal elements. Table 17-1 is a grid-like structure that can be used to guide the therapist's thinking when using the model in practice with a patient. The grid in Table 17-1 has not been

Table 17-1

Spirituality Model Assessment Grid

Spirituality Concept	Past	Present	Future	How?	Why?	Goals?
Level of Connectedness to Self	Level ___	Level ___	Level ___			
High connectedness = 3						
Moderate connectedness = 2						
Low connectedness = 1						
Neutral = 0						
Low disconnectedness = -1						
Moderate disconnectedness = -2						
High disconnectedness = -3						
Level of Connectedness to Others	Level ___	Level ___	Level ___			
High connectedness = 3						
Moderate connectedness = 2						
Low connectedness = 1						
Neutral = 0						
Low disconnectedness = -1						
Moderate disconnectedness = -2						
High disconnectedness = -3						
Level of Connectedness to the World	Level ___	Level ___	Level ___			
High connectedness = 3						
Moderate connectedness = 2						
Low connectedness = 1						
Neutral = 0						
Low disconnectedness = -1						
Moderate disconnectedness = -2						
High disconnectedness = -3						

Table 17-1, continued

Spirituality Model Assessment Grid

Spirituality Concept	Past	Present	Future	How?	Why?	Goals?
Level of Connectedness to a Greater Power High connectedness = 3 Moderate connectedness = 2 Low connectedness = 1 Neutral = 0 Low disconnectedness = -1 Moderate disconnectedness = -2 High disconnectedness = -3	Level _____	Level _____	Level _____			
Total Scores						
Horizontal Element (add self, others, and world scores and divide by 3)	Horizontal Element:	Horizontal Element:	Horizontal Element:			
Vertical Element (Greater Power score)	Vertical Element:	Vertical Element:	Vertical Element:			

tested in practice nor has it been researched for validity and reliability; it is simply a tool to help readers understand more fully the definition of spirituality and the three-dimensional model presented in this chapter.

To start with, a therapist wanting to broach the topic of spirituality with a patient for the first time can begin by saying something like, "Sometimes it helps people receiving services if we include spirituality in our interventions. I know spirituality is a personal topic and I was wondering if I could ask you some questions about yours to help me to better help you." If the person gives consent, then the therapist can ask a patient to reflect on and rate how connected he or she felt to self before receiving services (on a scale from -3 to +3); how he or she feels regarding connectedness to self now, and how he or she wants to feel in terms of connectedness to self in the future. The therapist can ask the following questions:

- "Why do you think you felt (feel) that way?"
- "How did you connect to yourself in the past?"
- "How do you want to connect to yourself in the future?"

From this kind of discussion with the person, client-centered collaborative goals and treatment plans can be written for the aspect of spirituality related to connectedness to the self. This same process can be repeated for the other aspects of connectedness to others, the world, and a greater ower, across linear time.

Rationale for the OT-QUEST

Now that spirituality has been defined, the next section of this chapter will focus on the OT-QUEST itself. The OT-QUEST was developed to meet a perceived need for a structured way to address spirituality in clinical practice. Persons with disabilities have stated that they would like their spirituality to be included when receiving rehabilitation services.[55] The *Framework* includes the spiritual context in the scope of practice for the profession.[48] However, before intervention can be provided, assessment must be done. Assessment tools were needed to be developed to appropriately measure and address spirituality in health care.[9] While there are spirituality assessments available for different professions, such as the Spiritual Health in Four Domains Index (SH4DI),[56] the Spiritual Well-Being Scale (SWBS),[57] and the Spiritual Experience Index–Revised (SEI-R),[58,59] the OT-QUEST is a spirituality assessment tool that offers therapists a way to assess spirituality that is specifically designed by an occupational therapist and for occupational therapy practice.

HISTORY AND DEVELOPMENT OF THE OT-QUEST

The first edition of the OT-QUEST was developed by the author as an assignment in an assessment course in the doctoral program at Texas Woman's University. It is based on Collins' Model,[60] and the Occupational Adaptation Frame of Reference.[49,50] The questions in the instrument were developed based on those models and modified after receiving feedback from an expert in the field. The first edition was comprised of 11 visual analog questions to gather quantitative data and 12 sentence completion questions to retrieve qualitative information from the participants. It was pilot tested as an anonymous survey in 1999 with a nonclinical population (n = 41). Participants were primarily Caucasian women ages 18 to 55. With one item removed, the OT-QUEST scored a Cronbach's alpha of .71, and factor analysis revealed four noncorrelated factors.

Table 17-2

Demographics of Older Adults With Low Vision

Gender

Category	N	%
Male	14	31%
Female	31	69%

Race

Category	N	%
White	35	78%
Black	10	22%

Marital Status

Category	N	%
Married	18	40%
Single	5	11%
Divorced	7	16%
Widowed	15	33%

Education

Category	N	%
< than 12th grade	16	36%
Graduated 12th grade	9	20%
Some college	10	22%
College degree	7	16%
Graduate degree	3	7%

Employment Status

Category	N	%
Retired	39	87%
Working	2	4%
Disability	4	9%

Income

Category	N	%
< $20,000	25	60%
$20,000-$39,000	11	26%
> = $40,000	6	14%

Medical Conditions[a]

Category	N	%
Arthritis	16	36%
Hypertension	15	33%
Cardiovascular disease	11	24%
Diabetes	8	18%
Hearing problems	6	13%
Balance problems	3	7%
Stroke/TIA	3	7%

Ocular Conditions[a]

Category	N	%
Cataract	35	78%
AMD	27	60%
Glaucoma	10	22%
Scotoma	10	22%
Diabetic retinopathy	6	13%
Hemianopsia	3	7%
Stargardt's disease	1	2%

[a]From chart audit

Depressive Symptoms (CESD)[b]

Mean Score	SD
17.56	7.98

Cognitive Status (SPMSQ)[c]

Mean Score	SD
0.84	0.60

[b]Score of 16-18+ = Possible depression

[c]Subjects had intact cognition

Table 17-2, continued
Demographics of Older Adults With Low Vision

Visual Functioning (NEI-VFQ)[d]

Category	Mean Score	SD
General health	36.67	27.49
General vision	30.67	17.37
Ocular pain	75.56	23.07
Near vision	30.28	23.74
Distance vision	37.41	26.06
Social functioning	54.72	29.83
Mental health	44.72	25.56
Role difficulties	31.94	26.99
Well-being/Distress	43.33	34.75
Driving[e]	95.83	36.71
Color vision	69.44	33.24
Peripheral vision	46.02	29.99

[d]Higher Score (1-100) = better functioning
[e]Only driving subjects responded to this item

Expectations and Goals: Areas for Treatment[a]

Activities of daily living
Communication device use
Community mobility
Financial management
Functional mobility
Home establishment and management
Improve vision/visual perception
Leisure
Meal preparation
Personal hygiene
Shopping
Social participation

[a]From chart audit

Research, Validity, and Reliability of the OT-QUEST

The OT-QUEST was modified for the second edition in order to make the instrument more specific in its wording. The resulting revised OT-QUEST includes 14 Likert scale questions and 15 open-ended questions. A Likert scale was used instead of a visual analog scale in the second edition to ease administration and scoring. A study was conducted in 2005 to determine the test-retest reliability, construct validity, and internal consistency of the second edition of the OT-QUEST with older adults with low vision.

Patients with low vision, aged 50+, were recruited from a clinic for this study (Table 17-2).

The intended design for this study was to recruit 120 subjects; however, due to time constraints, and a drop in clientele at the clinic, doing so was problematic. The study design called for two telephone interviews to be conducted prior to the subjects' first visit to the clinic to avoid bias. The second interview occurred 1 to 2 weeks after the first interview. However, some subjects only responded to the first survey; others changed appointment dates and could not be interviewed for the follow-up, resulting in a small n = 45. In the first interview, eight surveys were given: a demographic survey, then the OT-QUEST, followed by the SH4DI,[56] SWBS,[57] and the SEI-R[58,59] to ascertain the OT-QUEST's construct validity. Those surveys were followed by several others: The Center for Epidemiologic Studies Depression Scale (CESD),[61] which measured subjects' depressive symptoms; The National Eye Institute Visual Function Questionnaire (NEI-VFQ),[62] which addressed their visual functioning; and The Short Portable Mental Status Questionnaire (SPMSQ),[63] which measured their cognitive status. For the second interview, subjects only responded to the OT-QUEST to determine its test-retest reliability. A chart audit was done after the subjects attended the low vision clinic for the first time as new patients.

Results of the study indicated that the OT-QUEST had strong, significant test-retest reliability (Spearman's Correlation = .57; $p < .0001$) for items on the Likert scale, and moderate concurrence in the themes from the sentence completion questions (50% to 72%). It had significant moderate construct validity with the SWBS[57] (Spearman's Correlation = .35; $p = .0178$) and with the SH4DI56 (Spearman's Correlation = 0.34; $p = .0206$). Construct validity was nonsignificant and weak with the SEI-R[58,59] (Spearman's Correlation = -.22; $p = .1566$). Internal consistency was also weak (overall Cronbach's alpha = .68); Cronbach's alpha ranged from .59 to .70 for the six factors (Spiritual = .70, Being = .65, Meaning = .59, Expression = .65, Intention = .64, and Adaptation = .62).

Administration and Scoring

The next part of this chapter will describe the administration and scoring of the OT-QUEST. A case study will be presented also to illustrate how to score the instrument.

HOW THE TOOL IS ADMINISTERED

The OT-QUEST can be administered as a paper-and-pencil survey, or as 15 to 20 minute interview.

What Concepts Are Being Measured

The concepts measured by the OT-QUEST are the Five Key Factors within the person that relate to spirituality and quality of experience as found in Collins' Model[60]: Spiritual, Being, Meaning, Intention, and Expression; and also Adaptation as found in the Occupational Adaptation Frame of Reference.[49,50] Collins' Model[60] states that if people are having good quality of experience in their lives, then their spiritual selves are also well. According to Collins, evidence of patients having healthy spirituality becomes apparent to therapists if those patients exhibit the following qualities: positive renewal and acceptance (Spiritual Factor), awareness and understanding (Being Factor), purpose and discovery (Meaning Factor), motivation and will (Intention Factor), and exploration and causation (Expression Factor).[60] Collins developed questions for each of the Five Key Factors and their subcomponents.[60] Those questions were modified slightly in wording for the first edition of the OT-QUEST and some were expanded in the second edition for clarity. A question about adaptation and spirituality was included in the tool to measure whether spirituality was a factor when adapting to challenges for persons responding to the tool.

How Concepts Are Measured

As stated previously, the second edition of the OT-QUEST is comprised of 14 Likert scale questions (on a 5-point scale) and 15 open-ended questions.

HOW TO SCORE THE OT-QUEST

There are two to three Likert Scale questions for each of the Five Key Factors[60] and one item for Adaptation.[49,50] The mean score for the items for each Key Factor and the one score for the Adaptation item are used in scoring the Likert scale section; a range is set for low, medium, and high mean scores. An overall mean score is also calculated. A low overall score or a low score for one of the Five Key Factors indicates that the person may be struggling with spirituality and quality of experience in general (in the case of the overall score), or with that particular issue (in the case of the Factor). Further information about the Five Key Factors and Adaptation comes to light through the sentence completion section of the instrument, as those items closely relate to the Likert Scale questions. The sentence completion questions are not scored in a traditional sense; however, general themes can be written down to summarize issues the patient is having. Those themes are divided under two categories on the score sheet: Facilitators and Barriers.

GOAL WRITING USING THE OT-QUEST

Goal writing should be collaborative and client-centered and flow naturally from the findings of the assessment. It should be done in a collaborative conversation with the patient.

Case Study

T. L. is a woman in her 40s with three grown children who live out of state. She is currently living in the Midwest after recently moving from another part of the United States. She is going through a second divorce. She is recovering from a hairline ® hip fracture after a fall down the stairs and has Crohn's disease. She is having difficulty adjusting to her new living situation and is experiencing reactionary depression. She does not consider herself religious, but does consider herself to be spiritual and feels a strong connection to angelic beings. She enjoys doing crafts, volunteering to take care of babies with AIDS, and participating in the Society for Creative Anachronism; however, because of a series of traumatic events in her life over the past 4 years (death of family member, loss of two homes, divorce, bankruptcy, recent relocation to another state, stressful job), she no longer does these things. She completed the OT-QUEST as a survey. Her responses on the tool and scoring are shown in Table 17-3. Goal writing was completed in collaboration with her.

Table 17-3

T.L.'s Responses to the OT-QUEST

OT Quality of Experience-Spirituality Assessment Tool (OT-QUEST)

Instructions: Circle or state your response to each question.
(Note: T.L.'s responses are in brackets).

1. How important is an experience of inner peace to you?

1	2	3	4	[5]
Not at all important	Not very important	Somewhat important	Very important	Extremely important

2. Do you usually feel good about yourself?

1	2	[3]	4	5
Never	Rarely	Sometimes	Most of the time	Always

3. Do you regularly take the time to meet your own needs?

1	2	[3]	4	5
Never	Rarely	Sometimes	Most of the time	Always

4. How do you usually feel about the actions you have taken?

1	2	[3]	4	5
Not at all positive	Not very positive	Somewhat positive	Very positive	Extremely positive

5. How do you usually feel about the decisions you have made?

1	2	[3]	4	5
Not at all positive	Not very positive	Somewhat positive	Very positive	Extremely positive

6. Do you value being engaged in doing something?

1	2	3	4	[5]
Never	Rarely	Sometimes	Most of the time	Always

7. Is it important to you to express yourself in a manner that is uniquely you?

1	2	3	4	[5]
Not at all important	Not very important	Somewhat important	Very important	Extremely important

continued

Table 17-3, continued
T.L.'s Responses to the OT-QUEST

8. Does the physical environment around you have an impact on your ability to express yourself to the fullest degree possible?

1	2	3	[4]	5
No impact at all	Not a very strong impact	Somewhat of an impact	Very strong impact	Extremely strong impact

9. Do the people around you have an impact on your ability to express yourself to the fullest degree possible?

1	2	3	[4]	5
No impact at all	Not a very strong impact	Somewhat of an impact	Very strong impact	Extremely strong impact

10. Is it important to you to plan ahead what you will do in life?

1	2	[3]	4	5
Not at all important	Not very important	Somewhat important	Very important	Extremely important

11. How easy is it for you to follow through with plans?

1	2	3	[4]	5
Not at all easy	Not very easy	Somewhat easy	Very easy	Extremely easy

12. How easy is it for you to stay interested in an activity?

1	2	3	4	[5]
Not at all easy	Not very easy	Somewhat easy	Very easy	Extremely easy

13. Does spirituality have an important role in how you adapt to change?

1	2	3	4	[5]
Not at all important	Not very important	Somewhat important	Very important	Extremely important

14. How valuable is spirituality to you?

1	2	3	4	[5]
Not at all valuable	Not very valuable	Somewhat valuable	Very valuable	Extremely valuable

continued

Table 17-3, continued
T.L.'s Responses to the OT-QUEST

Instructions: Please finish the following sentences as briefly or as thoroughly as you wish. (Note: T.L.'s responses are in all caps.)

15. Spirituality to me is A PART OF MY LIFE.

16. I experience inner peace when I'M LISTENING TO MUSIC.

17. I feel most positive about myself when I CREATE SOMETHING.

18. I am best able to pay attention to my own needs when EVERYTHING IS QUIET.

19. I feel best about what I do when I'M THINKING POSITIVELY.

20. I feel best about my decisions when I GET POSITIVE FEEDBACK.

21. I am most engaged in an activity when MY MIND IS INVOLVED.

22. I am most able to express myself in my own unique way when COMMUNICATION IS EASY.

23. I am most able to express myself when the physical environment ALLOWS ME TO USE MY HANDS.

24. When I plan for the future I — THAT'S NOT SOMETHING I DO.

25. I am able to follow through with plans when I WRITE THEM DOWN.

26. I am able to stay interested in an activity when MY MIND IS ENGAGED.

27. When going through a difficult change or transition in my life, I usually adapt by GOING TO MY SPIRITUALITY.

28. I would define spirituality as THE WHOLE OF MY BEING AND MY ANGELS AROUND ME.

continued

Table 17-3, continued

T.L.'s Responses to the OT-QUEST

Factor	Likert Scale Questions	Add Scores	Divide by	Factor Score (Average)	LOW (Score of 1.0-2.3)	MEDIUM (Score of 2.4-3.7)	HIGH (Score of 3.8-5.0)
1. Spiritual (Renewal and Acceptance)	1 &14 1. How important is an experience of inner peace to you? 14. How valuable is spirituality to you?	Q1_5_ + Q14_5_	2	Factor 1 Score: _5_			X
2. Being (Awareness and Understanding)	2 & 3 2. Do you usually feel good about yourself? 3. Do you regularly take the time to meet your own needs?	Q2_3_ + Q3_3_	2	Factor 2 Score: _3_		X	
3. Meaning (Purpose and Discovery)	4, 5, & 6 4. How do you usually feel about the actions you have taken? 5. How do you usually feel about the decisions you have made? 6. Do you value being engaged in doing something?	Q4_3_ + Q5_3_ + Q6_5_	3	Factor 3 Score: _3.66_		X	

continued

Table 17-3, continued

T.L.'s Responses to the OT-QUEST

Factor	Likert Scale Questions	Add Scores	Divide by	Factor Score (Average)	LOW (Score of 1.0-2.3)	MEDIUM (Score of 2.4-3.7)	HIGH (Score of 3.8-5.0)
4. Expression (Exploration and Causation)	7, 8, & 9 7. Is it important to you to express yourself in a manner that is uniquely you? 8. Does the physical environment around you have an impact on your ability to express yourself to the fullest degree possible? 9. Do the people around you have an impact on your ability to express yourself to the fullest degree possible?	Q7 _5_ + Q8 _4_ + Q9 _4_	3	Factor 4 Score: _4.33_			X
5. Intention (Motivation and Will)	10, 11, & 12 10. Is it important to you to plan ahead what you will do in life? 11. How easy is it for you to follow through with plans? 12. How easy is it for you to stay interested in an activity?	Q10 _3_ + Q11 _4_ + Q12 _5_	3	Factor 5 Score: _4_			X

continued

Table 17-3, continued

T.L.'s Responses to the OT-QUEST

Factor	Likert Scale Questions	Add Scores	Divide by	Factor Score (Average)	LOW (Score of 1.0-2.3)	MEDIUM (Score of 2.4-3.7)	HIGH (Score of 3.8-5.0)
6. Adaptation (Spirituality and Adaptation)	13 13. Does spirituality have an important role in how you adapt to change?	Q13 _5_	1	Factor 6 Score: _5_			X
TOTAL	Add: Factor Scores 1-6 (1 _+2_ _+3_ _+4_ _+5_ _+6_) = 5 + 3 + 3.66 + 4.33 +4 + 5 = 21.99	******	6	TOTAL SCORE: 21.99	LOW (5 -13.3)	MEDIUM (13.4-21.8)	HIGH (21.9-30)

continued

Table 17-3, continued

T.L.'s Responses to the OT-QUEST

OT-QUEST Score Sheet – Sentence Completion Questions

Instructions: Using the themes found in the OT-QUEST sentence completion questions (15-28), and collaborating with your client, fill in the spaces below.

Factor Scores From Likert Scale and Ratings	Sentence Completion Questions	Facilitators of Client's Quality of Experience/ Spirituality	Barriers to Client's Quality of Experience/ Spirituality	Goals to Address
Factor 1: Spiritual ___X___ Lo Med Hi	15, 16 & 28 15. Spirituality to me is 16. I experience inner peace when 28. I would define spirituality as	MUSIC AND WHOLE SELF, ANGELS	MAKING TIME FOR MUSIC AND SELF	1. PUT ASIDE 30 MINUTES A DAY TO WRITE OUT DAILY SCHEDULE 2. AT THE END OF DAY WRITE IF SHE DID IT OR NOT IN HER JOURNAL
Factor 2: Being ___X___ Lo Med Hi	17 & 18 17. I feel most positive about myself when 18. I am best able to pay attention to my own needs when	QUIET ENVIRONMENT CREATIVE EXPRESSION (PAINTING, WRITING, SEWING)	NOT HAVING A PLACE OF QUIET SOLITUDE AND PRIVACY NOT HAVING A PLACE TO WORK NOT CREATING TIME	1. PUT ASIDE 15 MINUTES A DAY FOR CREATIVITY 2. CLEAR A SPACE FOR BASKET OF CRAFTS MATERIALS

continued

Table 17-3, continued

T.L.'s Responses to the OT-QUEST

OT-QUEST Score Sheet – Sentence Completion Questions

Factor Scores From Likert Scale and Ratings	Sentence Completion Questions	Facilitators of Client's Quality of Experience/ Spirituality	Barriers to Client's Quality of Experience/ Spirituality	Goals to Address
Factor 3: Meaning __X__ Lo Med Hi	19, 20, & 21 19. I feel best about what I do when 20. I feel best about my decisions when 21. I am most engaged in an activity when	THINKING POSITIVELY POSITIVE FEEDBACK FROM OTHERS MIND IS INVOLVED IN ACTIVITY	GETTING NEGATIVE FEEDBACK FROM PEERS OR SOMEONE IMPORTANT BEING PUT DOWN BY OTHERS UNJUSTLY BEING INTIMIDATED WHEN TRYING TO COMPLETE A THOUGHT OR ACTIVITY	1. PRACTICE TAKING A DEEP BREATH WHEN CONFLICT IS HAPPENING FOR 5 MINUTES A DAY IN FRONT OF A MIRROR 2. ALSO WITH A TRUSTED OTHER PERSON 1/X WEEK.

continued

Table 17-3, continued

T.L.'s Responses to the OT-QUEST

OT-QUEST Score Sheet – Sentence Completion Questions

Factor Scores From Likert Scale and Ratings	Sentence Completion Questions	Facilitators of Client's Quality of Experience/ Spirituality	Barriers to Client's Quality of Experience/ Spirituality	Goals to Address
Factor 4: Expression ___X___	22 & 23 22. I am most able to express myself in my own unique way when 23. I am most able to express myself when the physical environment	EASY COMMUNICATION EXPRESSION WITH HANDS (GESTURES)	HAVING PEOPLE WHO WANT TO HAVE THEIR OWN OPINIONS HEARD RATHER THAN HEARING MINE IF ENVIRONMENT IS TOO SMALL	1. PRACTICE ASKING PEOPLE TO LISTEN ALL THE WAY THROUGH 2. ONCE A WEEK FIND A SPACIOUS ENVIRONMENT TO EXPRESS SELF 3. VOLUNTEER HELPING WITH BABIES AND HOLDING THEM 1X/MONTH
Factor 5: Intention ___X___ Lo Med Hi	24, 25, & 26 24. When I plan for the future I 25. I am able to follow through with plans when 26. I am able to stay interested in an activity when	PLANNING DAY AND JOURNALING MIND ENGAGED LEARNING NEW THINGS OR MORE ABOUT OLD THINGS SOCIETY FOR CREATIVE ANACHRONISM ENGAGES HER MIND AND LEARNING	DOES NOT PLAN BECAUSE OF MAJOR STRESS & GRIEF IN A 4-YEAR PERIOD	1. DAILY USE OF JOURNAL 2. PLAN AN ACTIVITY WITH NEW SOCIETY GROUP

continued

Table 17-3, continued

T.L.'s Responses to the OT-QUEST

OT-QUEST Score Sheet – Sentence Completion Questions

Factor Scores From Likert Scale and Ratings	Sentence Completion Questions	Facilitators of Client's Quality of Experience/ Spirituality	Barriers to Client's Quality of Experience/ Spirituality	Goals to Address
Factor 6: Adaptation X Lo Med Hi	27 27. When going through a difficult change or transition in my life, I usually adapt by	SPIRITUALITY ANGEL ALTAR PRAYER AT ALTAR	NOT MAKING TIME FOR IT	1. PUT ASIDE 10 MINUTES A DAY TO MAKE TIME FOR PRAYER AT HER ANGEL ALTAR
TOTAL SCORE: X Lo Med Hi	N/A			

In looking at T.L.'s mean overall score, she is on the low-end cusp of the high range. However, when looking at her mean scores for the Five Key Factors, her lowest score is a medium score for the Being Factor (when averaging her responses to the two questions: Do you usually feel good about yourself? and Do you regularly take the time to meet your own needs?). The themes for Facilitators and Barriers that came up for her in the Sentence Completion questions related to the Likert Scale Being Factor items (I feel most positive about myself when; and I am best able to pay attention to my own needs when) clarified why she scored lower on Being, and goals were written to help her address this Factor. This process continued for all of the Factors.

Appropriate Populations for Use of the OT-QUEST

Appropriate populations for use of the OT-QUEST are adults who are able to answer abstract questions.

Strengths and Limitations of the OT-QUEST

The OT-QUEST has yet to be trialed with patients receiving occupational therapy services, so how it translates to practice is unknown. The weak internal consistency finding in the above study is of concern; however, it may be in part a result of the small n and the small number of items per subscale. Results of the above study also indicate that the OT-QUEST is a tool with good construct validity, which means that it appears to measure what it sets out to measure. It has strong test-retest reliability, which means that over time, it elicits consistent responses from people. It also offers therapists useful quantitative and qualitative information about the spiritual aspect of the person, which has the potential to lead to meaningful treatment goals, plans, and interventions for patients.

Further Research

The low number of subjects in the reliability and validity study decreased the power of the results. Therefore, replication of the study with a larger set of subjects is suggested. Further research is also needed to ascertain to which clinical populations it is best suited and how outcomes of occupational therapy intervention would be affected by using it in clinical practice.

Acknowledgments

The author would like to thank:

Kathlyn L. Reed, PhD, OTR, FAOTA, MLIS, AHIP, Visiting Professor, Texas Woman's University-Houston Center, Houston, TX, for inspiration, mentoring, and guidance provided to the author in developing The OT-QUEST;

Cynthia Owsley, PhD, Professor of Ophthalmology at the University of Alabama at Birmingham;

Gerald McGwin Jr., PhD, Associate Professor in the School of Public Health/Trauma/Ophthalmology at the University of Alabama at Birmingham; and

Donald Fletcher, MD, Director of Low Vision Clinic in the Department of Ophthalmology at the University of Alabama at Birmingham, for mentoring and collaboration provided to the author in the reliability and validity research on the second edition of The OT-QUEST.

References

1. Congdon JG, Magilvy JK. Themes of rural health and aging from a program of research. *Geriatr Nurs.* 2001;22(5):234-8.
2. Farrar JE. Addressing spirituality and religious life in occupational therapy practice. *Physical & Occupational Therapy in Geriatrics.* 2001;18(4):65-85.
3. Pulchalski CM. Spirituality and medicine. *The World & I Journal.* 1998;13(6):180-185.
4. Ross L. The spiritual dimension: its importance to patient's health, well-being and quality of life and its implications for nursing practice. *Int J Nurs Stud.* 1995;32(5):457-468.
5. Ziegler J. Spirituality returns to the fold in medical practice. *J Natl Cancer Inst.* 1998;90:1255-1257.
6. Chibnall JT, Videen SD, Duckro PN, Miller DK. Psychosocial-spiritual correlates of death distress in patients with life-threatening medical conditions. *Palliative Medicine.* 2002;16(4):331-338.
7. Ferrell BR, Smith SL, Juarez G, Melancon C. Meaning of illness and spirituality in ovarian cancer survivors. *Oncol Nurs Forum.* 2003;30:249-257.
8. Kirby SE, Coleman PG, Daley D. Spirituality and well-being in frail and nonfrail older adults. *J Gerontol B Psychol Sci Soc Sci.* 2004;59:123-129.
9. Lowry, LW, Conco, D. Exploring the meaning of spirituality with aging adults in Appalachia. *J Holist Nurs.* 2002;20(4):388-402.
10. Touhy TA. Nurturing hope and spirituality in the nursing home. *Holist Nurs Pract.* 2001;15:45-56.
11. Algado SS, Gregori JMR, Egan M. Spirituality in a refugee camp. *Can J Occup Ther.* 1997;64:138-145.
12. Christiansen C. Nationally speaking: acknowledging a spiritual dimension in occupational therapy practice. *Am J Occup Ther.* 1997;51:169-172.
13. Egan M, DeLaat MD. The implicit spirituality of occupational therapy practice. *Can J Occup Ther.* 1997;64:115-121.
14. Frank G, Bernardo CS, Tropper S, Noguchi F, Lipman C, Maulhardt B, Weitze L. Jewish spirituality through actions in time: daily occupations of young orthodox Jewish couples in Los Angeles. *Am J Occup Ther.* 199751:199-206.
15. Howard BS, Howard JR. Occupation as spiritual activity. *Am J Occup Ther.* 1997;51:181-185.
16. Kirsh B. A narrative approach to addressing spirituality: exploring personal meaning and purpose. *Can J Occup Ther.* 1996;63:55-61.
17. Low JF. Religious orientation and pain management. *Am J Occup Ther.* 1997;51:215-219.
18. Neuhaus BE. Brief or new: including hope in occupational therapy practice: a pilot study. *Am J Occup Ther.* 1997;51:228-234.
19. Peloquin SM. Nationally speaking: the spiritual depth of occupation: making worlds and making lives. *Am J Occup Ther.* 1997;51:167-168.
20. Toomey M. Reflections on...the art of observation: reflecting on a spiritual moment. *Can J Occup Ther.* 1999;66(4):197-199.
21. Unruh AM. Spirituality and occupation: garden musings and the Himalayan blue poppy. *Can J Occup Ther.* 1997;64:156-159.
22. Collins JS, Paul S, West-Frasier J. The utilization of spirituality in occupational therapy: beliefs, practices, and perceived barriers. *Occupational Therapy in Health Care.* 2001;14(3/4):73-92.
23. Engquist DE, Short-DeGraff M, Gliner J, Oltenbruns K. Occupational therapists' beliefs and practices with regard to spirituality and therapy. *Am J Occup Ther.* 1997;51:173-180.
24. Prochnau C, Liu L, Boman J. Personal-professional connections in palliative care occupational therapy. *Am J Occup Ther.* 2003;57(2):196-204.
25. Rose A. Spirituality and palliative care: the attitudes of occupational therapists. *British Journal of Occupational Therapy.* 1999;62(7):307-312.
26. Taylor E, Mitchell JE, Kenan S, Tacker R. Attitudes of occupational therapists toward spirituality in practice. *Am J Occup Ther.* 2000;54(4):421-426.
27. Udell L, Chandler C. The role of the occupational therapist in addressing the spiritual needs of clients. *British Journal of Occupational Therapy.* 2000;63(10):489-494.

28. Meraviglia, MG. Critical analysis of spirituality and its empirical indicators. *J Holist Nurs*. 1999;17:18-33.
29. Zinnbauer BJ, Pargament KI, Cole B, Rye MS, Butter EM, Belavich TG, et al. Religion and spirituality: unfuzzying the fuzzy. *J Sci Study Relig*. 1997;36:549-564.
30. Koenig HG, McCullough ME, Larson DB. *Handbook of Religion and Health*. London: Oxford University Press; 2001.
31. Bellingham R, Cohen B, Jones T, Spaniol L. Connectedness: some skills for spiritual health. *Am J Health Promot*. 1989;4:18-31.
32. Bosacki S, Ota C. Preadolescents' voices: A consideration of British and Canadian children's reflections on religion, spirituality, and their sense of self. *International Journal of Children's Spirituality*. 2000;5(2):203-219.
33. Burkhardt, MA. Becoming and connecting: Elements of spirituality for women. *Holist Nurs Pract*. 1994;8:12-21.
34. Dossey BM. Florence Nightingale. *J Holist Nurs*. 1998;16:111-163.
35. Dyson J, Cobb M, Forman D. The meaning of spirituality: a literature review. *J Adv Nurs*. 1997;26:1183-1188.
36. Hodge DR. Spiritual assessment: A review of major qualitative methods and a new framework for assessing spirituality. *Social Work*. 2001;46(3):203-214.
37. Hodge DR, Cardenas P, Montoya H. Substance use: spirituality and religious participation as protective factors among rural youths. *Social Work Research*. 2001;25(3):153-161.
38. Hungelmann J, Kenkel-Rossi E, Klassen L, Stollenwerk RM. Spiritual well-being in older adults: harmonious interconnectedness. *J Relig Health*. 1985;24:147-153.
39. Kessler R. Nourishing students in secular schools. *Educ Leadersh*. 1998;56(4):49-52.
40. Piedmont RL. Spiritual transcendence and the scientific study of spirituality. *J Rehabil*. 2001;67(1):4-14.
41. Pike M. Spirituality, morality, and poetry. *International Journal of Children's Spirituality*. 2000;5(2):177-191.
42. Do Rozario L. Ritual, meaning and transcendence: the role of occupation in modern life. *Journal of Occupational Science*. 1994;1:46-53.
43. Spencer J, Davidson H, White V. Helping clients develop hopes for the future. *Am J Occup Ther*. 1997;51:191-198.
44. Smith H. *The World's Religions: Our Great Wisdom Traditions*. New York, NY: HarperCollins; 1978.
45. Greene B. *The Fabric of the Cosmos: Space, Time, and the Texture of Reality*. New York, NY: Vintage; 2005.
46. Wolf FA. *Yoga of Time Travel: How The Mind Can Defeat Time*. New York, NY: Quest Books; 2004.
47. Nager B. *The Ego Identity Crisis: Handbook For Enlightenment*. Orlando, FL: RTN Publishing; 2005.
48. American Occupational Therapy Association. Occupational therapy practice framework: domain and process. *Am J Occup Ther*. 2002;56:609-639.
49. Schkade JK, Schultz S. Occupational adaptation: toward a holistic approach for contemporary practice. part 1. *Am J Occup Ther*. 1992;46:829-838.
50. Schultz S, Schkade JK. Occupational adaptation: toward a holistic approach for contemporary practice. part 2. *Am J Occup Ther*. 1992;46:917-926.
51. Schulz EK. The meaning of spirituality in the lives and adaptation processes of individuals with disabilities. Unpublished Doctoral Dissertation, 2002: Texas Woman's University, Denton, Texas.
52. Meyer A. The philosophy of occupational therapy. *Archives of Occupational Therapy*. 1922;1(1):1-10.
53. Csikszentmihalyi M. The flow experience and human psychology. In: Csikszentmihalyi M, Csikszentmihalyi IS. (Eds.) *Optimal Experience: Psychological Studies of Flow in Consciousness*. Cambridge, England: Cambridge University Press; 1998.
54. Csikszentmihalyi M, Csikszentmihalyi IS. *Optimal Experience: Psychological Studies of Flow in Consciousness*. Cambridge, England: Cambridge University Press; 1998.
55. Nosek MA. The defining light of Vedanta: personal reflections on spirituality and disability. *Rehabilitation Education*. 1995;9:171-182.
56. Fisher JW, Francis LJ, Johnson P. Assessing spiritual health via four domains of spiritual wellbeing: the SH4DI. *Pastoral Psychology*. 2000;49:133-145.
57. Paloutzian RF, Ellison CW. Loneliness, spiritual well-being and the quality of life. In: Peplau LA, Perlman D. (Eds.) *Loneliness: A Sourcebook of Current Theory, Research, and Therapy*. New York: Wiley-Interscience; 1982: 224-237.
58. Genia V. The Spiritual Experience Index: a measure of spiritual identity. *J Relig Health*. 1991;30:337-347.
59. Genia V. The Spiritual Experience Index: revision and reformulation. *Rev Relig Res*. 1997;38:344-381.
60. Collins M. Occupational therapy and spirituality: reflecting on quality of experience in therapeutic interventions. *The British Journal of Occupational Therapy*. 1998;61(6):280-284.
61. Schein RL, Koenig HG. The Center for Epidemiological Studies Depression (CES-D) Scale: assessment of depression in the medically ill elderly. *Int J Geriatr Psychiatry*. 1997;12(4):436.

62. Cole SR, Beck RW, Moke PS, Gal RL, Long DT. The National Eye Institute Visual Function Questionnaire: experience of the ONTT. Optic Neuritis Treatment Trial. *Invest Ophthalmol Vis Sci.* 2000;41(5):1017-1021.
63. Roccaforte WH, Burke WJ, Bayer BL, Wengel SP. Reliability and validity of the Short Portable Mental Status Questionnaire administered by telephone. *J Geriatr Psychiatry Neurol.* 1994;7(1):33-38.

Funding

The validity and reliability study conducted on the second edition of the OT-QUEST was funded by a Research to Prevent Blindness (RPB) grant from the University of Alabama at Birmingham, Department of Ophthalmology Clinical Research Unit and a matching grant from the Alabama at Birmingham, School of Health Related Professions, Department of Occupational Therapy.

PART VII:
COMPUTERIZED ASSESSMENTS

18

STRESS MANAGEMENT QUESTIONNAIRE

Franklin Stein, PhD, OTR, FAOTA

"For future research, it may be ideal to focus on the significance of single life events for an individual's goal system and to include measures of the effectiveness of coping strategies." Klumb PL, Bates M. (2004). Adverse life events in late life: their manifestation and management in daily life. Journal of Stress Management. 2004;11:3-20.

Introduction

Stress is defined as the arousal of physical and psychological responses in the individual that occur in reaction to daily experiences that make life difficult or create discomfort.[1] What is the origin of stress? What are the internal biological and psychological factors that are affected by stress? How does stress produce a breakdown in the body's functions? Can an individual develop resistance to stress? How can an individual manage stress? How can stress be measured?

In general, stress can be conceptualized as both a cause and an effect.[2] As a cause, stress can trigger symptoms such as depression, headaches, back pain, or anxiety. As an effect, demands on a job, pressure from family members to achieve, illness, or divorce can trigger a stress reaction. Stress precipitates a total response of the body to cope with the everyday demands of living. From a biopsychosocial perspective, stress is understood as the demands placed on an individual, the ability to withstand the pressure, and the resultant effects. In this conceptualization, there are stressors, copers, and symptoms. The *stressors* are the pressures and demands on the individual such as from a job, school, family, or from within the individual. *Copers* are the stress management strategies in which an individual engages to reduce the stress, such as walking, meditation, or music. Symptoms of stress are the physical, emotional, cognitive, and behavioral results that occur from stress, such as headaches,[3] anger,[4] inability to concentrate,[5] or difficulty sleeping.[6] For example, an individual working on an assembly line meeting standards of performance to produce a specified number of objects is under stress to succeed.[7] If the individual doesn't have the psychological or physical capacity to meet the demands, the stress is increased, as compared to the individual who is able to meet the production goals comfortably.[8] In this example, stress is caused by an inability to meet a job requirement. Other people may have too many things to do within a time period or feel inadequate in social situations. Stress may also be triggered by internal factors, such as worrying about relationships. As one of the major risk factors along with smoking, obesity, lack of exercise, and poor nutrition, stress increases the probability of the initial onset of a disease and the chances of recurrence. It is a significant problem throughout the world and contributes to cardiovascular, psychosocial, neurological, and joint disorders.[9] Stress can also interfere with the quality of work performance, accidents at work, and increase the use of health care services.[10] Research has presented overwhelming evidence that severe stress during prolonged periods has a detrimental effect on an individual's life. Unremitting stress can also exacerbate symptoms, such as in arthritis, multiple sclerosis, and Parkinson's disease.[11] Studies have linked stress with several diseases, such as hypertension and coronary heart disease,[12] stroke,[13] musculoskeletal disorders,[14] bronchial asthma,[15] depression,[16] anxiety,[17] headaches/migraines,[18] obesity type II diabetes,[19] gallbladder disease,[20] alcoholism,[21] substance abuse,[22] cancer,[23] rheumatoid arthritis,[24] gastrointestinal diseases,[25] skin disorders,[26] ulcerative colitis,[27] and a host of other infection and immune system disorders.[28]

How does stress affect one's psychophysiology? What is the difference between eustress and distress? The severity of the stress reaction will depend upon the coping skills and resources that an individual has to accomplish a task. Stress is a mind-body interaction that triggers a sympathetic nervous system response in the individual that was first identified by Cannon[29] in 1939 as a "flight or fight" reaction. Stress can be experienced as mild, moderate, or severe. Mild stress may be experienced when driving in light traffic. Moderate stress may be experienced while taking a weekly examination, and high stress may be experienced when losing a job. The ability to tolerate high amounts of stress varies with the individual and his or her ability to use copers to manage stress. Some individuals with a high tolerance for stress are able to self-regulate their stress through activities such as exercise and meditation. Other individuals may be vulnerable to even mild degrees of stress that may trigger psychophysiological symptoms. The ability to self-regulate stress or to minimize its effects on the body has been defined as *hardiness*.[30]

Not all stress is bad; mild to moderate amounts of stress can be a motivating force in an individual. This is called *eustress*.[31] Cognitive, physical, and emotional systems function efficiently in eustress, allowing the individual to perform maximally and to have the stamina to endure perceived challenges. On the other hand, severe, adverse, or negative stress is termed *distress*.

Stressors are specific to each person. There are external stressors that are generated by the environment; these can include crowds, noise, poor lighting, inadequate ventilation, and environmental pollutants. There are also internal stressors that are generated from within the person, such as worrying about a strained relationship, which can cause feelings of insecurity and fearfulness. The final category of stressors is *social* stressors. Social stressors could include major life changes, such as divorce, job loss, major illness, financial problems, family death, car breakdown, and accidents.[1]

The body reacts to stressors by producing physiological responses, such as increases in heart rate, blood pressure, perspiration, muscle tone, and cell metabolism. Other aspects of the body will be affected, for example, blood vessels will constrict, digestion will be slowed, and the endocrine system will release adrenaline to cause the body to be in a high state of arousal and vigilance. The body does this through activation of the sympathetic nervous system. If this response is too intense or prolonged, it can lead to symptoms or adverse reactions to the stress such as headaches, heartburn, blurring of vision, and numerous other problems. Severe stress can also impair one's thinking and disrupt one's emotions.[32] In addition to the immediate physiological effects, it has long been shown that prolonged stress can suppress the immune system.[33] The immune system includes the body's defense against infection, allergies, bacteria, viruses, cancer, and other pathogens.

In general, high or severe stress can cause wear and tear on bodily organs and become a risk factor for disease and injury. A stress management program can help the individual to lessen the effects of stress and to increase his or her tolerance for highly stressful situations.

Development of the Stress Management Questionnaire (SMQ)

A stress management instrument identifying stressors, symptoms, and copers can be helpful in developing a stress management program. Stress is unique to each individual. What one person perceives as being a manageable amount of stress may be too much for the next person to handle.[34] Likewise, situations and events may elicit different stress reactions in different people. The situations or events that precipitate or cause a stress reaction are known as stressors.[35] When an individual is unable to cope successfully with his or her perceived stressors, various symptoms may arise.

Stein,[36] then at the University of Wisconsin-Milwaukee, initially developed the Stress Management Questionnaire (SMQ) as a self-administered paper-and-pencil test. The major purpose of the questionnaire is to help the individual to gain insight into one's stress, how stress triggers symptoms, and the activities or occupations that can be used in managing the stress reaction. Three versions of the questionnaire were developed over a 20-year period with the help of undergraduate and graduate occupational therapy students at the University of Wisconsin-Milwaukee and the University of South Dakota. The test can be administered in a group or individually. The original paper-and-pencil questionnaire consists of 158 items and takes about 30 to 45 minutes to complete. The questionnaire uses a forced choice format for each item and a section for ranking the top 10 symptoms, stressors, or copers covered in each section. The purpose of the SMQ is to help the client identify the: 1) symptoms and problems precipitated by stress, 2) stressors in the individual's life that cause a stress response, and 3) coping activities that the individual currently uses to manage or alleviate stress. From these results, the client, with guidance from the therapist, would be able to incorporate the copers into his or her daily schedule as a means of alleviating stress.

Natz,[1] a graduate student in occupational therapy at the University of South Dakota, developed a computer version of the SMQ. This included a printout of the client's stress profile and a client database of scores obtained. The SMQ computer version was originally administered on IBM PS/2 model 30's with color displays, a keyboard, and a mouse used for input. The latest computer version of the SMQ[37] was published by Delmar Learning and is available in an individual or institutional version. It allows the client to complete the questionnaire in a clinic, work environment, or in the privacy of his or her own home or office. The computer version has the potential to be used in large corporations and health and wellness programs where individuals can have the opportunity to self-regulate their stress reactions.

A third version of the SMQ, the Sorting Out Stress (SOS) Cards, was devised at the University of South Dakota and published in 2003. It is a shortened version of the paper-and-pencil test and takes about 10 to 15 minutes to complete. It consists of three decks of color-coded cards representing symptoms, stressors, and copers that can be used by occupational therapists in a clinical setting. In a recent study, it has been shown to have good reliability and validity (r = .57 to .77).[38] The SOS Cards can be used with a variety of clinical populations to identify activities that promote healthy adjustment, lower anxiety, and to increase quality of life. The forced-choice format of the SOS Cards provides the opportunity for self-monitoring of symptoms, stressors, and copers. The format is somewhat similar to the principle of the Q-sort technique originally developed by Stephenson in 1953.[39]

The SMQ was originally designed through clinical research studies that are shown in Table 18-1. The format of these clinical studies included administration of the SMQ before and after intervention. A cognitive behavioral approach[47] was integrated into the clinical protocol. Usually, eight sessions were held, either individual or group. For example, the sessions included the following:

- First session: Establish rapport with clients and a climate of trust, administer SMQ, explain purposes of the Stress Management Group, introduce and demonstrate the Benson Relaxation Response[48]

- Second session: Discuss the relationship between stress and the onset of symptoms, introduce and demonstrate Progressive Relaxation[49]

- Third session: Discuss the everyday stressors, visual imagery, sleep hygiene

- Fourth session: Discuss copers and personal resources in managing stress, biofeedback, exercise

- Fifth session: Discuss pleasant occupation in one's everyday life, role playing stressful situations, food as enjoyment

- Sixth session: Set up individualized stress management program, discuss learning how to control feelings and activities to increase concentration

- Seventh session: Discuss the use of music, art, reading, and creative activities in managing stress, demonstrate Paradoxical Intention exercise[50]

- Eighth session: Closure activity, readministration of the SMQ, and qualitative evaluation of the experience.

During the eight sessions, the clients were encouraged to practice relaxation exercises as homework, and to keep a daily diary of the symptoms, stressors, and copers in their everyday living.

Components of the SMQ

The first set of descriptors in the SMQ describes the symptoms that individuals experience while under stress. These descriptors were generated in an open-ended questionnaire that asked the participants to list the symptoms that were experienced during stress, ie, "When I feel stressful, I experience the following symptoms, feelings or problems." From the original research, the specific symptoms and problems resulting from stress were organized into four factors:

1. *Physiological*: such as headaches, tremors, neck/low back pain

2. *Cognitive*: such as difficulty concentrating, remembering, decision making

3. *Emotional*: such as feeling angry, hopeless, tense, and sad

4. *Behavioral*: such as difficulty sleeping, eating, and speaking.

Table 18-1		
Clinical Studies of Stress Management Questionnaire		
Research Populations	**Settings**	**Dates of Study**
Psychiatric populations attending day treatment center[40]	Day One, Milwaukee	1985-1987
Case study of individual with schizophrenia[41]	Day One, Milwaukee	1987
Group of individuals with recovering alcoholism[42]	De Paul Rehabilitation Hospital, Milwaukee	1987-1988
Hospitalized group of individuals with schizophrenia[43]	Alberta Provincial Hospital, Canada	1986
Hospitalized individuals with depression[44]	Edmonton General Hospital, Canada	1986
Hospitalized individuals with depression[45]	Winnipeg Health Centre, Canada	1991-1993
Community group manic-depression society[46]	University of Manitoba	1993

In total, 72 descriptors were listed; 27 describe physiological symptoms, 8 are cognitive, 18 describe emotional, and 19 are behavioral.

The second set of descriptor choices on the SMQ identifies situations that cause the stress response. These stressors include arguments, criticism, encountering "red tape," and driving in heavy traffic. Stressors are those aspects of the environment that increase demands on the individual and tend to increase stress.[51] The stress inducing occurrences of daily events parallel major life changes in their potential to produce stress. The Survey of Recent Life Experiences (SRLE) is a measure that comprises a list of experiences to measure how much everyday stressors affect physical and mental health.[52] The 51-item scale of the SRLE incorporates four levels of intensity of the stress experience: not at all, only slightly, moderately, and very much. The SMQ includes a range of daily hassles under the stressors heading that is related to the SRLE. Everyday stressors precipitating stress reactions were grouped under nine factors:

1. *Interpersonal*: such as arguments with family members
2. *Intrapersonal*: such as low self-esteem
3. *Time demands*: such as meeting a deadline at work
4. *Mechanical breakdown*: such as dealing with a broken household appliance
5. *Performance*: such as taking a test
6. *Financial pressures*: such as loss of income
7. *Illness*: such as having the flu
8. *Environmental disturbance*: such as excessive noise
9. *Complex situations*: such as raising a child alone

Thirty-six items are included under the question: What are the everyday situations or thoughts that cause stress for you?

The third section of the SMQ lists coping responses, such as exercise, listening to music, and talking to a friend. Interactional theories emphasize the mediating role of coping and adaptive mechanisms in determining overall levels of stress. A related scale, the Health Promotion Lifestyle Profile (HPLP),[53] incorporates six areas as indicators of positive coping. Everyday activities that manage or reduce stress (copers) were organized in the SMQ into nine factors:

1. *Creative*: such as writing a poem
2. *Construction*: such as knitting a sweater
3. *Exercise*: such as walking
4. *Appreciation*: such as listening to music
5. *Self-care*: such as taking a bath
6. *Social*: such as talking to friends
7. *Plant and animal care*: such as having a pet
8. *Performance*: such as singing in a choir
9. *Sports*: such as swimming

Forty-eight items are included under the statement: List the following activities that help you relieve stress.

A final section of the questionnaire asks for demographic information and also poses questions concerning the experience of completing the questionnaire itself, such as:

- Was the questionnaire too long?
- Were the directions clear?
- Did the questionnaire accurately reflect your feelings?
- Did the questionnaire help you to become more aware of the stressors in your everyday life?
- Did you identify from the questionnaire any new methods to manage stress?
- Do you feel you would benefit from an individualized stress management program?

Reliability of the SOS Cards

A reliability study of the SOS Cards was conducted in 2001 at the University of South Dakota using a test-retest design. The SOS Cards were administered to participants between age categories 18 to 24, 24 to 44, 45 to 64, and 65+. Adult age categories were created based on the major career changes in a person's life. Folkman et al[54] described how age is related to the way individuals experience stress and in their coping mechanisms. Individuals 18 to 24 years old are graduating from high school, entering college, or graduating from college and transitioning to a full-time career. Those between 25 to 44 are usually starting careers, marriages, and families. Individuals 45 to 64 are consolidating their careers and preparing for retirement, and those 65+ are in the retirement stage. Each age category included 20 participants. Four graduate students from the University of South Dakota were assigned an age category and were responsible for recruiting 20 individuals for the SOS Card reliability study. Participants were recruited from general communities in South Dakota and surrounding areas. Participation was voluntary and each participant was informed about the nature of the study before signing an informed consent form. Participants were eligible for inclusion if they were 18 years or older with no clinical diagnosis and satisfactory function in the social milieu. Both men and women of various backgrounds and occupations were welcome to participate.

Eighty participants were individually tested. Each participant was asked to sort through three decks of descriptor cards—a symptoms deck, stressor deck, and a copers deck. Descriptors used on the SOS Cards were selected based on the previous research conducted on the SMQ. Based on responses, the researchers generated a list of items that were most frequently identified by respondents. The identified descriptors were used for the SOS Cards. The participant placed the individual descriptors into a yes, no, or maybe pile. After this, the participant was asked to decide from the maybe pile which ones selected belong in the yes or no pile. The no pile was then discarded. The participant was then asked to rank his or her top 5 responses in the yes pile, with 1 being the most troublesome symptoms, top stressors, and top copers. As a result of this, the participant had an individualized stress profile with a list of symptoms triggered by stress, stressors that cause stress, and the top copers that help in reducing stress.

Reliability of the SOS Cards was tested randomly. To determine which participants were to be retested, a simple process of assigning random numbers to each person and drawing names from a box was used. Twenty participants, five from each age category, were then randomly selected and retested within 2 weeks. Test administration was conducted in participants' homes, schools, a senior citizen center, and a nursing home located in South Dakota. Each test was administered in a quiet room that was free from distractions, with the test administrator and participant positioned at a table to allow proximal visual and physical contact. A table allowed adequate space for sorting the cards and for the tester to record the responses. Test administration took approximately 10 minutes for the first three age categories, and approximately 15 to 20 minutes for the age category 65+.

Data analysis was performed using congruence of agreements on test-retest reliability. Data from the two test sessions was compared. A match or congruence of agreement was an item selected and ranked in the first card session and selected and ranked in the second card session. Concurrent responses were an indicator of reliability. Test-retest reliability data ranged from .57 to .77 for symptoms, stressors, and copers. The results of the test-retest are described in Tables 18-2 through 18-7. Tables 18-2 through 18-5 display the rankings for the symptoms, stressors, and copers in each age category. Table 18-6 lists the overall ranking for the symptoms, stressors, and copers. Tables 18-7 through 18-11 describe the concurrence of agreement in a test-retest reliability for each age category.

The primary purpose of the SOS study was to measure the reliability of a shortened version of the SMQ that would be convenient and easy to use in a clinical setting. A shortened version of the SMQ was shown to be a reliable and valid tool for assessing individual symptoms of stress, stressors, and copers. By shortening the time it takes to complete the SMQ, test administrators will be able to obtain results quickly without compromising the validity or reliability of the SMQ. It takes about 10 minutes to complete the shortened card version of the SMQ, as compared to 20 to 45 minutes to complete the paper and pencil version of the SMQ. The results of this study indicate that the SOS Cards is a reliable test instrument, with test-retest reliability congruence of agreement scores, of a stratified age sample, ranging from 57% to 77% for all symptoms, stressors, and copers.

Table 18-2

Rankings for Age Group 18 to 24

Symptoms	Stressors	Copers
Rank	Rank	Rank
1 Irritable	1 Financial situations	1 Hot shower/bath* Analyze Situations*
2 Moody* Fatigue*	2 Criticism by others	2 Talk to a friend
3 Muscle tension* Headaches*	3 Not having any free time for oneself or friends	3 Listen to music
4 Anxious	4 Having no control over a situation	4 Watch TV
5 Neck\low back pain* Low tolerance to others* Trouble concentrating* Tense*	5 Being unprepared (date, test, guests, speaking, etc.)	5 Relax (lie down)

*Tied Ranks

Table 18-3

Rankings for Age Group 25 to 44

Symptoms	Stressors	Copers
Rank	Rank	Rank
1 Moody	1 Financial situations	1 Talk to a friend
2 Irritable	2 Having too many things to do with not enough time	2 Analyze situation
3 Tense	3 Having no control over a situation	3 Listen to music* Watch TV*
4 Anxious	4 Being unprepared (date, test, guests, speaking, etc.)	4 Exercising
5 Low tolerance to others* Fatigue*	5 Gaining or losing weight* Criticism by others* Feeling too much pressure at school, work, or at home*	5 Hot shower/bath* Meditate or pray*

*Tied Ranks

Table 18-4

Rankings for Age Group 45 to 64

Symptoms	Stressors	Copers
Rank	Rank	Rank
1 Tense	1 Having too many things to do with not enough time	1 Analyze situation
2 Anxious	2 Having no control over a situation	2 Talk to a friend
3 Irritable* Nervous*	3 Being unprepared (date, test, guests, speaking, etc)* Financial situations*	3 Meditate or pray
4 Headaches* Low tolerance to others* Problems with sleeping*	4 Not having any free time for oneself or friends	4 Walking* Read for pleasure
5 Neck/low back pain* Moody* Problems with eating	Feeling too much pressure at school, work, or home	5 Watch TV Listen to music Exercising* Relax (lie down)* Crying*

*Tied Ranks

Table 18-5

Rankings for Age Group 65 and Up

Symptoms	Stressors	Copers
Rank	Rank	Rank
1 Nervous	1 Having too many things to do with not enough time Lack of confidence in oneself*	1 Meditate or pray
2 Problems with sleeping	2 Having no control over a situation* Criticism by others*	2 Watch TV* Listen to music*
3 Irritable* Tense*	3 Gaining or losing weight	3 Analyze situation Talk to friend*
4 Anxious	4 Feeling too much pressure at school, work, or home	4 Relax (lie down)
5 Neck/low back pain* Muscle tension* Restless*	5 Financial situations	5 Read for pleasure

*Tied Ranks

Table 18-6

Combined for All Age Groups

Symptoms	Stressors	Copers
Rank	Rank	Rank
1 Irritable	1 Financial situations	1 Talk to a friend
2 Tense	2 Having too many things to do with not enough time	2 Analyze situations
3 Anxious	3 Having no control over a situation	3 Meditate or pray
4 Moody* Fatigue* Nervous*	4 Criticism by others	4 Listen to music
5 Problems with sleeping	5 Being unprepared (date, test guests, speaking, etc.)	5 Watch TV

*Tied Ranks

Table 18-7

Percentage of Concurrence on the Sorting Out Stress Cards on a Test-Retest Reliability Study

Major Areas	Percentage of Agreement
Symptoms and problems resulting from stress	57%
Everyday stressors precipitating the stress response	66%
Everyday coping activities that manage stress	77%

Table 18-8

Percentage of Concurrence on the Sorting Out Stress Cards on a Test-Retest Reliability Study: Age 18 to 24

Major Areas	Percentage of Agreement on Rank-Ordered Items
Symptoms and problems resulting from stress	44%
Everyday stressors precipitating the stress response	72%
Everyday coping activities that manage stress	56%

Females = 18
Males = 2

Table 18-9

Percentage of Concurrence on Sorting Out Stress Cards on a Test-Retest Reliability Study: Age 25 to 44

Major Areas	Percentage of Agreement on Rank-Ordered Items
Symptoms and problems resulting from stress	76%
Everyday stressors precipitating the stress response	80%
Everyday coping activities that manage stress	92%

Females = 9
Males = 11

Table 18-10

Percentage of Concurrence on the Sorting Out Stress Cards on a Test-Retest Reliability Study: Age 45 to 64

Major Areas	Percentage of Agreement on Rank-Ordered Items
Symptoms and problems resulting from stress	64%
Everyday stressors precipitating the stress response	76%
Everyday coping activities that manage stress	88%

Females = 17
Males = 3

Table 18-11

Percentage of Concurrence on the Sorting Out Stress Cards on a Test-Retest Reliability Study: Age 65+

Major Areas	Percentage of Agreement on Rank-Ordered Items
Symptoms and problems resulting from stress	44%
Everyday stressors precipitating the stress response	36%
Everyday coping activities that manage stress	72%

Females=17
Males=3

One aspect observed in these results is that the degree of concordance between rankings of a person's most significant symptoms, stressors, and coping activities varied between the two administrations of the SOS Cards; this was also noted in previous studies involving the SMQ. There is some indication of agreement on identifying the symptoms, stressors and coping activities; however, there is little evidence of stability in the relative rankings of the individual components over time.

Summary

Based on the results of this research, it is thought that the game-like presentation of the SOS Cards offers an innovative and interesting alternative to the paper and pencil version of the SMQ. This version of the SMQ provides a more appealing opportunity for individuals to identify their individual symptoms of stress, stressors, and copers. This instrument encourages the person to become a more active participant in identifying these stress-related aspects of his or her life. Once these aspects are identified, clinicians can then use this information to develop individualized stress management programs in concert with the client. This approach is consistent with client-centered treatment.[55] In general, the SOS Cards are intended to help in development of personal stress profiles, which will help people to identify stressors and to reduce resultant symptoms by incorporating individual copers into their everyday lives. It is envisaged that the SOS Cards will have wide potential for self-monitoring symptoms, stressors, and copers as part of a holistic stress management program. This test can serve as a comprehensive interactive measuring instrument for guided self-understanding and healthy lifestyle planning, as in health promotion and disease prevention programs in school and work environments. Information provided by stress management tools such as the SMQ or SOS Cards would be of great benefit to health care professionals such as occupational therapists. Occupational therapists frequently develop individualized stress management programs, and employ stress management techniques as important aspects of many occupational therapy interventions.[56] They do this by identifying with the client meaningful and purposeful activities that can be incorporated into his or her daily routine. The occupational therapy profession emphasizes the importance of helping clients to develop activity strategies that can be used on an everyday basis to better cope with stressors that trigger stress reactions and subsequent symptoms. Information generated by the SMQ or SOS Cards may be incorporated into the development of individualized stress management programs that could help clients self-regulate their stress by incorporating coping activities into their daily lives as part of a comprehensive cognitive behavioral approach.[57]

Further research is needed to establish general reference norms and to determine concurrent and discriminative validity for the SMQ and SOS Cards. Research is also needed to determine the reliability of the SOS Cards with different diagnostic populations. Also, future studies should be expanded to include a greater geographical distribution, and possible cross-cultural investigations. Another potential area for future investigations would be to compare particular score levels, especially of coping activities, with levels of success in managing stress. The final recommendations are to incorporate more males into future research studies in order to create equivalence to current population demographics, and to further investigate the applicability of the SMQ and SOS Cards to older clients.

The SOS Cards is a reliable and valid stress management instrument that could potentially be a very valuable asset to clinicians, particularly occupational therapists, in identifying activities that promote a healthy lifestyle, lower anxiety, and improve a person's overall quality of life.

References

1. Stein F, Bentley D, Natz M. Computerized assessment: the stress management questionnaire. In: Hemphill-Pearson B. *Assessments in Occupational Therapy Mental Health: An Integrative Approach.* Thorofare, NJ: SLACK Incorporated; 1999:301-317.
2. Seyle H. *The Stress of Life.* New York: McGraw-Hill; 1956.
3. Davis GC, Grassley JS. Measurement of the experience of living with primary recurrent headache. *Pain Manag Nurs.* 2005;6:37-44.
4. Wofford JC. Meta-analysis of relations of stress propensity with subjective stress and strain. *Psychology Reports.* 2002;9,:1133-1136.
5. Sandstrom A, Rhodin IN, Lundberg M, Olsson T, Nyberg L. Impaired cognitive performance in patients with chronic burnout syndrome. *Biol Psychol.* 2005;69:271-2799.
6. Spoormaker VI, van den Bout J. Depression and anxiety complaints; relations with sleep disturbances. *Eur Psychiatry.* 2005;20:243-455.
7. Sanders M. Minimizing stress in the workplace: whose responsibility is it? *Work.* 2001;17:263-265.
8. Stein F. Occupational stress, relaxation therapies exercise and biofeedback. *Work.* 2001;17:235-245.
9. Stress. (n.d.). Retrieved November 2, 2005, from http://www.stress.org
10. Kalia M. Assessing the economic impact of stress—the modern day hidden epidemic. *Metabolism.* 2002;51:49-53.
11. Sapolsky RM. *Why Zebras Don't Get Ulcers: An Updated Guide to Stress, Stress-related Diseases, and Coping.* New York: W.H. Freeman and Company; 1998.
12. Rozanski A, Blumenthal JA, Kaplan J. Impact of psychological factors on the pathogenesis of cardiovascular disease and implications for therapy. *Circulation.* 1999;101:177-178.
13. Bowler D. "It's all in your mind": the final common pathway. *Work.* 2001;17:167-173.
14. Warren N. Work stress and musculoskeletal disorder etiology: the relative roles of psychosocial and physical risk factors. *Work.* 2001;17:221-234.
15. Sandberg S, Paton J, Ahola S, McCann D, McGuinness D, Hillary C, Oja H. The role of acute and chronic stress in asthma attacks in children. *Lancet.* 2000;356:982-996.
16. Day G. Stress prevention, not cure. *Director.* 1998;52:46.
17. Leonard B, Song C. Stress and the immune system in the etiology of anxiety and depression. *Pharmacology, Biochemistry & Behavior.* 1996;54:299-303.
18. Hoodin F, Brines B, Lake A, Wilson J, Saper J. Behavioral self-management in an inpatient headache treatment unit: Increasing adherence and relationship to changes in affective distress. *Headache.* 2000;40:377-383.
19. Bjorntorp P, Rosmond R. Visceral obesity and diabetes. *Drugs.* 1999;58:75-82.
20. Shafer A, Ashley J, Goodwin C, Nanagas V, Elliott D. A new look at the multifactoral etiology of gallbladder disease in children. *Am Surg.* 1983;49:314-319.
21. Pohorecky L. The interaction of alcohol and stress. *Neurosci Biobehav Rev.* 1981;5:209-229.
22. McMahon R. Personality, stress, and social support in cocaine relapse prediction. *J Subst Abuse Treat.* 2001;21:77-87.
23. Panzer A. Depression or cancer: the choice between serotonin or melatonin? *Med Hypotheses.* 1998;50:385-387.
24. Zautra A, Hamilton N, Potter P, Smith B. Field research on the relationship between stress and disease activity in rheumatoid arthritis. *Ann N Y Acad Sci.* 1999;876:397-412.
25. Collins S. Stress and the Gastrointestinal Tract IV. Modulation of intestinal inflammation by stress: basic mechanisms and clinical relevance. *Am J Physiol Gastrointest Liver Physiol.* 2001;280:G315-318.
26. Singh L, Pang X, Alexacos N, Letourneau R, Theoharides T. Acute immobilization stress triggers skin mast cell degranulation via corticotropin releasing hormone, neurotensin, and substance P: A link to neurogenic skin disorders. *Brain Behav Immun.* 1999;13:225-239.
27. Fergus S. Pathogenesis of ulcerative colitis. *Lancet.* 1993;342:407-412.
28. Goldberger L, Breznitz S. *Handbook of Stress.* 2nd ed. New York: Macmillan; 1993.

29. Cannon WB. *The Wisdom of the Body*. New York: Norton; 1939.
30. Huang C. Hardiness and stress: a critical review. *Matern Child Nurs J*. 1995;23:82-89.
31. Selye H. *Stress Without Distress*. Philadelphia: J.B. Lippincott; 1974.
32. Orioli EM. *Stress Map. Personnel News*. San Francisco, CA: Essi System, Inc.; 1992.
33. Ader R, Cohen N. Psychoneuroimmunology: conditioning and stress. *Annu Rev Psychol*. 1993;44:53-85.
34. Giles GM, Neistadt ME. Treatment for psychosocial components: Stress management. In: Neistadt ME, Crepeau EB, eds. *Willard and Spackman's Occupational Therapy*. 9th ed. New York: Lippincott; 1998: 458-463.
35. Stein F, Roose B. *Pocket Guide to Treatment in Occupational Therapy*. San Diego, CA: Singular Publishing Group, Inc; 2000.
36. Stein F. Reliability and validity of the stress management questionnaire. Unpublished manuscript. University of Wisconsin-Milwaukee; 1986.
37. Stein F, Grueschow D, Hoffman M, Natz M, Taylor S, Tronback R. *Stress Management Questionnaire: An Instrument for Self-Regulating Stress, Individual Version*. Clifton Park, NY: Thomson Delmar Learning; 2003.
38. Stein F, Grueschow D, Hoffman M, Taylor S, Tronback R. The Sorting Out Stress Cards—a version of the SMQ: A reliability study. *Occupational Therapy in Mental Health*. 2003;19:41-59.
39. Anastasi A, Urbina S. *Psychological Testing*. 7th ed. New York: Prentice Hall; 1996.
40. Stein F. Group and individual stress management techniques with schizophrenic patients. American Occupational Therapy Association Annual Conference, Phoenix, Arizona, April 17, 1988.
41. Stein F, Nikolic S. Teaching stress management techniques to a schizophrenic patient. *Am J Occup Ther*. 1989;43:162-169.
42. Stein F, Neville SA. Biofeedback, locus of control and reduction of anxiety in alcohol dependent adults. Unpublished manuscript. University of Wisconsin-Milwaukee; 1987.
43. Stein F. Stress and schizophrenia. *Alberta Psychology*. 1987;16:10-11.
44. Stein F, Smith J. Short-term stress management program with acutely depressed in-patients. *Can J Occup Ther*. 1989;56:185-192.
45. Stein F, Cutler S. *Psychosocial Occupational Therapy: A Holistic Approach*. 2nd ed. Clifton Park, NY: Thomson Delmar Learning; 2002.
46. Stein F. Psychosocial Occupational Therapy. World Federation of Occupational Therapy Congress, Stockholm, Sweden, June 23, 2002.
47. Dobson K, Block L. Historical and philosophical bases of the cognitive-behavioral therapies. In: Dobson KS, ed. *Handbook of Cognitive-Behavioral Therapies*. New York: Guildford; 1988:3-38.
48. Benson H. *The Relaxation Response*. New York: William Morrow; 1975.
49. Jacobson E. *Progressive Relaxation*. Chicago, IL: University of Chicago; 1929.
50. Frankl V. *Man's Search for Meaning*. Boston, MA: Beacon; 1967.
51. Derogatis LR, Coons HL. Self-Report measures of stress: In: Goldberger L, Breznitz S, eds. *Handbook of Stress: Theoretical and Clinical Aspects*. 2nd ed. New York: Free Press; 1993: 200-233.
52. Kohn PM, MacDonald JE. The survey of recent life experiences: a decontaminated hassles scale for adults. *J Behav Med*. 1992;15:221-236.
53. Walker SN, Sechrist KR, Pender NJ. The Health-Promoting Lifestyle Profile: development and Psychometric characteristics. *Nursing Research*. 1987;36:76-81.
54. Folkman S, Lazarus RS, Pinely S, Novacek J. Age differences in stress and coping processes. *Psychol Aging*. 1987;2:171-184.
55. Canadian Association of Occupational Therapists (CAOT). *Occupational Therapy Guidelines for Client-Centered Mental Health Practice*. Toronto, ON: Author; 1993.
56. Courtney C, Escobedo B. A stress management program of inpatient-to-outpatient. continuity. *Am J Occup Ther*. 1990;44:306-310.
57. Stein F. Stress management. In: Carlson J. *Complementary Therapies and Wellness Practice Essentials for Holistic Health Care*. Upper Saddle River, NJ: Prentice Hall; 2003:295-303.

OT FACT APPLICATION IN MENTAL HEALTH: AN UPDATE

Roger O. Smith, PhD, OT, FAOTA

"Laws of computer programming: Any given program, when running, is obsolete." Computers and Programming. Retrieved April 5, 2006. http//www.health.uottawa.ca/biomech/csb/laws/computer. htm.

Introduction

The conceptualization of OT FACT and its initial development stages began in 1985 with a small seed grant from the American Occupational Therapy Foundation (AOTF).[1] Since that time, that initial work—not only the OT FACT instrument, but the test and measurement theory from which the OT FACT data collection process is grounded—has matured. OT FACT differs from most traditional assessments. Like several newer assessments, OT FACT is based on modern test and measurement theory, derived from the decision sciences and health outcomes assessment rather than on traditional psychological and educational testing. Consequently, a significant portion of this chapter describes the theoretical basis and structure of OT FACT. To appropriately apply OT FACT, the user should have a solid understanding of both traditional and newer measurement theories.

The instrument itself is a functional assessment approach that is designed into software. The assessment has three aspects, each of which will be discussed separately. The first aspect is the taxonomy of questions and the theory in which it is framed. The second aspect is the software, which uses a questioning methodology called Trichotomous Tailored Sub-Branching Scoring (TTSS). The TTSS method is made feasible through its computer presentation. (OT FACT data collection is not practical using traditional paper-and-pencil administration.) The third aspect is the OT FACT software, which includes a number of features to assist in data collection for patient-progress documentation, program evaluation, and outcomes research.

These three aspects introduce OT FACT. This chapter describes the psychometric aspects of OT FACT, including its theoretical foundation, reliability, and validity.

The OT FACT Taxonomic Organization: Human Occupational Performance Practice Integration Theory (HOPPIT)

OVERVIEW OF HOPPIT

OT FACT is structured around a human performance theory that is based on occupational therapy practice. This theory describes the relationships between different functional areas, provides the foundation, and explains how OT FACT tallies the scores and how results are interpreted.

The HOPPIT model is organized as a hierarchy of four levels that depict the individual's functional areas (Figure 19-1). The first level, Integrated Roles of Performance, includes such items as role balance, continuity of roles across time, and meeting role expectations of others and is at the top of the hierarchy. Successful role performance, however, is dependent upon performance in these activities. Activities of Performance is the second level, underneath the integrated roles. Personal maintenance areas of activity and occupational role-related activities fall into this level of function. Categories within the personal maintenance area address basic self-care skills, such as toileting, eating, and other traditional activities of daily living (ADLs). Included in the occupational role-related activities are areas typically described in the gerontological literature as instrumental activities of daily living (IADLs), such as meal preparation, household safety, and community mobility. Additionally, categories such as educational, vocational, caregiving, and religious activities are encompassed in role-related activities.

How well individuals perform these activities depends on yet a third level called Integrated Skills of Performance. This third level includes such items as problem solving, hand function, and management of maladaptive behavior. The lowest level on this hierarchy is Components of Performance, which is the most fundamental level and enables the Integrated Skills of Performance. The component level includes such items as memory, ability to initiate a task, ability to terminate a task, endurance, and pain.

These four levels are arranged in a dependency hierarchy, as each is believed to contribute to the functions above it. HOPPIT, however, acknowledges that individual function is dependent on outside influences (Figure 19-2). Therefore, on the perimeter of the individual's function, beyond these four hierarchical levels, lie the Environment and Therapeutic Interventions. The domains of the Environment are physical and social-cultural areas. The domain of Therapeutic Interventions includes all potential therapeutic methods. Both the Environment and the Therapeutic Interventions can target any of the four levels of individual performance. For example, in the Environment, an individual in a wheelchair may encounter an inaccessible bathroom, which would directly impact the Activities of Performance. Or a lack of social support systems in the Environment could directly impact several levels of the person's functional performance. Likewise, Therapeutic Interventions can address the specific areas of functional performance. For example, a list of steps that could be used for someone who has difficulty sequencing tasks could be created as an assistive-technology intervention. This could help with several of the categories within the Components of Performance domain. As another example, social interaction strategies that impact social functional performance in the Integrated Skills of Performance domain could be taught to individuals.

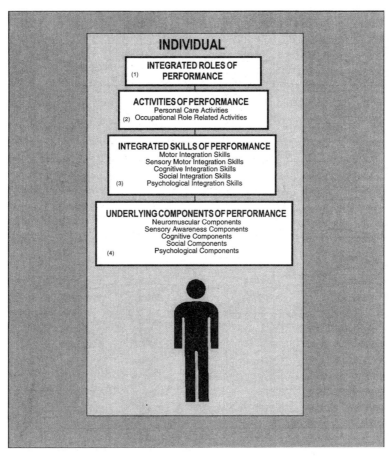

Figure 19-1. Relationship of the functional performance level of an individual.

One additional important domain lies over the Activities of Performance level, resulting in a three-dimensional HOPPIT model. This functional-activity domain is the Co-Variates of Performance, which includes two major types. The first is the skill/component type, representing every category on the Integrated Skills of Performance and the Components of Performance levels of the HOPPIT model. For example, whether or not an individual is functional in self-care activities might be dependent on the component of pain. The importance of the Co-Variate domain to the HOPPIT model is that functional performance can be scored by OT FACT for any given co-variate. A specific component, such as an individual's delusional or hallucinatory processes, can be viewed as a skill/component co-variate. The result of this co-variate scoring is the percent contribution of a thought process impairment to functional performance deficits.

The second type of co-variate is the Task Attribute. Task Attributes include factors that contribute to functional performance, such as the quality of performing an activity, the speed in completing an activity, or the safety with which an activity is completed. Figure 19-3 highlights how these two types of co-variates overlay each of the Activities of Performance categories. OT FACT integrates this HOPPIT model and makes each of these co-variates scorable assessments in themselves.

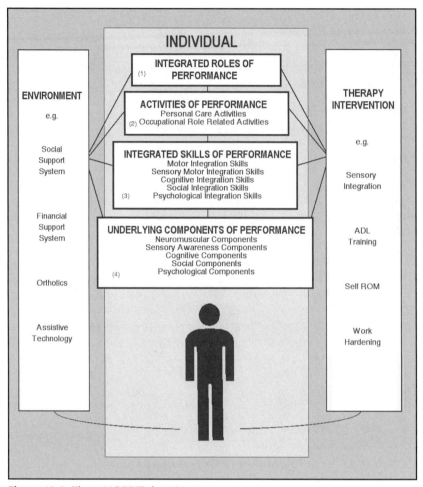

Figure 19-2. Three HOPPIT domains.

HOPPIT Development

The HOPPIT was initially developed in the mid-1980s and underwent many revisions through the 1990s. The hierarchical relationships of the four functional performance levels were developed through extensive discussion and review by occupational therapists. The development of the taxonomy was initiated with the first edition of AOTA's *Uniform Terminology*[2] and further developed in conjunction with the revisions included in *Uniform Terminology II*.[3] AOTA's *Uniform Terminology III*[4] added the context domain that includes environmental and temporal types of considerations already framed into the HOPPIT model.

The importance of viewing the HOPPIT in this way is to identify an individual's functional capacities and the relationships of these capacities across levels. It also clearly recognizes the two domains outside intrinsic performance and how they interact with a person's functional performance outcome.

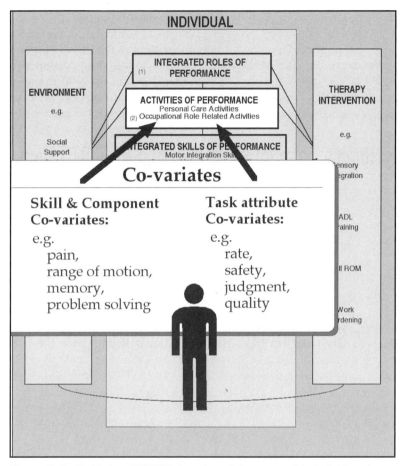

Figure 19-3. Co-Variate HOPPIT domain as it interacts with Activities of Performance.

The development of *Uniform Terminology* versions and the development of the OT FACT taxonomy also have run parallel to other major efforts. The National Center for Medical Rehabilitation Research's Taxonomy[5] and the Institute of Medicine Taxonomy[6] have modeled human performance as well. All of these taxonomies have many commonalities. The HOPPIT model, however, retains the gestalt scope yet incorporates functional performance detail. This model provides the foundation for the current version of OT FACT.

The Number of Categories in the OT FACT Taxonomy

The approximately 1,000 categories in version 2.03 of OT FACT create the potential questions for occupational therapy practitioners to use. The large number of categories is designed to accommodate the prominent areas of occupational therapy practice—physical disabilities, pediatrics, and mental health practice. Practitioners, however, may want to skim over the detail of many OT FACT categories that are specific to specialty areas of practice other than their own. For example, practitioners working in mental health may want to avoid the depth required in range of motion, sensory testing, or strength, which are desirable in physical disability settings. Therefore, while OT FACT includes 1,000 categories, the software provides a mechanism to customize the depth of questioning to de-emphasize the detail of practice areas less relevant to a given population or setting. In this way, OT FACT is packaged for a comprehensive occupational therapy program assessment across disability types, diagnoses, and practice settings, while its customization of questions allows the detail required for specialty areas of practice.

Mental Health Categories Within the OT FACT Taxonomy

While the philosophy of OT FACT and the HOPPIT model support the concept that all occupational therapists assess the same generic categories of human functioning, primary areas of practice do have focuses. Thus, while occupational therapists working in mental health must acknowledge a cursory review of neuromuscular, skeletal, and sensory functioning, they do not need to delve into detail. On the other hand, more detailed categories specific to mental health issues fall within various levels and domains. Excerpts of categories from OT FACT relating to mental health are included as Appendix U.

TTSS: The Software Question Methodology of OT FACT

OT FACT uses a trichotomous scale. All the questions throughout the instrument follow the same format. A score of 2 is given if an individual has met all of the criteria in the category, basically having no deficit in that area. A score of 0 is given to a person in the category if none of the criteria are met for that particular question, indicating that an individual has a total deficit in that area. A score of 1, partial deficit, is given for all situations where an individual has some function in a given area but the function is neither complete nor totally dysfunctional.

The scoring of TTSS is tailored by tallying "non-applicable" for a category of function. Many questions in other tests and assessments are dependent on gender, age, vocation, culture, or other individual characteristics that might render a given question inappropriate for the particular person being assessed. The TTSS approach allows a category to be omitted from the total scoring process when it is irrelevant. The result of this customization of questions is that the total scores obtained using the TTSS approach are comprised only of questions relevant to individuals in their particular contexts. Therefore, 100% performance of people using a TTSS strategy is 100% performance of these individuals for their particular needs in their particular situations. The implications of this are profound. The question set for any individual may differ from that of other individuals, as the question set is no longer standard across every person. This also has implications for the validity of the question set to an individual's needs. The questions, uniquely gathered to those of other types of tests and measures, are specifically selected because they are deemed valid to an individual's functional areas of concern.

Sub-branching is the characteristic of scoring that moves the questioning process from one category to the next, depending on how the previous question was answered. The use of a computer for TTSS allows this quick and efficient presentation of questions. Generally, the algorithm used by TTSS is simple. If an individual scores a 2 or a 0, then the TTSS process goes on to the next category in the same level of questioning. If a score of 1 is obtained, and a person is identified as having some deficit in an area, then TTSS

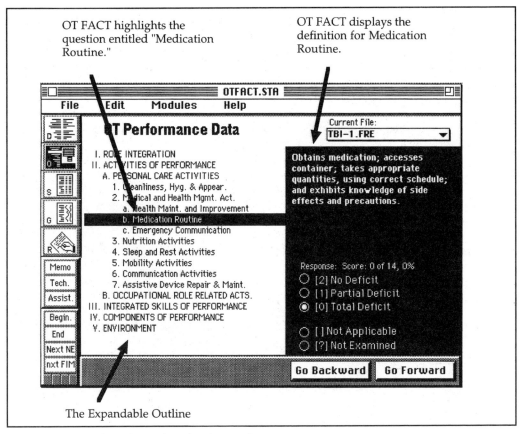

Figure 19-4. TTSS branching of medication routine.

branches into further detailed categories to follow this line of questioning. In this way, every question is a screening question. If there is no deficit or a total deficit in the area, then no further questioning is required. However, if some deficit has been identified, then the TTSS asks, "Tell me more about this deficit." Figures 19-4 through 19-6 highlight this branching process, using medication routine as the category of focus.

The result of this sub-branching process is to make the questioning procedure more efficient. Indeed, the TTSS methodology used in the OT FACT taxonomy of questions can result in a practitioner scoring less than 100 questions or as many as 1,000. The detail prompted by the software is totally dependent on an individual's particular needs, which must be assessed and determined by the scope of his or her deficits.

OT FACT Software Features

DATA ENTRY AND DATA USE

All of the data that are entered into OT FACT are available for merging into reports. Various types of reports can be printed, saved to disk, or compiled into databases. The

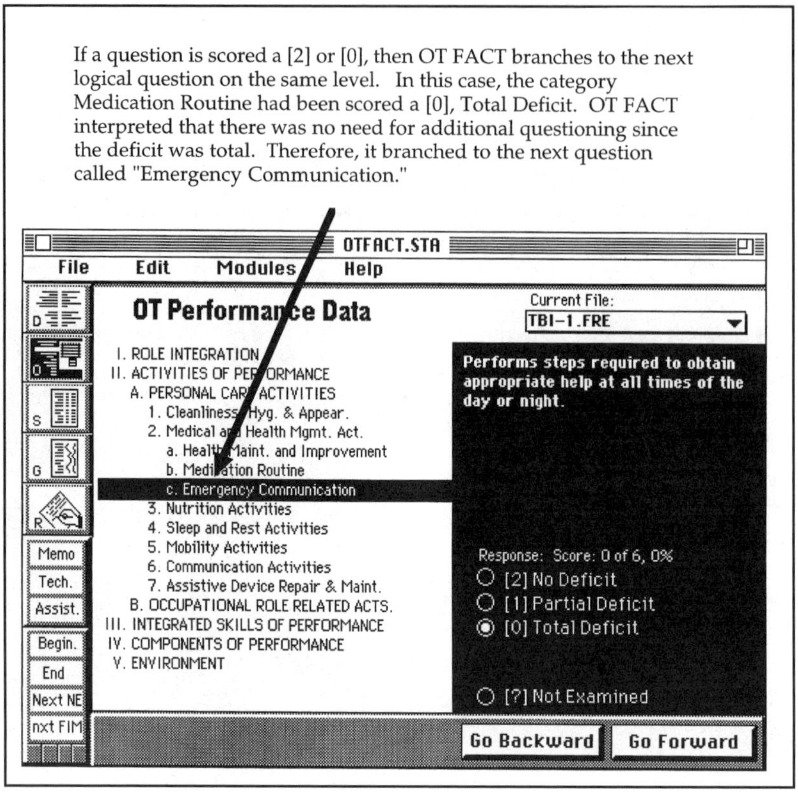

If a question is scored a [2] or [0], then OT FACT branches to the next logical question on the same level.   In this case, the category Medication Routine had been scored a [0], Total Deficit. OT FACT interpreted that there was no need for additional questioning since the deficit was total. Therefore, it branched to the next question called "Emergency Communication."

Figure 19-5. TTSS question progression if no or total deficit.

standard reports include data summaries or prose. Any data of any type entered into OT FACT can be included in a report. Once the performance data have been collected, OT FACT allows viewing of the information in summary tables or graphs. Up to three given administrations of OT FACT can be compared side by side. For example, data collected for an initial evaluation, a progress note, and a discharge summary can be placed side by side.

Many different types of comparisons can be made. The previous example of initial progress and discharge assessments is a method of comparing across time. Comparisons also can be made between perspectives. For example, an individual's perspective of his or her performance, a practitioner's perspective of performance, and a family member's perspective of performance can be compared. Comparisons can be made across interventions. For example, a person's performance in self-care skills when at home alone can be compared to his or her self-care skills when at home with a supportive family member. These two could be examined side by side to view the impact of family support. OT FACT will also calculate the differences between any two data sets.

DEMOGRAPHICS

OT FACT has three types of demographic data that allow a practitioner to collect administrative information: (1) dates of assessments, admissions, and the frequency of OT sessions; (2) patient information, such as name, diagnoses, and prior living status; and

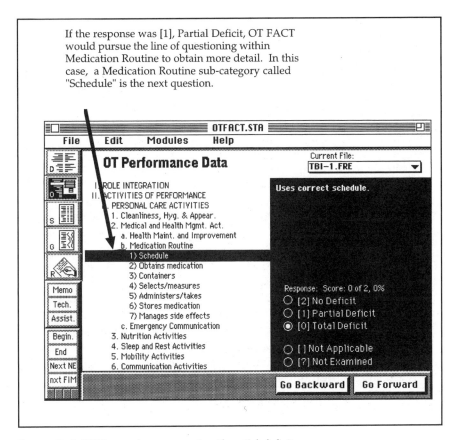

Figure 19-6. TTSS question progression if partial deficit.

(3) extended demographics, such as other disciplines involved in intervention, sources of payment, primary language, socioeconomic status, and education completed. None of the demographic fields are required, but all are available.

FILE TYPES

OT FACT data have many uses. OT FACT data can be collected for a number of purposes and using various frames of reference. Purposes can include initial assessments, progress assessments, discharge assessments, goal setting, or other data collection. If other data collection purposes are identified, the practitioner can enter a specific description. There are also several scoring types that can be selected in OT FACT. These include environment-free, indicating a person's performance without any support systems; environment-adjusted, indicating that some accommodations are made in the environment; environment-assisted, indicating that personal assistance is provided; self-satisfaction, portraying how an individual feels about his or her performance; co-variate scoring, specifying co-variates to be described such as safety and judgment; or other types of scoring, as delineated by the software user.

REPORT WRITING

OT FACT includes a report generation module. This module contains features that help the practitioner write a report. One feature uses a form-merging mechanism. OT FACT allows a practitioner to develop a form, including codes that incorporate OT FACT demographic and performance data, into the prose text in the report. Thus, once a form has been developed, the practitioner saves time by selecting the form and simply pressing a button labeled, "Fill in data." This process merges the data from the OT FACT assessments and drops the information into the report using the previously designed format. These reports can be printed as paper copy or saved as an electronic text file. Refer to Appendix V for an example of a case study and reporting data.

PICK LISTS, MEMOS, AND TEMPLATES: ADDITIONAL DATA COLLECTION AND REPORT STRATEGIES

Pick lists are simply lists of text items that can be selected and pasted into a report. These may be lists of such commonly used goals as interventions and interpretations. OT FACT also makes available areas in which practitioners can attach memoranda information to any question or category being assessed. For example, if an individual has extreme difficulty organizing time, and the chosen intervention being tried is an electronic scheduler, the details of this scheduler could be described in the assessment itself using a memo category. All memos can automatically be merged into the report.

Templates are simply prewritten parts of the data collection process. For example, if another assessment is commonly used in an intake assessment, this form can be built directly into the OT FACT data collection process by placing the intake data collection categories into OT FACT memo areas. It is essential to recognize, however, that many of these extended features of OT FACT, like any significant software package, demand time to learn and customize.

Program Evaluation and Outcomes Research

OT FACT includes a mechanism for compiling large data sets so that information can be placed into a spreadsheet or a statistic package for an examination of group data. While OT FACT generates no specific program evaluation or outcomes report, it does have a plug-in available that allows the data to be compiled for additional investigative research studies.

Psychometric Aspects of OT FACT

CRITERION-REFERENCED

OT FACT is a criterion-referenced assessment. Many occupational therapy assessments are based on normal distributions and compare individual scores to a mathematical mean by examining standard deviations or standard scores. OT FACT does not subscribe to the concept of normal functional performance. Moreover, OT FACT does not even suppose that there are normal functional areas that must be assessed to determine whether an individual is functional. OT FACT is criterion-referenced and founded on the concept that individuals can range from being able to perform 100% of the specific tasks and life activities they need to perform, to being totally unable to perform any of the specific tasks and life activities. Thus, the score represents a person's function in the tasks, not a comparison to any normative group.

NOMOTHETIC VERSUS IDIOGRAPHIC APPROACH

In addition to the OT FACT criterion-referenced orientation, the tasks and activities assessed specifically target the needs of the individual. Again, this sets OT FACT apart from most assessments used in occupational therapy practice. The items in the OT FACT assessment may differ from one person to the next, as previously described in the tailoring aspect of the TTSS approach. Traditional test and measurement instruments, even criterion-referenced tests, tend to use a standard set of questions enabling a nomothetic application. OT FACT individualizes the questioning process to better match the concept of an idiographic assessment approach.[7] The construct that OT FACT targets is the functional performance of individuals in their own environmental, physical, social, cultural, and developmental contexts.

DATA-BASED THEORY VERSUS DECISION-BASED THEORY

The measurement theory closest to OT FACT methodology is called decision-based theory, as opposed to data-based theory. *Data-based* theory collects data and obtains distributions of data to which an individual's score is compared. Typically in classical test and measurement theory, the assumed distribution is a bell-shaped curve, which sets the backdrop for comparing an individual's score to the normal distribution.

Recognizing non-bell-shaped distributions, however, has become more popular in recent years. For example, the types of assessments that use item-response theory can assume non-normal distributions that have been obtained from prior data sets.[8] Item-response theory applications, including Rasch Scale Measurement,[9] use item difficulty to ascertain distributions. These distributions are often not normal but are consistent with assessments created from data-based theory, as they require previously collected group data for proper interpretation. Data-based theory can also drive the selection of items within a given assessment. For example, Rasch Scaling analysis methods allow the omission of a test question because previously collected data has documented the item difficulty of each question. Rasch Scaling allows for the interpretation of the meaning of an individual's score by simply adjusting the "difficulty" ruler.[10]

OT FACT is one assessment used in mental health and occupational therapy for which use and interpretations do not depend on prior data, thus reflecting a *decision-based* theoretical perspective. In OT FACT, questions are included in the assessment and scores interpreted specific to the individual. Additionally, OT FACT, like other decision-based assessments, relies heavily on subjective information, subjective weighting of question items, and adaptive interrogation. Question selection is dependent on the individual and his or her answers to prior questions. Many mental health assessments that collect data using the interview technique are similarly based on this type of theoretical perspective.

Validity and Reliability Design Implications of TTSS

Inherent in the fundamental structure and design of the TTSS approach is an attempt to optimize reliability and validity. For example, the branching component of TTSS theoretically increases the reliability of response. In most assessments, when an individual response is being elicited and the individual administering the assessment does not know the answer because of a poor understanding of the question or an ambiguity in the definition, the practitioner must respond by either guessing or leaving data missing. In the case of the TTSS data collection methodology, if an individual does not understand a given question or how an individual should be scored in that category, the proper scoring response is 1. The TTSS software then proceeds to expand the question into more detail, breaking down the particular construct of the question category. The more detailed questions explain the question construct with more concrete behaviors and make it easier to provide an accurate response. In this way, the TTSS methodology allows the data collector to clarify questions for consistency of response.

Additionally, the TTSS design attempts to increase reliability throughout its trichotomous scale. The trichotomous scale provides only three options, allowing the data collector to quickly and confidently tally a score. The more common assessments, which have a 5-point or 7-point scale, require more data collection deliberation, as there are more intermediate points on the scale. Often, these types of assessments require special training sessions for data collectors.

A third characteristic of the TTSS approach that helps optimize reliability is its number of questions. The trichotomous and sub-branching aspect of TTSS permits rapid data collector response. Thus, the data collector can efficiently answer many more questions in a similar amount of time as would be used with a complicated scaling system. The Spearman-Brown formula statistically proves that increasing the number of questions on a test increases its reliability.

The TTSS methodology also attempts to maximize the validity of functional performance assessment in three ways.

- First, the TTSS structure enables a prompting system. The comprehensive nature of the OT FACT taxonomy presents functional performance categories to the data collector for consideration of each area. While a given question may not be applicable, the range of questions offered allows appropriate questions to be completed for an individual's assessment of functional performance. Thus, fewer questions are left out due to inadvertent omissions or an assessment's attempts to standardize questions across the population (many assessments lose richness of detail as the questions move toward the lowest common denominator).

- Second, validity also is addressed with nonapplicable questions. Not only does the OT FACT taxonomy prompt a comprehensive performance review, but the ability to omit questions as nonapplicable individualizes the question set. The resulting process performs a mini-validation of each question to match the needs and diversity of people with disabilities.

- Third, the validity of the TTSS methodology is forwarded by the methods with which the OT FACT taxonomy was generated. The taxonomy of questions was developed from field research and multiple iterations of feedback from occupational therapy practice from more than 30 feedback sessions. Two national field tests supplemented early taxonomies that were based on practice from AOTA's *Uniform Terminology*.

A number of small reliability and validity studies have been performed during the development of OT FACT. Some of these studies were performed early to identify whether the TTSS process was going to be sufficiently robust; other studies are confirmation. Table 19-1 charts the overall results of these studies. While these studies are just beginning

Table 19-1
Results of Reliability and Validity Studies

Type of Reliability or Validity Activity	N	Procedure	Statistical Outcome	Interpretation	Reference
Content Validity Development		Began with AOTA *Uniform Terminology*; design team worked with AOTA Uniform Terminology II in parallel development.		OTFACT taxonomy of questions based on practice-accepted uniform terminology.	
Rater Reliability Development		Up-front deliberate design		Scoring procedure designed to minimize rater error. Discussed in more detail in chapter.	Smith, 1991
Construct Validity Development	41 surveys from workshops	Likert-style survey on paper-and-pencil version	Wide range depending on question.	Predominantly positive about the conceptualization of the instrument. Skepticism about paper-and-pencil version being the right tool for their particular area of practice. Specific question asking whether the tool should be computerized resulted in overwhelming agreement that it should.	Smith, unpublished
Content Validity Development	>30 regional workshops and group feedback sessions	Informal focus group discussion		Seven major versions were generated. Two major version of taxonomy in software.	Smith, 1990; Smith, 1998

continued

Table 19-1, continued
Results of Reliability and Validity Studies

Construct Validity Development		Development of theory as foundation		The HOPPIT model was developed and is discussed in the chapter in more detail.	Various
Content Validity Development		National field-test computer version 1.0		Comments on taxonomy and procedures. Resulted in new versions.	
Alternate Form	national field data of N = 127	Pearson and Spearman Correlations	All r > .97	Short form and long form virtually identical.	Smith & Rust, 1992
Content Validity	national field data of N = 127	The above analysis also subjects the test to interval scaling analysis.	As above	The score of 1 (average) to be equidistant between 2 and 0.	Smith & Rust, 1992
Content Validity	25 patients with multiple sclerosis	Krippendorf coefficients and rater agreement	0.89 five 5 OT raters; agreement between OT raters and patients 94%; 86% agreement with patients 10 days later	OTFACT categories highly correlated with Activity Configurations used in practice.	Bhasin & Goodman, 1992
Interrater Validity	13 pairs of diversely trained therapists	Pearson Correlations, Spearman Correlations, Item Agreement	Fifteen of twenty-four of the correlations resulted in p values of <.005. Nine of twenty-four r values >.9, eight additional >.7. Percent exact agreement of summed categories ranged from 62% to 92%.	Strong indications that the TTSS/ OTFACT approach demonstrated a high degree of inter-rater reliability.	Smith, 1998

continued

Table 19-1, continued					
Results of Reliability and Validity Studies					
Rater Reliability	Two sets of true data were used for this analysis. For 7-point scaling there were 3,456 primary data cells (24 questions* 144 tests), and for TTSS there were 13,064 (21 branches and 21 bottom-level leaves totaling 92 questions* 142 tests).	Sensitivity Analysis	Almost zero resulting error below 30% forced rater error. Over 30% forced rater error explodes resulting error substantially.	Assuming that OT FACT raters produce less than the 30% error tolerance, rater reliability is excellent. Traditional 7-point scale was not stable at error levels below 30% tolerate error as well.	Smith, 1993

to identify the usefulness of OT FACT, they are viewed as indicators of the potential of software data collection.

Contemporary Reliability and Validity

In the early 1990s, it became apparent that the TTSS process was developing innovative types of dynamic scaling that traditional reliability research methods were only partially able to address. TTSS is not an instrument for which we can confirm or reject reliability. It is a scaling approach. Unfortunately, traditional test and measurement methodology is attuned to examining instruments, not approaches. Therefore, to investigate the reliability of TTSS, which is a decision-based theory method, one study used a decision-theory technique. The TTSS approach was examined by sensitivity analysis, comparing it to the traditional 7-point scale.[11] The results of this study showed that the TTSS method was more stable than a 7-point scale method. The study examined how rater error affected the true score. The results showed that when a rater was within 30% of the true score, the TTSS method was extremely stable compared to the 7-point scale method. When rater error exceeded 30% of the true score, however, the TTSS scale became volatile, resulting in an exaggerated amount of error. In contrast, under the scenario of high rater error, the traditional 7-point scale method was more stable. Given the features of the TTSS design to improve the inherent reliability of data collectors highlighted earlier, and the high correlations of preliminary inter-rater reliability studies,[1] it seems quite plausible that occupational therapy raters would remain within the 30% tolerance. Therefore, the TTSS scaling structure could very well be viewed as more likely to score the true functional abilities of an individual than the traditional 7-point scale method. Obviously, additional studies are required, but these initial steps to validate the method seem promising.

Use of OT FACT to Teach Holistic Physical and Mental Health Perspectives in Occupational Therapy

Since the HOPPIT taxonomy is comprehensive, it allows a unique way for professionals entering occupational therapy to view disability and individual functional performance of people with disabilities. Several university and college programs training occupational therapy students have used the OT FACT software to help students review and document functional performance across all domains relevant to occupational therapy. While specialization in occupational therapy fragments functional assessment into areas of practice, it becomes important for occupational therapy students to view practice from a much wider perspective. OT FACT allows students to consider all aspects of human dysfunction and human performance abilities in one data collection scheme to frame a mental model that encapsulates all of occupational therapy.

Use of the HOPPIT model can frame curricular content to ensure appropriate coverage and help students identify where the different areas of coursework apply to overall human performance. The OT FACT software has assisted students in Level I and Level II fieldwork placements, as the prompting of categories helps teach practitioners-in-training to avoid inadvertent omission of important assessment and intervention areas.

Past, Present, and Future Contribution of Occupational Therapy to Measurement

The development of OT FACT, over more than a decade of maturation, has provided a concerted effort to optimize reliability and validity in every step of the design process. This is attempted through careful attention in design to unique methods of scaling, its comprehensive approach, and its theory-grounded approach to the construct of function. One might ask why, when measurement of people's disabilities has been around for decades, this type of approach has been suggested only recently. Interestingly enough, the answer to this question is two-fold. First, occupational therapists have only become interested in measurement in recent decades. As a profession and a discipline of occupational science, occupational therapy is relatively new and has not been ready to propose new ways of looking at measuring human performance and the functioning of people with disabilities. The literature and chapters in this text highlight much of the interest in assessment and measurement in occupational therapy, as interest has risen in recent decades. Only recently have the occupational therapy profession and the occupational sciences discipline been ready to offer and contribute functional assessment and holistic approaches to disability. Second, the technology and instrumentation potential used in

OT FACT was not ready for computerized implementation until the 1990s. Computer power and costs have only recently become practical for daily use in occupational therapy. The computerized, complex assessment schemes offered by the TTSS method and the OT FACT taxonomy have only become possible in the past decade.

Future Use of OT FACT

The availability of computer technology to occupational therapists in recent years made OT FACT possible. Computer portability, price, and accessibility has finally made computerized assessment realistic in occupational therapy practice. OT FACT, with the customization potential to tune its use across many applications, is a comprehensive tool for occupational therapists. While it is able to customize to specific, specialized areas in occupational therapy practice, the unique contribution of OT FACT is its ability to view patients from a comprehensive and holistic perspective based on a practice theory generated from the field. The software provides a consistent method for collecting data and merging the data into various types of reports.

Although the OT FACT software is no longer available for use through the AOTA, its theoretical foundation and new measurement methods deserve serious examination and comparison with other assessment approaches. OT FACT still offers a fresh model for assessment. Plus, other applications of OT FACT are being explored. For example, the OT FACT structure is being viewed as a possible mechanism for teasing out the specific impact of assistive technology and its contribution to overall functional performance.[12-15]

While OT FACT's innovativeness continues to require intensive research efforts to validate specific applications within areas of occupational therapy practice, it remains a model for versatile measurement, documentation, and reporting for occupational therapy practice and represents an innovative tool for the profession.

Occupational therapy practice is comprehensive in scope. It spans diagnostic populations and stretches across a full spectrum of practice settings. This extremely wide scope of practice is unique to occupational therapy and provides a rich basis for organizing a scheme to assess the degree and outcome of disability. This extraordinary perspective of the occupational therapy profession is the foundation of OT FACT. Through the use of computerized data collection, this scheme has become feasible to apply. OT FACT brings together a practice theory model of human performance, modern test theory, and technology.

Summary

This chapter provides an overview of the OT FACT data collection software, the theory underlying its scoring methodology, and its use. The scaling approach, Trichotomous Sub-Branching Scoring, is described as a data collection method that has only become feasible with the use of computer technology in the practice setting. The chapter also summarizes the psychometric characteristics of the instrument. Excerpts of OT FACT psychosocial categories and definitions, as well as an OT FACT profile, have been included in Appendices U and V.

References

1. Smith RO. OT FACT, version 2.0, version 2.03. [Computer software and manual]. Rockville, MD: American Occupational Therapy Association Inc; 1998.
2. American Occupational Therapy Association. *Occupational Therapy Product Output Reporting System and Uniform Terminology for Reporting Occupational Therapy Services*. Rockville, MD: Author; 1979.
3. American Occupational Therapy Association. *Uniform Terminology for Occupational Therapy*. 2nd ed. *Am J Occup Ther*. 1989;43:808-815.
4. American Occupational Therapy Association. *Uniform Terminology for Occupational Therapy*. 3rd ed. *Am J Occup Ther*. 1994;48(11):1047-1054.
5. National Center for Medical Rehabilitation Research. *Research Plan for the National Center for Medical Rehabilitation Research*. Washington, DC: US Dept of Health and Human Services, Publication No. 93-3509; 1993.
6. Institute of Medicine. Models of Disability and Rehabilitation. In: Brandt J, Edward N, Pope AM, eds. *Enabling America: Assessing the Role of Rehabilitation Science and Engineering*. Washington, DC: National Academy Press; 1997.
7. Silva F. *Psychometric Foundations and Behavioral Assessment*. Newbury Park, CA: Sage Publications Inc; 1993.
8. Hambleton RK, Swamihathan H, Rogers HJ. *Fundamentals of Item Response Theory*. Newbury Park, CA: Sage Publications Inc; 1991.
9. Wright BD, Masters GN. *Rating Scale Analysis*. Chicago, IL: Mesa Press; 1982.
10. Fisher W. Scale-free measurement revisited. *Rasch Measurement Transactions*. 1993;7(1):272-273.
11. Smith RO. Sensitivity Analysis of Trichotomous Tailored Sub-Branch Scoring (TTSS) and traditional Scales. Unpublished PhD dissertation. University of Wisconsin-Madison; 1993.
12. Smith RO. Using the Occupational Therapy Comprehensive Functional Assessment (OTCFA) to Evaluate the Efficacy of Technological Intervention in Rehabilitation. Paper presented at the RESNA '87. Washington, DC; 1987.
13. Smith RO. Assessing the Impact of Assistive Technology Using OT FACT Version 2.0. Paper presented at the RESNA '93. Arlington, VA; 1993.
14. Davel N, Smith RO. Functional Impact of Assistive Technology on People With Hemiplegia From Stroke. Paper presented at the RESNA '96. Salt Lake City, UT; 1996.
15. Bhasin CA. Review of OT FACT. In: Vitaliti LU, ed. *RESNA Resource Guide for Assistive Technology Outcomes: Assessment Instruments, Tools, and Checklists From the Field*. Arlington, VA: RESNA; 1998;2:22-31.

PART VIII:
ADDITIONAL ASSESSMENTS

A SUMMARY OF ASSESSMENTS IN WELLNESS

Virginia K. White, PhD, OTR, FAOTA
Kathlyn L. Reed, PhD, OTR, MLIS, FAOTA

"Wellness is a way of life and life style a person designs to achieve an optimal potential for well being." Travis JW, Ryan RS. Wellness Index. *Berkeley, CA: Celestial Arts; 2004.*

Introduction

Within the profession of occupational therapy, several authors have described *wellness.* Johnson[1] describes wellness as a way of adapting patterns of behavior to lead to improved physical, emotional, and spiritual health, and heightened life satisfaction. White[2] describes the concept of wellness as the result of a lifestyle for well-being that a person chooses, regardless of the presence or absence of disabling conditions, to reach optimum potential. Swarbrick[3] suggests that "wellness is a lifestyle that incorporates a good balance of health habits, such as adequate sleep and rest, productivity, exercise, supportive thought processes, and social resources" that influence social roles and associated activities. Burkhardt[4] describes wellness simply as good health that includes those aspects contributing to the maintenance of health. In the current edition of *Willard & Spackman's Occupational Therapy,*[5(p1035)] wellness is defined as "actions that lead to a healthy lifestyle, including nutrition, exercise, stress reduction, and other strategies."

Taber's Cyclopedic Medical Dictionary[6(p2110)] defines wellness as "the condition of being in good health, including the appreciation and the enjoyment of health. Wellness is more than a lack of disease symptoms; it is a state of mental and physical balance and fitness." Cammack and Eisenberg[7(p124)] state that wellness is "a process for living that one follows in order to achieve one's optimum potential," and that wellness is a dynamic process to be achieved, regardless of the presence of illness and disability. Wellness is also defined as a dynamic state of health in which an individual progresses toward a higher level of functioning, achieving an optimum balance between internal and external environments.[8(p1665)] Finally, Travis and Ryan[9] provide several definitions that form a summary of assumptions about wellness:

1. Wellness is a choice or decision a person makes to move toward optimal health.
2. Wellness is a way of life and lifestyle a person designs to achieve the highest potential for well-being.
3. Wellness is a (dynamic adaptive) process for developing awareness that there is no end point, but that health and happiness are possible in each moment, here and now.
4. Wellness is an efficient channeling of energy that is received from the environment, transformed within the person, and sent on to affect the world outside (to create a dynamic balance between internal and external factors).
5. Wellness is the integration of body, mind, and spirit—the appreciation that everything a person does, thinks, feels, and believes has an impact on the state of his or her health.
6. Wellness is the loving acceptance of the self.

The descriptions of wellness suggest the conditions and situations that facilitate or contribute to the maintenance of wellness, but do not provide an assessment or an intervention approach to assist people in achieving a dynamic state of wellness. In particular, the descriptions of wellness do not provide the framework for organizing a practice model or intervention approach that draws upon the unique contribution of occupational therapy to the attainment of occupational wellness as an outcome and goal.

What Is Occupational Wellness?

Occupational wellness links occupation to wellness, and by so doing creates a concept that has the potential for introducing a new practice model. First, it is necessary to define terms. *Occupation* involves "groups of activities and tasks of everyday life, named, organized, and given value and meaning by individuals and a culture; occupation is everything people do to occupy themselves, including looking after themselves (self-care), enjoying life (leisure), and contributing to the social and economic fabric of their communities (productivity)."[10(p181)] This definition was modified for the *Occupational Therapy Practice Framework*.[11] In addition, occupation may be viewed as "the highest level of complexity of human function that provides longitudinal organization of time and effort in a person's life. Occupation defines and organizes a sphere of action over a period of time and is perceived by the individual as part of her/his personal and social identity."[12(p55)] In other words, occupation frames a person's, group's, or institution's satisfaction and quality of life by providing meaning, mission or purpose, and enjoyment to actions. Occupation permits the participation in family, economic, and social life. It contributes to the promotion, maintenance, and recovery of health and sense of well-being. Occupation organizes groups of activities into patterns and routines within a temporal framework of past, present, and future; it may facilitate the achievement or attainment of a sense of efficacy and competence, and of self-actualization and high-level wellness over a span of years. The attributes of occupation create the foundation for the practice of occupational therapy. The complexity of occupation creates a wide variety of options for occupational therapists to use when interacting with individuals.

PHILOSOPHY, ASSUMPTIONS, AND CONCEPTS

The philosophy, assumptions, and concepts of occupational wellness were designed to support the development of an assessment and intervention model for use in occupational therapy. Occupational wellness is defined as "the process of organizing daily life patterns into units of occupation that individuals perform in a manner that is meaningful, purposeful, and satisfying. The units of occupation contribute to maintaining health and wellness and to avoiding those that represent substantial risk factors."[13] In developing the concept of occupational wellness, several philosophical statements were identified by drawing from the literature on wellness, but integrating the concept of occupation. Occupational wellness:[13]

1. Addresses individual or personal issues, rather than group or institutional issues.

2. Builds on the tradition of health promotion and prevention, rather than the remediation or "patching up" of illness or disability.

3. Addresses the need for intervention in physical, cognitive, mental, social, and spiritual disorders that have a major impact on a person's lifestyle and participation in society over a period of months and years, not just hours or days.

4. Enables a person to create a satisfying lifestyle that uses occupation as a focal point for attaining a level of wellness that is independent of any disabling condition.

5. Stresses what a person can do to organize and live a lifestyle by selecting occupations that are effective in achieving satisfaction and quality of life.

6. Is a dynamic, interactive process that is achieved by the individual through knowledge and performance of the socially expected occupations, the health-maintaining and -promoting occupations, and the play-leisure occupations in a balanced state acceptable to the individual.

7. Is a dynamic process that changes over a lifetime, although certain themes or interests may appear again and again, such as love of the outdoors, creative crafts, or cooking and baking. The process can be influenced by physical, social, and cultural contexts.

8. Is an internal mechanism that is acquired through participation with the environment and by making conscious choices about action taken that the person finds pleasurable and enjoyable. Actions may be planned well in advance or may appear to occur on a whim but with the person's knowledge and willingness to participate.

9. Requires the person to be actively involved, an active agent, in the choice of occupations that are engaged in to create a balance of occupation in harmony and rhythm with the individual's life situation.

10. Requires the person to feel and believe the self to be a significant part of the action, activity, or task inherent within the occupation.

11. Incorporates a present and future time perspective as opposed to dwelling on or living in the past.

12. Must be developed from within the person because it is a state of mind and a belief system. Occupational wellness cannot be forced upon a person. Self-initiation and self-efficacy are essential, although others may suggest ideas and methods directly or indirectly that the person adopts or adapts to his or her own purpose.

13. Results in a value system that values the self as an occupational being who is able to engage and participate in occupation, regardless of the actual or perceived state of health, illness, dysfunction, disorder, disease or condition.

Other assumptions further refine the beliefs and values about occupational wellness. These are:[13]

1. The individual is able to achieve and maintain a balance between socially expected health maintenance and play-leisure occupations that are personally satisfying.

2. The individual is an active agent in the choice of occupations performed and the occupational activities or tasks in which the individual engages.

3. The individual is an active agent in determining the spatial and temporal components in which the occupational activities or tasks are performed.

4. The individual is able to change the performance of occupations into different units of space and time; that is, perform the occupations in different geographical space and at different times of the day, week, etc.

5. The individual demonstrates a degree of mastery or competence in the performance of the occupations in which the individual engages.

6. The individual demonstrates a sense of pride in achieving the performance level of at least some occupational activities or tasks that are performed.

7. The individual engages in self-selected occupational activities or tasks on a routine basis that result in a recognizable pattern of daily performance of occupation.

8. The individual derives a sense of self-worth and self-efficacy by identifying with the selection and performance of occupations and the achievement of occupational wellness.

9. Occupational therapists are able, through their knowledge, skills, and values, to assist individuals in the attainment of occupational wellness through observation, interview, and self-report of the individual and the application of selected strategies and management of an intervention program using socially expected, health-promoting and -maintaining, and play-leisure occupations.

Concepts

The essential concepts of the Occupational Wellness Model include occupation, values, and sense of personal control. These concepts also require definition. Occupation is further defined as the ordinary and familiar things that people do every day.[14] Occupation is not limited to one's job, position, or work, although the term does encompass aspects of employment or service for pay. Occupation can be divided into three subcategories: socially expected, health-promoting and -maintaining, and play-leisure. *Socially expected* occupations are those that the individual performs as a result of attaining a certain age or stage of life, such as going to school, working for a living, being a marriage partner, caring for young children, or being a retiree. *Health-promoting* and *-maintaining* occupations are those self-care and domestic tasks that promote and maintain physical, mental, and spiritual health, such as eating, sleeping, brushing one's teeth, taking a bath or shower, finding and using shelter from the weather, keeping the shelter free of human waste and rotting food, and attending religious services. *Play-leisure* occupations are those that the individual chooses to perform because of personal values or interests, rather than in response to social expectation. Kielhofner[15(p46)] defines *values* as "a coherent set of convictions that assign significance or standards to occupations, creating a strong disposition to perform accordingly." He summarizes values as "images of what is good, right and/or important."[15(p509)] *Sense of personal control* is defined as an internal mechanism that enables individuals to feel they can change the outcome of situations in which they participate.[15]

Subcategories of Occupation

The subcategories of occupation create additional concepts related to occupation: balance of occupation and occupational activities. A *balance of occupation* involves engagement in occupation that leads to a sense of well-being. For example, the balance may be among physical, mental, and social occupations; between chosen and obligatory occupations; between strenuous and restful occupation; or between doing and being.[16] Balanced occupation is idiosyncratic; the individual must determine what constitutes a balance of occupation for him or her. However, the occupational therapist can provide examples and opportunities to try different groupings of occupational activities. *Well-being* is "a subjective sense of overall contentment, thought to be defined by affective state and life satisfaction."[17(p606)]

Occupational activities are activities that are part of, or concerned with, the performance of an occupation.[18] *Activities* are recognizable sequences of actions taken together in a particular context.[19] *Tasks* are a means of accomplishing an activity.[19] Occupational activities and tasks are external to the individual. The individual develops skills to accomplish occupational activities and tasks.

Values

One value often mentioned by clients is health. The World Health Organization defines health as "a complete state of physical, mental, and social well-being and not just the absence of disease or infirmity."[20(p29)] Health has also been described in the professional literature as involving four different models: clinical, role performance, adaptive, and eudaemonistic.[21] The clinical model is concerned with remediating disease and is not, therefore, of primary interest to the model of occupational wellness. However, the role performance, adaptive, and eudaemonistic models are pertinent. *Eudaemonism* is that system of ethics that defines and enforces moral obligation by its relation to happiness or personal well-being.

The *role performance* model considers health as the state of optimum capacity of the individual for the effective performance of roles and tasks within the social environment. If the person can perform the roles and tasks, the person is considered healthy.

The *adaptive* model considers the environment as a central factor in which the individual can engage in effective interaction with both the physical and social environment. Illness is an inability to cope with changes in the environment. Therefore, adaptive behavior is characterized by the ability to interact effectively with the changing environment.

The *eudaemonistic* model extends the definition of health to include well-being and self-realization; it characterizes the value of life in terms of happiness and the achievement of the individual's best aspirations.

These three models of health are pertinent to the concept of lifestyle in which a pattern of daily occupations over time becomes stable and predictable and forms the framework through which an individual expresses his or her identity.[22] Lifestyle often changes due to chronic disability. In such cases, lifestyle may be amenable to the concept of *health promotion,* in which programs are put in place to promote the physical, mental, and social well-being of the person including a focus on the individual's ability to function optimally in his or her environment.

Another important value for many people is the achievement of life satisfaction and/or quality of life. Life satisfaction is defined as an overall positive perception or feeling about the quality of one's own life.[23] Life satisfaction is similar to quality of life, which is an individual's perception of overall satisfaction with one's living circumstances, including physical status and abilities, psychological well-being, social interactions, and economic conditions.[17] Both life satisfaction and quality of life are partly determined by participation, which involves an internal sense of being "in the middle of" planning and executing occupation, and an external, social recognition that the individual is actively engaged in a particular occupational environment. In addition, the person achieves a balance in mind, body, and spirit across all of life's experiences.[22]

Control

Closely related to sense of control are the concepts of mastery and competence. *Mastery* is defined as the achievement of skill to a criterion level of success.[22] In the occupational wellness model, mastery defines a personal criterion level of skill. *Competence* is achievement of skill equal to the demands of the environment.[22] Competence is used to define the socially expected level of skill.

Also related to sense of control are the concepts of self-efficacy and self-worth. *Self-efficacy* involves judgments about one's own capabilities to organize and execute the course of action required to attain a designed type or types of performances.[23] *Self-worth* is a subjective judgment or appraisal of being a worthwhile human being. A person who recognizes his or her own worth tends to also have a high degree of self-acceptance and self-esteem.[23] It is also assumed that self-efficacy that results in successful performance of actions in occupations would contribute to a positive sense of self-worth.

Developing a Practice Model Based on the Conceptual Model of Occupational Wellness

To actuate the conceptual model of occupational wellness in a practice model for occupational therapy, an assessment instrument and suggested intervention approaches needed to be developed. An assessment instrument needs to be based on the major elements of the concept of occupational wellness. In the case of the Occupational Wellness Model, the research project that created the assessment instrument facilitated the identification of the model's essential concepts.

INSTRUMENT DEVELOPMENT

The Occupational Wellness Assessment (OWA) was developed through a research project completed in cooperation with the Veterans Affairs Medical Center (VAMC) in Houston, Texas. The research questions were:

1. What are the meaningful engagements in activities that comprise lifestyles, health values, beliefs, and attitudes of older veterans with disabilities?

2. How do these veterans perceive the quality of their lives?

3. What is the nature of an occupational wellness assessment based on the veterans' profiles that would be the outcome of the interviews with the veterans?

Given these questions, the research objectives were to: (1) develop an occupational wellness profile of older veterans with disabilities, based on the findings from interviews and quality of life assessment; and (2) design an OWA to reflect the uniqueness of veterans with disabilities.

Methods

Subjects were identified by occupational therapists in the rehabilitation department at the VAMC. Although the intent was to include both males and females in the study, only male veterans met the criteria for selection during the time allotted for the study: hospitalized with a stroke, 50 years of age or over, and able to respond to questions during an interview that would take about an hour of their time. As a result, only nine veterans and eight family members were available. Each veteran was asked to designate a family member who would be willing to respond to questions similar to those given to the veteran.

The study was conducted in two phases: Phase 1 was profile development, and Phase 2 was instrument development. Both qualitative and quantitative research methods were used. Qualitative interviews of nine veterans and eight family members were conducted by student research assistants, using a guided interview schedule of questions based on descriptors from the occupational wellness model. Additional descriptors were identified from life stories about elders found in the literature. A schedule was developed containing questions about veterans' health beliefs and practices, satisfaction with the quality of their lives, their present state of life, and history of occupational engagements leading up to the time of the interview. Sample questions were:

- How would you describe a typical day before you were hospitalized?
- What do you do that you believe keeps you healthy?
- What is it about a veteran that is different from someone who is not a veteran?
- Who do you have that you can depend on when you need someone?
- If you were to describe the quality of your life to someone, what would you say?
- What difficulties or obstacles do you experience in your daily life?

The schedule was adapted for the family member so that information about the veteran could be obtained from the viewpoint of the family member.

An additional data source was the Quality of Life Profile, Senior Version (QOLPSV), short form, which elicits information about an individual's being, belonging, and becoming.[24] *Being* refers to physical, psychological, and spiritual arenas; *belonging* refers to physical, social, and community areas of being; *becoming* refers to practical, leisure, and growth areas. Gathering data from three different sources (interviews with the veteran and family member, along with the QOLPSV) added to the trustworthiness and credibility of the data, a process referred to by Creswell[25] as *triangulation*.

Data from the interviews were transcribed verbatim, then "chunked" to reduce the volume of information using open coding, which is the naming and categorizing of phenomena through close examination of the data related to the interview schedule.[26] Summaries of each veteran's and family member's interviews were written as narrative studies, and from these, themes were identified across all cases. Based on the findings, a profile of each informant was developed to guide the framing of the OWA. Those wellness themes were compared with ones found in the literature. Analysis of the data in the QOLPSV yielded numerical and descriptive data that indicated the level of satisfaction of the informants in nine areas of life. These data, along with the veterans' and family members' narratives and identified themes, were sent to a panel of experts for oversight review. The panelists had expertise in areas such as instrument development, lifestyles of community elders, occupational science, and research methodology. They provided conceptualization oversight concerning interviews and literature both in and out of occupational therapy, and critiqued individual and set data of veterans and family members for themes, similarities, and differences.

Questions were developed to expand on the themes of occupation, values, and sense of personal control. Versions of questions were reviewed by practicing occupational therapists at two different conferences. Consideration was given both to the information each question could elicit, as well as to the length of the total interview. Consensus was reached that 12 questions in each area should be used. Thus, the research edition of the OWA is composed of the three subject areas, 12 questions in each, for a total of 36 items. The amount of time needed for the client interview would depend on the client's responsiveness to the questions, but was expected to average about 30 to 45 minutes.

USING THE OCCUPATIONAL WELLNESS ASSESSMENT

The OWA (see Appendix X) is an interview format containing 36 questions that are divided equally into three themes: control, occupation, and values. Control, or sense of control, is the person's perception of his or her ability to take control or be in control of performing the occupation, or directing the situation according to personal desire or need. Occupation is the chunks of daily life activities and tasks that the person performs. Values are the personal belief system about the worth or significance of the occupation or situation. The scoring system ranges from 0 to 4 for each item, depending on the number of responses the person gives to each question. Three questions are scored in reverse, because fewer responses are considered more positive toward achieving a higher level of occupational wellness. Interviews are performed one-on-one and range from 30 to 50 minutes, depending on the person's amount and speed of responses. The OWA has been pilot-tested and revised to improve the clarity of the questions and scoring criteria.

Recent Studies

The OWA has been used in a recent study with patients having early Parkinson's disease. This study summarized four student studies that are part of a larger project designed to increase the knowledge about the Occupational Wellness Model developed by White, Davidson, and Reed and to standardize the OWA. As previously noted in this chapter, the Occupation Wellness Model and the OWA provide information on three major concepts: the types of occupation clients do, the value of those occupations in the clients' lives, and the extent of control the clients feel they have over the performance of those occupations in the past, present, and future.

The primary purpose of the study was to gather data on the effectiveness (construct validity) of the OWA to collect data relevant to each of the major concepts in the Occupational Wellness Model. Additional purposes were to assess the need to reword questions to improve the data-gathering potential of the assessment as a practice-oriented assessment, to establish inter-rater reliability, and to establish concurrent validity with a quality of life instrument. Only data related to the first purpose is reported here.

A total of 20 subjects were interviewed: 10 subjects from an outpatient support group at the VAMC in Houston, Texas and 10 from the Houston Area Parkinson's Society (HAPS). There were 18 men and two women, ranging in age from 59 to 83. All were living in their own homes. Eighteen were married, one was single, and another divorced. All signed consent forms agreeing to be interviewed by student researchers as part of the students' graduation requirement to complete a project or thesis. Four students, working in pairs, interviewed five subjects each. One student observed, while the other interviewed. Because the students were novice investigators, all interviews were recorded and transcribed to increase accuracy.

A summary of the results from the interviews is organized under the themes of occupations, values, and control.

- *Occupations*: All subjects had participated in self-care, work, and leisure activities in the past. At the time of the interviews, all were retired, although several did volunteer work. Most subjects commented about increasing difficulty in performing self-care and leisure activities. Future occupations included a variety of leisure and volunteer activities, although two expressed interest in working again in a limited capacity.

- *Values*: Common values were marriage, having children, graduating from college, being good Christians, and various achievements in sports (men) and crafts (women).

- *Control*: Major issues in control were getting dressed independently, decreasing the risk of falling, difficulty with walking and shuffling gait, lack of energy, loss of driver's license, and difficulty with hand dexterity because of shakiness and tremor. Most interviewees said they were still able to perform occupations and tasks important to them, but were slower and needed more time and assistance.

The implications for occupational therapy, based on the interviews in this study, are that people with early stage Parkinson's could benefit from consultation, education, evaluation, and short-term intervention by occupational therapists. These categories covered all of the intervention processes listed in the *Framework*,[11] except for the Therapeutic Use of Self.

ASSESSMENT OF WELLNESS INSTRUMENTS

As noted previously, the concept of wellness differs among various professions. Some emphasize ways to maintain a healthy body, others emphasize living the good life. In occupational therapy a more comprehensive view has developed. Johnson[1(p129)] defines wellness as a "context for living" that includes six elements:

1. The capacity for expressiveness or ability to communicate
2. A sense of connectedness or caring and concern for others
3. A recognition of something sacred to which one has a commitment
4. The creation of roles that are important in one's life
5. A caring for one's body
6. An ability to handle the ups and downs of life without becoming overwhelmed.

In the study, the analysis of wellness yielded nine themes:
1. Adaptation
2. Context

3. Health

4. Health promotion

5. Occupational performance

6. Prevention

7. Quality of life

8. Role competence

9. Spirituality

These are viewed as independent and not organized in a hierarchy. These themes are defined alphabetically below to emphasize that one is not more important than another to wellness as a concept, although one theme may predominate as a focus of concern for a particular person, at a particular time, and in a particular situation.

- *Adaptation*: A change a person makes in his or her response when the person encounters an occupational challenge. This change is implemented when the individual's customary responses are found inadequate for producing some degree of mastery over the challenge.[11,27] The key element is change. The person must evidence a change in behavior toward a desired goal related to wellness.

- *Health*: A complete state of physical, mental, and social well-being, and not just the absence of disease or infirmity.[20] Health is viewed as a current state that may include positive and negative aspects related to wellness.

- *Health promotion*: Process of enabling people to increase control over and improve their health.[28] Health promotion is viewed as learning and taking action that will have a positive result on wellness in the future. Health promotion is a process to be attained, but never completely achieved.

- *Occupational performance*: The ability to carry out activities of daily life (areas of occupation activities) such as activities of daily living (ADL), instrumental activities of daily living (IADL), education, work, play, leisure, or social participation.[11] Occupational performance includes doing or performing a task, activity, or occupation in one or more of the seven areas of occupation.

- *Prevention*: Anticipation and forestallment of harm, disease, or injury.[6] Prevention occurs when an undesirable or adverse event or behavior does not occur or ceases to occur. A vaccination prevents a disease from occurring; a person may stop smoking and, thus, lessen or eliminate his or her risk of contracting lung disease.

- *Quality of life*: A person's dynamic appraisal of his or her life satisfaction, health and functioning, and socioeconomic factors.[11] Quality of life includes the perception of leading the "good life" or statements suggesting that the person is satisfied with life as it is being lived.

- *Role competence*: The ability to effectively meet the demands of roles in which the client engages.[11] Examples include preschooler, student, homemaker, employee, or retired worker.

- *Spirituality*: Includes contemplation, meditation, prayer, reflection, and activities fostering self-growth and connection with others and with nature.[6]

In most cases, the definitions and descriptions were taken from the *Framework*.[11] The exceptions were health promotion, prevention, and spirituality. Health promotion and prevention are not viewed in this chapter as synonyms, as the definition in the *Framework* would suggest. Health promotion improves the state of a person's overall health, and may include a variety of actions to increase the level of health. Prevention focuses on maintaining health by avoiding as much as possible those known risk factors that decrease health, such as harm, disease, or injury. Spirituality is not discussed in the *Framework*, although spiritual is mentioned as a context. Spirituality is attained through a variety of actions, whereas spiritual is a general motivator without specific actions.

The ideas of action and doing are central to the themes defined within wellness. Since most assessment instruments rely on behavior that can be observed or on verbal or written narrative, the action orientation seemed appropriate. Such descriptors as beliefs, values, attitudes, affect, or feelings are inherent in many actions, but may also be present without being acted upon. Assessment requires that the client provide some action.

EVALUATING THE WELLNESS ASSESSMENTS

Since wellness includes several themes, there are many assessments that could have been reviewed within this chapter, such as functional assessments of daily living tasks, role performance, work-related, and health status. Such assessments tend to be based on one dimension of wellness rather than a broader view. The decision was made to focus on assessments that appeared to focus on the broader scope of wellness. Wellness as a term for identifying assessments produced limited results. Therefore, a decision was made to broaden the search by using additional terms. Typical synonyms and related ideas appeared to be psychological well-being, life satisfaction, and quality of life. Additional assessments could be readily identified using the three terms. Those selected for review include assessments identified as having an occupational therapy author, assessments well-known in the research literature, and those by authors outside the field. Another selection factor was availability of a sample of the assessment or a good description. In addition to determining if the nine factors were included in the assessment, an attempt was made to determine the extent of coverage. Minimal coverage meant the subject was mentioned but very little detail was included. Moderate coverage meant that about half of the content related to the concept was included. Comprehensive coverage meant that all or nearly all of the content related to the concept was covered.

The result of these criteria is a review of 14 assessments: seven with authors from other fields (Table 20-1) and seven with occupational therapy authors (Table 20-2).

The review is summarized in Tables 20-1 and 20-2. Two assessments meet eight of the nine criteria: one with an occupational therapy author and one with a non-occupational therapy author. The best overall coverage in occupational therapy was the Quality of Life Profile: Senior, Full Version.[24] The other assessment was the Lifestyle Assessment Questionnaire, which is based on the work of Dr. William Hettler at the University of Wisconsin.

The assessments by occupational therapists were not as consistent as those by non-occupational therapy authors in covering five of the subject areas: context, health, health promotion, prevention and role competence. Occupational therapy authors tended to cover the subjects of occupational performance and adaptation better than non-occupational therapy authors. Coverage of quality of life and spirituality was judged to be about the same. In general, coverage of adaptation, prevention, and role competence was judged as poor by all authors. Health, occupational performance, and quality of life were most completely covered. Comprehensive coverage was judged in six subjects within four assessments. The Quality of Life Profile[24] covered health and quality of life comprehensively. The Wellness Index[9] covered health promotion and spirituality comprehensively. The Life Satisfaction Index covered quality of life comprehensively and the Lifestyle Assessment Questionnaire covered health promotion comprehensively.

Table 20-1

Amount of Coverage of Wellness Themes in Assessments Not Developed by Occupational Therapists

Assessments:	GWS	LAS	LSI	QoL	WI-1	WI-2	WoW
Adaptation							
Context		Min			Min	Mod	Min
Health	Mod	Min		Mod	Mod	Mod	Mod
Health Promotion		Com				Com	
Occupational Performance		Min		Min	Min	Min	Mod
Prevention		Min				Min	
Quality of Life	Min	Min	Com	Min	Mod		Min
Role Competence		Min					Min
Spirituality		Min			Min	Com	Min

Assessments: General Well-being Schedule (GWS), Lifestyle Assessment Questionnaire (LAS), Life Satisfaction Index (LSI), Quality of Life Index (QoL), The Wellness Index, Slivinske, Fitch, & Morawski(WI-1), Wellness Index, Travis & Ryan (WI-2), Wheel of Wellness (WoW)

Min=Minimal coverage, Mod=Moderate coverage, Com=Complete coverage, Blank=No coverage

Dupuy HJ. The General Well-being Schedule. In: McDowell I, Newell C, eds. *Measuring Health*. Oxford: Oxford University Press; 1977: 206-213.

Hattie JA, Myers JE, Sweeney TJ. A factor structure of wellness: Theory, assessment, analysis, and practice. *Journal of Counseling & Development*. 2004;82:354-364.

Institute for Lifestyle Improvement. Lifestyle Assessment Questionnaire. In: Waltz CF, Strickland OL, eds. *Measurement of Nursing Outcomes. Volume 1: Measuring Client Outcomes*. New York: Springer Publishing; 1980: 362-376.

Myers JE, Sweeney TJ, Witmer JM. *The Wellness Evaluation of Lifestyle*. Greensboro, NC: Authors; 1998.

Neugarten BL, Havighurst RJ, Tobin SS. The measurement of life satisfaction (Life Satisfaction Index A). *J Gerontol*. 1961;16:134-143.

Slivainski LR, Morawski DP. The Wellness Index: Developing an instrument to assess elders' well-being. *J Gerontol Soc Work*. 1996; 25(3/4):185-204.

Spitzer WO, Dobson AJ, Hall J, et al. Measuring the quality of life of cancer patients: A concise index for use by physicians. *Journal of Chronic Diseases*. 1981; 34, 585-597.

Table 20-2

Coverage of Themes in Assessments Developed by Occupational Therapists

Assessments:	LSQ	MLQ	MNSS	NSAI	QOT	QoLP	SPSQ
Adaptation					Min	Mod	
Context		Min	Min			Mod	
Health	Min				Min	Com	
Health Promotion			Min		Min	Mod	
Occupational Performance	Mod	Mod		Min	Min	Mod	Mod
Prevention						Mod	
Quality of Life	Min	Mod	Min	Min	Min	Com	
Role Competence							
Spirituality		Min	Min		Mod	Mod	

Assessments: Life Satisfaction Questionnaire (LSQ), Mayer's Lifestyle Questionnaire (MLQ), Modified Need Satisfaction Schedule (MNSS), Need Satisfaction of Activity Interview (NSAI), Qual OT (QOT), Quality of Life Profile (QoLP), Revised Satisfaction with Performance Scaled Questionnaire (SPSQ)

Min=Minimum coverage, Mod=Moderate coverage, Com=Complete coverage, Blank=No coverage

Fugl-Meyer AR, Bränholm I-B, Fugl-Meyer KS. Happiness and domain-specific life satisfaction in adult northern Swedes. *Clin Rehab.* 1991;4:25-33.

Mayers CA. The development and evaluation of the Mayers' Lifestyle Questionnaire (2). *British Journal of Occupational Therapy.* 2003; 66(9):388-395.

Raphael D, Renwick R, Brown I. *Quality of Life Profile: Seniors (Full Version).* Toronto: University of Toronto: Centre for Health Promotion; 1996.

Robrett RH, Gilner JA. Qual-OT: A quality of life assessment tool. *OTJR.* 1995;15(3):198-214.

Tickle L, Yerxa EJ. Need satisfaction of older persons living in the community and in institutions, Part 1, The environment (Modified Need Satisfaction Schedule). *Am J Occup Ther.* 1981; 35(10):644-649.

Tickle L, Yerxa EJ. Need satisfaction of older persons living in the community and in institutions, Part 2. Role of activity. (Need Satisfaction of Activity Interview). *Am J Occup Ther.* 1981; 35(10):650-655.

Yerxa EJ, Burnett-Beaulieu S, Stocking S, Azen S. Development of the Satisfaction with Performance Scaled Questionnaire. *Am J Occup Ther.* 1988;42:215-221.

Summary

The assessment of occupational wellness appears to be a work in progress. The concept of wellness needs further refinement and definition. Two categories of instruments currently exist: those that measure wellness in relation to health status, and those that measure wellness as a topic for personal development, learning, and counseling. Occupational therapists need to decide what focus the profession of occupational therapy should take and develop assessments based on that perspective. Health status does not require intervention, but development and learning suggest that intervention is a consideration. Development and learning require change and adaptive behavior. If occupational therapists are interested in wellness as an outcome, then attention to change processes and adaptive behavior need to be addressed in greater detail than appears in current assessment instruments.

References

1. Johnson J. Wellness and occupational therapy. *Am J Occup Ther.* 1986;40:753-758.
2. White VK. Guest editorial – Promoting health and wellness: a theme for the eighties. *Am J Occup Ther.* 1986;40:743-738.
3. Swarbrick P. Wellness model for clients: Mental Health Special Interest Section Quarterly. 1997;20(1):1-4.
4. Burkhardt A. Occupational therapy & wellness. *OT Practice.* 1997;2(6):28-35.
5. Crepeau EB, Cohn ES, Schell BAB, eds. *Willard & Spackman's Occupational Therapy.* 10th ed. Philadelphia, PA: Lippincott Williams & Wilkins; 2003;1035.
6. Thomas CL, ed. *Taber's Cyclopedic Medical Dictionary.* 18th ed. Philadelphia: F.A. Davis; 1997.
7. Cammack S, Eisenberg MG, eds. *Key Words in Physical Rehabilitation: A Guide to Contemporary Usage.* New York: Springer Publishing Co;1995:124.
8. Anderson KN, Anderson LE, Glanze WD, eds. *Mosby's Medical, Nursing, & Allied Health Dictionary.* 4th ed. St. Louis, MO: Mosby;1994:1665.
9. Travis JW, Ryan RS. *Wellness Index.* Berkeley, CA: Celestial Arts; 2004.
10. Townsend E, ed. *Enabling Occupation: An Occupational Therapy Perspective.* Ottawa, Ontario: CAOT; 1997; 181.
11. American Occupational Therapy Association. *Occupational Therapy Practice Framework.* Bethesda, MD: Author; 2002:628.
12. Creek J, ed. *Occupational Therapy and Mental Health.* Edinburgh: Churchill Livingstone; 2003:55.
13. Reed KL. Occupational wellness definition. Houston, TX: Texas Woman's University-Houston Center. (unpublished paper); 1998.
13. Reed KL. Occupational wellness. Unpublished manuscript. Houston, TX: Texas Woman's University; 1997.
14. Christiansen C, Clark R, Kielhofner G, Rogers J. Position paper: Occupation. *Am J Occup Ther.* 1995;49:1015-1018.
15. Kielhofner G. *Model of Human Occupation: Theory and Application.* Baltimore, MD: Willliams & Wilkins; 1995.
16. Wilcock A. *An Occupational Perspective of Health.* Thorofare, NJ: SLACK Incorporated; 1998:257.
17. Christiansen C, Baum C. *Occupational Therapy: Enabling Function and Well-Being.* Thorofare, NJ: SLACK Incorporated; 1997:606.
18. Reed KL. *Models of Practice in Occupational Therapy.* Baltimore, MD: Williams & Wilkins; 1984: 501.
19. Townsend E, Christiansen C. *Introduction to Occupation: The Art and Science of Living.* Upper Saddle River, NJ: Prentice-Hall; 2004: 275.
20. World Health Organization. Constitution of the World Health Organization. *Chronicle of the World Health Organization.* 1947;1:29-43.
21. Smith JA. The idea of health: doing foundational inquiry. In: Munhall PL, Oiler CJ, eds. *Nursing Research: A Qualitative Perspective.* Norwalk, CT: Appleton-Century-Crofts; 1986.
22. Jacobs K, Jacobs L. *Quick Reference Dictionary for Occupational Therapy.* 4th ed. Thorofare, NJ: SLACK Incorporated; 2004: 129, 102, 136.

23. Corsini RJ. *The Dictionary of Psychology*. New York: Bruner-Routledge; 2002; 548, 877, 880.
24. Raphael D, Renwick R, Brown I. *Quality of Life Profile. Senior version*. Toronto, Canada: University of Toronto, Centre for Health Promotion; 1998.
25. Creswell JW. *Qualitative Inquiry and Research Design: Choosing Among Five Traditions*. Thousand Oaks, CA: Sage; 1998.
26. Strauss AS, Corbin J. *Basics of Qualitative Research*. Newbury Park, CA: Sage; 1990.
27. Schultz S, Schkade J. Adaptation. In: Christiansen C, Baum C, eds. *Occupational Therapy: Enabling Function and Well-Being*. Thorofare, NJ: SLACK Incorporated; 1997:474.
28. World Health Organization. *Ottawa Charter for Health Promotion*. Ottawa, Ontario: Canadian Public Health Association; 1986.

PEDIATRIC ASSESSMENTS USED IN MENTAL HEALTH

Sandra Edwards, MA, OTR, FAOTA

"There is always one moment in childhood when the door opens and lets the future in." Greene G. The Power and the Glory. *New York, NY: Penguin Classics; 1940.*

The purpose of this chapter is to discuss mental illness in childhood and the assessments used in public sectors such as schools, hospitals, private clinics, and homes. The chapter begins with an overview of the incidence of mental illness in childhood, and applies this information to occupational therapy. Selected assessments for children up to puberty are summarized. These instruments are used to assess children with mental illness to support their strengths and identify deficits for intervention.

Introduction

Approximately one in five children in this nation will experience mental health problems during their childhood at any given time.[1] A report on mental illness in children, cited in the first ever report on mental health in Americans by the US Surgeon General, reported that 9% to 13% of all children have substantial emotional illness.[2] Childhood offers no protection from mental illness. Children with psychosocial problems suffer from this disturbance, causing problems in their major occupations at home and school. The majority of children identified as emotionally disturbed demonstrate failure in the classroom, among peers in social interactions, and low self-esteem and value to the community.[3] These conflicts within themselves and with others can cause failure at school, increased school dropout rates, family conflict, substance abuse, violence, and even suicide. Mental disorders have specific criteria published in the *Diagnostic and Statistical Manual of Mental Disorders—Fourth Edition* (DSM-IV), and the selection of assessments can be used to address these criteria.[4] The selection of assessments needs careful analysis in order to properly assess and provide accurate and successful treatment for the child.

A recent study found that only 21% of children between 6 to 17 years old who were diagnosed with mental illness received the proper support for their mental illness, leaving some 7.5 million children without proper intervention. This lack of service affects children from minority groups more severely, including uninsured children and pre-schoolers.[5] Because children from minority groups attend public schools, and because public schools are among the largest employers of occupational therapists, schools are the most likely arena for the occupational therapists to identify children from minority groups with mental illness. Social stigma, lack of education and services, as well as limitations placed on mental health insurance are some of the reasons that children with psychosocial needs and their families do not get the treatment they require and deserve.

Occupational therapists offer important contributions to the early evaluation and identification of childhood mental disorders in the community, school, and home. However, in occupational therapy practice, it is often more comfortable to focus on motor skills versus the psychosocial, communication/interaction, and process skills of these children because of the ambiguity of the latter and the more comfortable, sharper definition of the former. A skilled occupational therapist providing a thorough evaluation will include a well-balanced selection of assessments representing both the wide perspective of the top-down approach and the detailed perspective of the bottom-up assessment.

Because parents are usually the ultimate experts on their children and the responsible "case managers," it is my practice to summarize the final report verbally using the written report to highlight charts or scores and to provide the parents with a copy of the written report for their records. To begin with verbal explanations is often a more gentle way for parents to receive news that their child is delayed and/or ill. The written report provides a document for future review. If your facility can supply the service of video samples of the child's behaviors to use during the explanation of your assessment results, it is a highly effective way of transmitting understanding of the child's behaviors and development to the parent. A skilled, caring clinician can always find the strengths of a child and the family that need to be highlighted in the results of the assessment. It has been my observation that if the clinician always focuses on what is wrong with a client, the clinician will build contempt. However, if the clinician focuses on what is positive, the clinician builds compassion. Most assessments cannot stand alone, and are best used as part of an interdisciplinary process to assist in the proper evaluation of the child and ultimately to provide successful intervention.

Rationale for the Selection of Assessments

The rationale used for the selection of the assessments in this chapter was based on the quality of the assessment's standardization, such as validity and reliability, usefulness in the school and clinical setting, and in determining intervention. Assessments that provided a continuum for intervention were selected because children with mental illness often require long-term intervention. Another consideration in the selection process was whether the assessment was top-down from a broad perspective, ie, using interview or an assessment of activities of daily living (ADL), or bottom-up with a more specific focus, ie, fine and gross motor coordination. Selections of assessments were made that include the caregiver and the client. The term *evaluation* will refer to the process, and the term *assessment* will refer to the instrument or tool used within the evaluation process of the child. It is rare to have one assessment that is complete and thorough, which compels the therapist to use a combination of assessments. Also, there is no one assessment that is universally applicable. Therefore, a variety of 17 assessments have been selected for review.

Sensory Processing Assessments

Assessments for sensory processing are designed to determine the rate and quality of the child's ability to process the reception of physical stimulus, and convert that stimulus into a neurological and perceptional experience of sensation. These combinations of processes are important because they are prerequisites for the child to learn, perceive, and act in his or her environment.[6] Multiple studies indicate that people with mental illness, such as schizophrenia, have sensory processing and integration problems.[7-9] Some of their deficits include hyper- or hyposensitivity to stimuli or an inability to modulate sensory input.

Attention deficit hyperactivity disorder (ADHD) is among the most prevalent psychiatric disorders in childhood and adolescence,[10] and sensory processing deficits can be characteristic of these children.[11] Preschool children with ADHD appear to have more risk of problems with sensory processing abilities beyond the core symptoms of ADHD.[12]

Another diagnostic group of children with sensory processing deficits are those with Autism Spectrum Disorders.[13] This group of disorders comprises Pervasive Developmental Disorders (PDDS) Autism, Asperger Syndrome, and Pervasive Developmental Disorder–Not Otherwise Specified (PDD-NOS).[1] Autism is the most well-known of these disorders and is associated with intense sensory processing problems. Early identification and treatment of children with PDD has been associated with positive outcomes.[14]

Some assessments that provide information about the child's sensory processing from the parent's and teacher's perspective for both diagnostic groups of ADHD and Autism Spectrum Disorders are the Sensory Profiles. The various Sensory Profiles are described below.

INFANT/TODDLER SENSORY PROFILE (AGES BIRTH TO 36 MONTHS)

This test serves as a standard measure of young children's sensory processing. A caregiver who has daily contact with the child is the source for the questionnaire-based assessment. A therapist with expertise in sensory processing scores and interprets the child's threshold responses as high or low or a combination of both. The therapist then determines how the child's functional activities of daily life are affected by his or her processing experience.[15]

The test is divided into two sections—birth to 6 months, and 7 to 36 months. There are 36 items divided between general, auditory, visual, tactile, and vestibular in the infant section, and 48 items divided into the same categories, plus oral sensory in the toddler section. It takes approximately 15 minutes for the caregiver to fill out the test and 15 minutes for the therapist to score it.[15]

SENSORY PROFILE (AGES 3 TO 10 YEARS)

The Sensory Profile is constructed to provide understanding of the child's ways of receiving and using sensory stimuli. Winnie Dunn created the rationale, theory, and development of the Sensory Profile. A strength of the assessment is that it can test children from infancy/toddler through to adolescence/adulthood, providing an important continuum in assessment and intervention. This assessment uses a combination of sensory processing and neuroscience frame of reference and embraces a family-centered philosophy by including information gathered from a caregiver. The tool was developed based on research of 1,000 children including those with disabilities, such as ADHD and autism. Research has demonstrated that it discriminates children both with and without disabilities. Children with disabilities were accurately classified into their respective disability categories.[16,17] The parent or caregiver completes a 125-question profile that identifies his or her perception of the child's responses to a variety of sensory experiences. The clinician then uses the Summary Score Sheet and Factor Grid to summarize the child's sensory processing into the following groups:

- Sensory seeking
- Emotional reactive
- Low endurance/tone
- Oral sensory sensitivity
- Inattention/distractibility
- Poor registration
- Sensory sensitivity
- Sedentary
- Fine motor/perceptual

The Sensory Profile needs to be combined with other evaluation information from the clinician, and possibly the teacher, to get a thorough picture of the child's need for diagnostic and treatment planning. For a more efficient assessment of sensory processing, there is a Short Sensory Profile, which can be used on a Personal Digital Assistant (PDA) or with a computer.[18]

SENSORY PROFILE SCHOOL COMPANION (AGES 3 TO 11 YEARS)

This tool is a standardized assessment that gathers data from the teacher's perspective of the child's sensory processing skills. The test provides information as to how the teacher observes the child's sensory processing affecting his or her classroom behavior and academic performances. It is constructed from Winnie Dunn's Model of Sensory Processing. The instrument is easy to administer and score, requiring approximately 30 minutes for both. The interpretation of the results is accompanied by case studies for better understanding and clarity, and the manual of instruction also provides intervention planning.[19]

Play Assessments

Play is a major occupation of children and can offer insights into their function and participation. As a primary role of childhood, occupational therapists have embraced play as an important outcome of therapy. According to the *Occupational Therapy Practice Framework*, play and leisure are the areas the occupational therapist identifies as playing with age-appropriate toys, and engaging in age-appropriate games and leisure activities such as art, music, sports, and after-school activities.[20] Occupational therapists can use the play of children to gain insight into their psychosocial health. When children cannot articulate their emotions or state of being, an assessment of play with objects and/or with others can assist with understanding the child's inner feelings. Researchers examined the play of preschool children with autism and discovered that play can be used to improve social behaviors.[21] Play assessments can also be used to observe factors related to sensory processing such as organization, sequencing, and praxis.

Play assessments can include: (1) direct observation, (2) video recording of play and then analysis, (3) retrospective video (home videos of such activities as birthday parties), and (4) interview of the parent, child, teacher, or other caretaker. Some instruments, such as the Test of Playfulness[22] and the Knox Preschool Play Scale,[23] offer standardized assessments of play that include observation of children playing. Retrospective video analysis, which is the use of video of a child's naturalistic settings or environment, can provide objective data of play of real life events. Taxonomy of object play from ages 2 to 30 months has been published for use with retrospective video of play. The taxonomy and retrospective video can be used clinically to assist in the description of levels of object play of children with autism and developmental delays.[24]

TEST OF PLAYFULNESS

This test was designed by Anita Bundy, an occupational therapist, and published in 1997. The purpose of the standardized tool is to assess the child's approach and attitude while playing. According to Bundy, playfulness is how the child approaches activities of play. The purpose of the assessment is to observe and measure the interactions of the child with activities and the environment and evaluate the child's role as a player.[22] It does not assess the skills of play, which are important, but emphasizes the child's approach and attitude during play. It objectively measures playfulness for children ages 15 months to 10 years and across diagnostic groups. It is useful to the occupational therapist for identifying delayed areas for intervention. It has 60 items that measure internal control, intrinsic motivation, and freedom to suspend reality. The internal control portion includes initiation, modification, and engagement in challenges while playing. Observations are recorded of the child's exuberance, persistence, and engagement while playing. These measurements give insight into the child's motivation. Observations are made of how the child pretends, engages in clowning or mischief as measures of suspending reality.[22]

KNOX PRESCHOOL PLAY SCALE

Susan Knox, an occupational therapist, designed this test. It is a criterion referred observation assessment of children's play skills designed for ages birth to 6 years. It assesses the child's ability to manage his or her space, management of the materials, the use of pretend or symbolic play, and participation in play.[22] Observing and analyzing how the child plays can provide the clinician with an important understanding of the child's abilities in communication, physical development, symbolism, and social maturity.[22]

School Setting Assessments

SCHOOL FUNCTION ASSESSMENT (SFA)

The School Function Assessment (SFA) has five authors. The lead author is Wendy Coster, an occupational therapist. Using a top-down approach, this tool assesses the child's overall process of participation in a naturalistic setting of the elementary school. This instrument can assess and monitor the child's performance in the academic and social environment of the school setting. It is designed for elementary school children, kindergarten through 6th grade. Children with psychosocial disorders need to be understood by their abilities to participate in the physical, temporal, and sociocultural features of their environment. The occupational therapist often uses the bottom-up approach to assess children with psychosocial disorders, measuring such skills as fine motor coordination, muscle strength, manipulation skills, and dressing. However, an important perspective of how the child is functioning within the context of his or her social environment using a standardized assessment can offer successful strategies for intervention. The occupational therapist can use the SFA to identify how the child is functioning in the educational programs and activities expected of their peers and identify limitations of the child. Using this instrument, the occupational therapist can get structured data on how the child can participate in tasks that support academic and social activities in school. The tool also provides an objective rating of the child's behavior on a variety of functional life tasks.[25]

- Part I: Participation, focuses on participation in six school activity settings. These settings are classrooms, both special education and regular, playground or recess, transportation back and forth to school, bathroom activities, transitions between classes, and lunch or snack time.[25]

- Part II: Task Supports, examines task supports for physical and cognitive/behavioral tasks. This section focuses on the assistance required by adults and adaptations such as specialized equipment or adapted materials necessary for the child to participate in the school program.

- Part II: Activity Performance, includes assessment of the physical tasks and cognitive/behavioral tasks such as movement in the classroom and school, social interactions, following rules, and communicating needs.[25]

Assessments Related to Eating Disorders: Tests for Physical Activity, Body Image, and Self-Esteem in School Children

The Center for Disease Control and Prevention has declared obesity as an epidemic in the United States. Statistics show 15% of children and teens are overweight; this is approximately a three-fold jump since 1980.[26] Children's leisure activities are becoming more sedate with the use of new technology, particularly electronic games and computers, and parents driving them to and from activities rather than the children walking or riding their bikes. A study of preschool children who have televisions in their bedrooms showed that they were 30% more likely to be overweight than other children because they were more likely to spend their time watching television than engaging in physical activities.[27]

Disordered eating is a complex problem; however, studies indicate body image, self-esteem, and physical activity are consistent features that correlate with eating disorders.[28] Obesity is calculated using the child's body mass index or BMI-for-age, which is the child's height divided by his or her weight, with the result applied to an age- and gender-specific growth chart. BMI-for-age can be used by clinicians to assess whether the individual ages 2 to 20 years old is underweight, overweight, or at risk for being overweight. The body fat of children fluctuates as they grow and there are gender differences also. The charts designed for children and adolescents are provided by the Center for Disease Control's National Center for Health Statistics[29] and provide a series of curved lines indicating

Table 21-1

Normal BMI Ratings

Name: Age:
Weight of child
Height of child
Underweight   BMI-for-age below 5th %
Normal   BMI-for–age 5th % to below 85th %
At risk of overweight   BMI-for age 85th % to below 95th %
Overweight   BMI-for age above or at 95th %

Adapted from the Center of Disease Control's National Center for Health and Statistics.

BMI = w/h2
w = weight in kilograms (or pounds divided by 2.2)
h = height in meters (or inches divided by 39.37)

specific percentiles. Occupational therapists can use the data in Table 21-1 for cutoffs to identify underweight and overweight children.

Occupational therapists have an opportunity to contribute to the arrest and prevention of this epidemic of obesity in children by using assessments and intervention to address this significant area of children's development. Preadolescent children, especially girls, demonstrate body image awareness, and anxieties appear before puberty.[30] Intervention among prepubescent girls and boys may assist in prevention of eating disorders such as bulimia, anorexia, and obesity. Some suggested assessments that may contribute to successful intervention are listed below.

PHYSICAL PARTICIPATION AND ACTIVITY CHECKLIST

The checklist shown in Table 21-2 can be developed by the clinician to measure frequency, duration, intensity, and context of physical activity of the child. The clinician can record levels of involvement in organized and informal activities such as soccer, swimming, and dance, both during and after school. Family support of physical activities is important information for the clinician to gather, such as whether the child has transportation to activities, and if there is demonstration of physical activity by the adults.

THE BODY IMAGE SCALE

This scale is designed to gather information from children about their current/actual perception of themselves. Seven body types representing his or her sex are presented in profile to the child. These profiles range in size from thin to solid/chunky. The children are asked to respond to five statements about their perceptions of themselves, their ideal image, how their mother would rate their present and ideal image, and the image the children would not like to look like. The results of the test give a score that is labeled "body dissatisfaction score."[30]

Table 21-2

Physical Participation and Activity Checklist

Name: Age: Date: Therapist:

Physical Activity	Frequency	Duration	Intensity	Alone or Group
Gross Motor				
Walking/running				
Jumping/hopping				
Playing ball				
Swimming				
Soccer				
Dance				
Other				
Summary				
Fine Motor				
Video games				
Drawing				
Musical instrument				
Computer games				
Board games				
Building, eg, blocks				
Other				
Summary				
Family support Comments				
Total Summary Fine, gross motor activity				

Copyright Sandra Edwards 2005

THE SELF-ESTEEM QUESTIONNAIRE

This assessment is a measure of self-esteem using a self-worth subscale asking the children to respond to "What I am like" by using six paired opposing statements that are indicating feelings about themselves.[31] For example, "some kids are popular with others their age; other kids are not very popular." The children respond with a range of "really true for me" or "sort of true for me." The subscales scores are tallied and range in points from 6 to 24, with the higher self-esteem reflected by the higher score.[31]

PIERS–HARRIS 2 CHILDREN'S SCALE

This assessment, subtitled The Way I Feel About Myself, is designed to measure a child's attitudes and behaviors in order to understand his or her self-concept. The tool is for children from age 7, with a minimum of a second-grade reading skill level, to adolescents up to 18 years old, or grades 4 through 12. Self-concept is developed primarily via interactions with the child's environment and from his or her primary caretakers, as well as the behaviors and attitudes of others. The scale's theoretical base is the assumption that a person's self-concept develops in childhood and remains consistent. Self-concept is important for motivation and organizing function in a child's life.[32] This tool consists of statements that express how the child may feel about him- or herself. Some examples of statements are "My classmates make fun of me," or "I am a happy person." Six domain scales are used to sort specific areas of self-concept. These domain scales are Behavioral Adjustment, Intellectual and School Status, Physical Appearance and Attributes, Freedom From Anxiety, Popularity and Happiness, and Satisfaction.[33]

The questionnaire contains 60 yes or no items in a booklet. Two types of forms are available: one form is completed by the client and scored manually by the clinician; the other form is completed and scored on the computer, and a report is generated from the publisher, Western Psychological Services. The test is available in English or Spanish. Administration of the test takes about 10 to 15 minutes using either of the two forms described. It can be used individually or in a classroom to screen for further psychological testing. The test is designed to be combined with other sources of data about the child's self-concept, such as clinical observations, prior history, child interview, school records, nonclinical observations, and other assessments.

Scoring is relatively simple and gives both a raw score and cluster score. The total score can range from 0 to 60. The high total score demonstrates a positive self-concept and the opposite for a low self-concept.

This instrument is easy to administer and score. It is nonthreatening to children and considerations are taken to decrease false scores. In order to represent different cultures in the test, a more diverse representation of subjects is needed in the sample size. Overall, it is a good screen for psychological treatment.[34] It was standardized using over 1,000 subjects and the validity and reliability can be analyzed using the manual.[33]

Projective Assessments

HOUSE-TREE-PERSON (HTP) PROJECTIVE DRAWING TECHNIQUE

This test has a long and distinguished history. It was developed by John N. Buck, first published in 1948, and again in a revised interpretive manual in 1993 by W.L. Warren. It has been widely used by health care professionals. Occupational therapists can use it with clients in elementary school. It is widely used because it is easy to administer and offers a lot of clinical information. The child simply draws pictures of a house, a tree, and a person. He or she is invited to describe, define, and explain the drawings. The activity of drawing can assist with rapport-building and clinicians report that it is an effective test to administer first in a series of psychological tests because it does reduce tension. It is a method of obtaining clinically relevant information in a nonthreatening way. This assessment can be successfully administered to young clients who are from a variety of cultures and educational levels, developmentally delayed, or non-English-speaking. It is a tool that can be used in the most challenging clinical situations, such as with clients who are autistic or extremely hyperactive.[35]

This test is especially well-designed for clients who are unable to communicate their feelings.[36] It is used with children over the age of 8 and is used most often with adolescents.[37] Through the use of drawings, clients can reveal concerns or conflicts in their lives and their environment. The author wanted to design a test that would establish and encourage trust, comfort, and interest between the therapist and client. In order to create a positive relationship between the client and therapist, the clinical diagnostic technique was to use an unstructured procedure. The drawings can display a disorder in spite of the child being unaware or trying to hide it. This author's theory was based on the assumption that children will express their inner feelings more readily with drawings than with words.[36]

Administration of the test takes about 30 minutes. It is administered in a quiet room with a desk and two chairs. Standardized drawing forms are used. The client is first given a form with the word HOUSE and a pencil, then a form with the word TREE, and finally a form with the word PERSON. The therapist observes and records observations. The second part of the test is to talk to the client about the meaning of the drawings and allow the client to express his or her feelings. In another part of the test, the client is asked to draw all three items, but is allowed to select from an assortment of crayons.

Scoring and interpretation require training and caution. There are over 475 characteristics that are identified to assist in interpreting the client's drawings. Some examples of these characteristics are regression, feelings of inadequacy, schizoid conditions, immaturity, and obsessive–compulsive conditions. This assessment is published by Western Psychological Services and comes in a kit with the drawing forms, manual with illustrated diagnostic handbook, and drawing/interpretation booklet. As mentioned above, W.L. Warren added an extensive new manual on the use and interpretations of the HTP in 1993. Interest is high among researchers as to the validity of these interpretations. Although this tool has application for children, it was originally designed for adults and used for the approximation of intelligence.[37]

Sample drawings of Draw-a-Person of a child with abuse and ADHD and a child with typical growth are shown in Figures 21-1 and 21-2, respectively. Some of the drawn items to observe are the details of facial features, hair, eyes, ears, nose, eyebrows, number of fingers, one or two dimensions of arms and legs, size of drawing, and narrative of child's explanation of body parts and figure.

Infant/Preschool Assessments

BAYLEY SCALES OF INFANT DEVELOPMENT II (BSID II), SECOND EDITION

The Bayley Scales of Infant Development II was revised in 1993 and is published by The Psychological Corporation. The revised tool includes an expanded representative sample of 1,700 children; revision of the content of The Infant Behavior Record, now referred to as Behavior Rating Scale (BRS); improved psychometrics; added color and redesigned materials; and added data that includes children with diagnoses such as Down's syndrome and prenatal drug exposure.[38] The test now has increased clinical

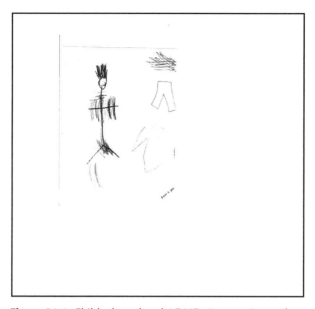

Figure 21-1. Child, abused and ADHD, 8 years, 3 months.

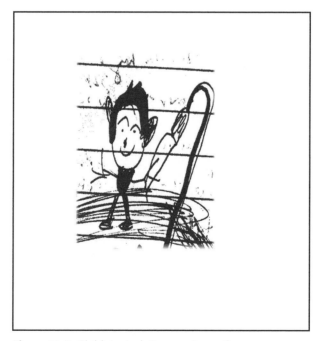

Figure 21-2. Child, typical, 5 years, 3 months.

validity because the items address children who might be at risk or are suspected to be at risk of impaired development. The clinician calculating the child's gestational age makes adjustments. The clinician uses adjusted items if the child is premature or postmature, rather than administering items at his or her chronological age.

This instrument is well-respected by health professions for clinical and research purposes to assess children ages birth to 42 months using three scales: mental, motor, and behavior. These scales are described in more detail below.

- *Mental scale* examines areas of cognition such as sensory-perceptual abilities, discriminations, object constancy and memory; problem solving, learning; verbal development, generalization, and classification.
- *Motor scale* assesses fine and gross motor coordination.
- *Behavior rating scale* assesses areas of attitude, interest, energy, activity, response to stimuli, and emotion.[38]

Some descriptions for administering the BSID II are really model testing procedures that can be used by clinicians for optimum results. Some of these procedures are as follows:[38]

1. Prepare by reading the manual several times; if you are a new examiner, observe while a trained examiner administers the BSID II.
2. Arrange an environment that is quiet, with floor lighting, not overhead lighting that shines in the infant's eyes, and a room large enough for testing.
3. Explain the test to the parent or caregiver at the beginning of the period.
4. Explain what is expected of the parent; do not encourage the parent to participate in the assessment.
5. Alternate easy and difficult items to maintain participation of the child.
6. Stay positive, enthusiastic, and emotionally connected, praising the child for his or her efforts even when the child fails. Do not give specific feedback about the success or failure of an item.
7. If a child becomes fussy or restless, the BSID II can be given in other situations, such as:
   - Seating the child in the mother's lap at an adult-height table
   - Seating the child in a child-sized chair at a child-sized table, with the adults at the child's height
   - Seating the child on the floor

BAYLEY SCALES OF INFANT AND TODDLER DEVELOPMENT (BSID-III), THIRD EDITION

This revision contains new normative data based on 1,700 children stratified by age and based on the US Census from 2000. The tests have five core scales: (1) Cognition, (2) Motor, (3) Language, (4) Social-Emotional, and (5) Adaptive Behavior. The first three scales are interactive with the child and scales 4 and 5 are questionnaires for the parent or caregiver. There is also a Behavior Observation Inventory that is a scale used to validate the perceptions of the parent/caregiver and the examiner of the child's responses. An interdisciplinary team of professionals dividing the test among their expertise can use this test. It takes about 30 to 90 minutes to administer the test, depending on the age of the child.[39]

Important additions to this assessment are the Social-Emotional scale, authored by Stanley Greenspan, who is an expert in early child development and the Adaptive Behavior scale. There is also a screening test to determine if further testing is needed. The revisions have improved the test by making the instrument more user-friendly with simplified scoring, more parent/caregiver participation, and size and weight reductions of the kit itself.

MILLER ASSESSMENT FOR PRESCHOOLERS (MAP)

When Public Law 94-142, the Education for All Handicapped Children Act, was passed in 1975 (now called Individuals with Disabilities Education Act [IDEA]), it increased occupational therapists' responsibilities for early childhood screening. There were considerable frustrations among occupational therapists caused by either inadequate or absent testing instruments for children in this target age group. In 1971, Lucy Jane Miller started designing and constructing a new standardized instrument that would predict school-related problems. She published the Miller Assessment for Preschoolers (MAP) in 1982.[40]

This assessment serves as a screening tool and indicates to the examiner a need for further assessment for young, emotionally disturbed children. It addresses children ages 2 years 9 months to 5 years 8 months. The tests contains 27 core items that were carefully researched and selected from an original 800 field-tested items, involving more than 4,000 children. These final 27 items are divided into classification groups:

- *Sensory and Motor Abilities* testing such areas as sense of position and movement, sense of touch, and basics of movement such as flexion, extension, and rotation. The coordination items combine sensory and motor components for complex oral, fine, and motor coordination testing activities.

- *Cognitive Abilities* have both verbal and nonverbal indices. The verbal items assess memory, sequencing comprehension, association and expression in verbal context. The nonverbal items test memory, sequencing, visualization, and mental manipulations that are nonverbal.

- *Combined Abilities* examines the child's abilities to integrate sensory, motor, and cognitive abilities including interpretation of visual-spatial information.

The materials required for the assessment are the examiner's manual, cue sheet, item score sheet (filled out based on behavior observed during testing), record booklet, drawing booklet, scoring transparency, scoring notebook and card notebook, and test kit materials. It is described in the manual as taking 20 to 30 minutes to administer and score, but extensive clinical experience has demonstrated that it takes closer to 40 to 50 minutes. The results are reported in norms for children in percentile ranks that can be used for developing individualized family service plans (IFSP) or individualized education programs (IEP) for school occupational therapists.[40]

MAP Supplemental Observations

Supplemental observations are provided to accompany the MAP using further assessment of the child. The manual indicates that these supplemental observations require specific workshop training and are to be administered by clinicians specifically trained in the use of this tool. These observations focus on the quality of language, vision, touch, movement, and Draw-a-Person.

Behavior During Testing

This section of the MAP is a form that accompanies the 27 core MAP items and pertains, as the title indicates, to the behavior of the child during testing. This section acknowledged the important component of behavior in identifying children with learning disabilities and predicting their academic success. Some of the specific behaviors that Miller listed in the behavior section are attention, social interaction, and sensory reactivity.[40]

Screening Assessments

When properly applied, screening assessments for preschool children with mental illness can assist with early identification of children with developmental delays. Screening tests can direct the clinician to do further in-depth testing, which can lead to improved outcomes because the child receives proper and early treatment. Children with a variety of mental diagnoses, such as autism, emotional/behavioral, and ADHD often go unrecognized until they reach school age. Without early intervention, the problems worsen and helpful intervention may be missed. Research has demonstrated that children with these mental disorders who receive early treatment have more successful academic experiences and are more likely to graduate from high school.[41]

DENVER DEVELOPMENTAL SCREENING TEST

The Denver Developmental Screening Test (DDST) is widely known and used nationally and internationally by pediatricians and early interventionists. This screening assessment was developed in 1967 for children ages birth to 6 years to screen their developmental progress. The revised version in 1990 expanded the number of children to include representation from areas all over the nation, rather than only Colorado. The improved data has less class and race bias, and improved sensitivity. The developmental areas tested are:

- Personal-Social
- Fine Motor
- Language
- Gross Motor
- Behavior Checklist

The form for the items is on one page and efficiently arranged. The caregiver can answer some of the items. It requires approximately 20 minutes to administer with easy-to-follow instructions for administration and scoring in the manual. The test consists of a small kit that contains the standardized items.[42]

This instrument is useful to give before preparing for more complex assessments because it gives the clinician a good estimate of the child's developmental level in order to prepare for more in-depth assessments.

TEMPERAMENT AND ATYPICAL BEHAVIOR SCALE

The Temperament and Atypical Behavior Scale (TABS) was designed by an interdisciplinary team of special educators and psychologists to identify dysfunctional behavior quickly. It is a 15-item questionnaire filled out by the parent or caregiver who knows the child's daily behaviors relating to temperament and self-regulation. It is also called the TABS Screener. It targets children ages 11 to 71 months. The scoring is simple and used to determine if the child needs further assessment. The materials needed are only the form that the parent fills out and the manual that has the information for administration, scoring, and interpretation. This assessment takes about 5 or fewer minutes to complete and score.

TABS is a norm-referenced assessment that can be administered following the Screener TABS or if the child has been referred because he or she demonstrates atypical behaviors. The tool is a questionnaire for parents or caretakers and has 55 items that are divided into four areas relating to temperament and self-regulation. These four areas are: 1) detachment, which is associated with autism spectrum; 2) hypersensitivity/activity, associated with ADHD; 3) under-reactive, commonly linked with children with brain injury; and 4) dysregulation, associated with children that may have difficulty with such things as crying, sleeping, or inconsolability. It takes the parent about 15 minutes to fill out. It is easy to score; the calculations are straightforward and simple. The interpretation requires some statistical knowledge. The materials for this tool are the questionnaire and the manual for scoring and interpretation. This assessment has the benefit of being used for IFSPs or IEPs and wraparound mental health behavioral support plans.[43]

Motor Assessments

Children with mental illness have multiple symptoms; among them are motor coordination problems, which can be assessed by occupational therapists.

Children with autism spectrum disorders are reported to have poor motor coordination.[44] In another study, a group of over 200 first- to fourth-grade students were referred to a school mental health project; they were then assessed as having substantial problems with coordination.[45] In an interesting study, videotapes of 265 children, ages 11 to 13 years old, revealed that preschizophrenia children demonstrated both social and neuromotor deficits specific to children who develop schizophrenia in adulthood.[46] The most important occupations of children, including play, work, and self-care, all depend on adequate hand skills, which are intimately associated with motor coordination.[47] It is the coordination of the hand and manual dexterity that assists children in fulfilling many of their developmental milestones.[48] This section presents several well-designed assessments to be used to assess gross and fine motor coordination of children with mental illness.

PEABODY DEVELOPMENTAL MOTOR SCALES II (PDMS II) (AGES BIRTH TO 5 YEARS)

This standardized instrument is designed to assess early childhood gross and fine motor development. The gross motor section consists of items that assess reflexes and locomotion. The fine motor section consists of items that assess grasping, object manipulation, and visual-motor-integration.

The subtests can be used for school reports, parent conferences, and research. The scores are reported in quotients for gross motor, fine motor, and total for both. The kit materials are easy to handle and child friendly. The manual is organized well and has clear instructions for administration, scoring, and interpretation.[49]

Studies suggest caution in selection of this assessment by early interventionists. A study indicates that direct handling of the high–risk infant required for reflex testing can be less effective in the PDMS II than the practical advantages of a tool that allows structured observations of motor items, as required by the PDMS II.[50] Also, caution is advised for professionals to not over-refer or deny services for young children due to poor choice in assessment tools, but to be aware of validity studies in order to accurately select the best assessment or assessments.[51]

BRUININKS-OSERETSKY TEST OF MOTOR PROFICIENCY

This popular assessment tool is widely used by occupational therapists in many schools, clinics, and private practices to assess children ages 4 years 6 months to 14 years 6 months. The purpose of the assessment is to examine the fine and gross motor development of typical children or discern children with motor dysfunction. The battery has both a screening and complete version. The screening takes approximately 20 minutes to administer 14 items and the complete battery has 46 items and takes about 60 minutes to administer. The assessment has eight subtests, which are as follows:[52]

Gross Motor

1. Running speed and agility
2. Balance
3. Bilateral coordination
4. Strength (arm, shoulder, abdominal, and leg)

Fine Motor

1. Upper-limb coordination
2. Response speed
3. Visual-motor control
4. Upper-limb speed and dexterity[51]

This assessment affords the opportunity to make additional clinical observations while the child is in action. Areas of sensorimotor development can also be assessed, such as motor planning during the ball throwing activities, bilateral integration, vestibular integrity during balance items, posture and grasp maturity during the fine motor items.

The kit comes in a canvas bag that is somewhat easy to transport. The assessment does take about 30 minutes to set up and requires a considerable amount of space for the gross motor items, such as running speed. The results are reported in stanines, percentiles, and age levels, so these measures can be understood by a variety of audiences, such as teachers, parents, or administrators. It can be used and understood by an interdisciplinary team as well as and parents.

It has been suggested that the knowledgeable use of this assessment based on examination of its usefulness as a descriptive or diagnostic and evaluative or changes over time be used in specific ways. Therapists can detect more change in children with mental illnesses when using the raw scores because they reflect more subtle change over time than standard scores and standard scores.[53]

Bruininks-Oseretsky Test of Motor Proficiency Second Edition (BOT-2)

The revised assessment has an expanded age range from 4 to 21 years 11 months old, which makes it usable with school-age children who come under the eligibility of IDEA.

Some improvements include an easel administration format, child friendly tasks, simple verbal instructions, photos that accompany instructions, and expanded norms based on the US Census data. It is designed to be a thorough test of a child's proficiency in gross and fine motor development.

The assessment has the following 7 subtests:

1. Fine Motor Precision includes seven items such as cutting out a circle.
2. Fine Motor Integration includes eight items such as copying shapes.
3. Manual Dexterity includes five items such as sorting, transferring, and stringing materials.
4. Bilateral Coordination includes seven items such as jumping jacks, tapping foot and finger.
5. Running Speed and Agility includes five items such as running timed, one-legged side hop.
6. Upper-Limb Coordination includes seven items such as throwing a ball at a target and catching a tossed ball.
7. Strength includes five items such as standing long jump and sit-ups.

Composite scores are for fine manual control, manual coordination, body coordination, strength, and agility. In addition, there is a total motor composite score that provides an overall perspective of the child's motor proficiency.

The interpretation of the scores provides the clinician with information to assess the child's strengths and weaknesses, a record booklet for clinical observations, and validity studies for autism and developmental coordination disorder (dyspraxia).[54]

Summary

This chapter has summaries of 17 assessments that can be used in private practice, hospitals, schools, and outpatient clinics. These assessments can be used in the evaluation process of children with mental illness. It is in the expert selection of assessments, administration, scoring, and interpretation of the information that afford successful intervention. It is our professional responsibility to remain current, maintain high standards of evaluation expertise, and seek the resources for purchase of the best assessments to serve children with mental illnesses.

References

1. American Psychiatric Association. *Diagnostic and Statistical Manual of Mental Disorders*. 4th ed., Text rev. Washington, DC: Author; 2000.
2. US Department of Health and Human Services. *Mental Health: A Report of the Surgeon General*. Rockville, MD: Author; 1999.
3. Combrinck-Graham L. The development of school-age children. In: Lewis M, ed. *Child and Adolescent Psychiatry: A Comprehensive Textbook*. 2nd ed. Baltimore, MD: Williams & Wilkins; 1996: 271-278.
4. Holladay J. Pediatric psychosocial therapy. In: Wagenfeld A, Kaldenberg J, eds. *Foundations of Pediatric Practice*. Thorofare, NJ: SLACK Incorporated; 2005.
5. Kataoka SH, Zhang L, Wells KB. Unmet need for mental health care among US children: variation by ethnicity and insurance status. *Am J Psychiatry*. 2005;159:1548-1555.
6. Kandel ER, Schwartz JH, Jessell TM. *Principles of Neural Science*. 4th ed. New York: McGraw-Hill; 2000.

7. Brown C, Tolefson N, Dunn W, Cromwell R, Filion D. The Adult Sensory Profile: Measuring patterns of sensory processing. *Am J Occup Ther.* 2001;55(1):75-82.

8. Doniger G, Dilipo G, Rabinowica EJ, Javitt D. Impaired sensory processing as a basis for object-recognition deficits in schizophrenia. *Am J Psychiatry.* 2001;158(11):1818-1826.

9. Blakeney A, Strickland LR, Wilkinson J. Exploring sensory integrative dysfunction in process schizophrenia. *Am J Occup Ther.* 1983;37(6):399-407.

10. American Academy of Child and Adolescent Psychiatry. Practice parameters for assessment and treatment of children, adolescents, and adults with attention-deficit/hyperactivity disorder. *J Am Acad Child Adolesc Psychiatry.* 1997;36(10suppl):855-1215.

11. Mangeor SD, Miller LJ, McIntosh DN, McGrath-Clarke J, Simon J, Hagerman RJ, et al. Sensory modulation dysfunction in children with attention deficit hyperactivity disorder. *Dev Med Child Neurol.* 2001;43:399-406.

12. Yochman A, Parush S, Ornay A. Responses of preschool children with and without ADHD to sensory events in daily life. *Am J Occup Ther.* 2004;58:294-302.

13. Smith KA, Gouze KR. *The Sensory-Sensitive Child.* New York: HarperCollins Publishers Inc; 2004.

14. Baird G, Charman T, Baron-Cohen S, Swettenham J, Wheelwright S, Drew A. A Screening instrument for autism at 18 months of age: A 6 year follow up study. *J Am Acad Child Adolesc Psychiatry.* 2000;39:694-702.

15. Dunn W. *Infant/Toddler Sensory Profile: User's Manual.* San Antonio, TX: The Psychological Corporation; 2002.

16. Dunn W, Bennett D. Patterns of sensory processing in children with attention deficit hyperactivity disorder. *The Occupational Therapy Journal of Research.* 2002;22:4-15.

17. Ermer J, Dunn W. The sensory profile: a discriminant analysis of children with and without disabilities. *Am J Occup Ther.* 1998;52(4):283-90.

18. Dunn W. *Sensory Profile: Examiner's Manual.* San Antonio, TX: The Psychological Corporation; 1999.

19. Dunn W. *Sensory Profile School Companion Manual.* San Antonio, TX: The Psychological Corporation; 2006.

20. Swinth Y. Educational activities. In: Crepeau EB, Cohen ES, Schell BAB. *Willard & Spackman's Occupational Therapy.* Philadelphia: Lippincott Williams & Wilkins; 2003.

21. Rastall G, Magill J. Play and preschool children with autism. *Am J Occup Ther.* 1994;48(2):113-120.

22. Bundy AC. *Test of Playfulness Manual* (Version 3). Ft. Collins, CO: Colorado State University; 2000.

23. Knox S. Development and current use of the Knox Preschool Play Scale. In: Parham LD, Fazio LS, eds. *Play in Occupational Therapy for Children.* St. Louis, MO: Mosby; 1997: 35-51.

24. Baranek GT, Barnett CR, Adams EM, Wolcott NA, Watson LR, Crais ER. Object play in infants with autism: Methodological issues in retrospective video analysis. *Am J Occup Ther.* 2005;59:20-30.

25. Coster W, Deeney T, Haltanger J, Haley S. *School Functional Assessment.* San Antonio, TX: The Psychological Corporation; 1998.

26. Newman C. Why are we so fat? *National Geographic.* August 2004:46-61.

27. Dennison BS, Erb TA, Jenkins PI. Television viewing and television in bedroom associated with overweight risk among low-income preschool children. *Pediatrics.* 2002;109(6):1028-1035.

28. Gralen S, Levine Pl, Smolak L, Murnen S. Dieting and disordered eating during early and middle adolescence: do the influences remain the same? *Int J Eat Disord.* 1990;9:501-512.

29. Center for Disease Control. National Center for Health Statistics. BMI Calculator for Child and Teen. Available at http://apps.nccd.cdc.gov/dnpabmi/Calculator.aspx

30. Sands R, Tricker J, Sherman C, Armatas C, Maschette W. Disordered eating patterns, body image, self-esteem, and physical activity in preadolescent school children. *Int J Eat Disord.* 1997;21:159-166.

31. Harter S. The perceived competence scale for children. *Child Dev.* 1982;53:87-97.

32. Piers EV, Harris D. *Piers-Harris Children's Self-Concept Scale* (revised). Los Angeles, CA: Western Psychological Services; 1984.

33. Piers EV, Herzberg D. *Piers-Harris 2 Children's Self-Concept Scale.* Los Angeles, CA: Western Psychological Services; 2002.

34. Stewart DJ, Crump WD, McLearn JE. Response instability on the Piers-Harris Children's Self-Concept Scale. *J Learn Disabil.* 1979;12(5):351-5.

35. Jegede RO, Bamgboye EA. Intellectual maturity in Nigerian primary school children. *South African Journal of Psychology.* 1981;11:88-89.

36. Buck JN, Revised by Warren WL. *The House-Tree-Person Projective Drawing Technique. Manual and Interpretive Guide.* Los Angeles, CA. Western Psychological Services; 1993.

37. Abell SC, Horkheimer R, Nguyen SE. Intellectual evaluations of adolescents via human figure drawings: an empirical comparison of two methods. *J Clin Psychol.* 1998;54(6): 811-815.

38. Bayley N. *Bayley II Scales of Infant Development*. New York: Psychological Corporation; 1993.
39. Bayley N. *Bayley III Scales of Infant Development*. San Antonio, TX: Harcourt Assessment, Inc; 2005.
40. Miller LJ. *Miller Assessment for Preschoolers*. San Antonio, TX: Harcourt Assessment Inc; 1982.
41. Stoppler M. Developmental screening—critical for every child. *General Health Newsletter*. 2005;6:21.
42. Frankenberg WK, Dodds J, Archer P, et al. Denver II screening manual. Denver, CO: Denver Developmental Materials; 1990.
43. Neisworth JT, Bagnato SJ, Salvia J, Hunt F. *TABS Manual for the Temperament and Atypical Behavior Scale*. Baltimore, MD: Paul Brookes Publishing Company; 1999.
44. Wing L. Autistic spectrum disorders. *BMJ*. 1996;312:327-328.
45. Cowen EL, Weissberg RP, Guare J. Differentiating attributes of children referred to a school mental health program. *J Abnorm Child Psychol*. 1984;12(3):397-409.
46. Schiffman J, Walker E, Ekstrom M, Schulsinger F, Sorensen H, Mednick S. Childhood videotaped social and neuromotor precursors of schizophrenia: a prospective investigation. *Am J Psychiatry*. 2004;161:2021-2027.
47. Edwards S, McCoy-Powlen J, Buckland-Gallen D. Hand development. In: Wagenfeld A, Kaldenberg J, eds. *Foundations of Pediatric Practice*. Thorofare, NJ: SLACK Incorporated; 2005.
48. Edwards S, Buckland D, McCoy-Powlen J. *Developmental and Functional Hand Grasps*. Thorofare, NJ: SLACK Incorporated; 2002.
49. Folio MR, Fewell RR. *Peabody Developmental Motor Scales*. 2nd ed. Austin, TX: Pro-ED Inc.; 2000.
50. Bean J, Breaux E, Hymel E, et al. Concurrent validity of the Alberta Infant Motor Scale (AIMS) and the Peabody Developmental Motor Scales II (PMDS II). *Pediatr Phys Ther*. 2004;16(1):49-50.
51. Provost B, Crowe TK, McClain C. Concurrent validity of the Bayley Scales of Infant Development II Motor Scale and the Peabody Developmental Motor Scales in two-year-old children. *Phys Occup Ther Pediatr*. 2000;20(1):5-18.
52. Bruininks RH. *Bruininks-Oseretsky Test of Motor Proficiency*. Circle Pines, MN: American Guidance Service Inc; 1978.
53. Wilson BN, Polatajko HJ, Kaplan BJ, Faris P. Use of the Bruininks-Oseretsky test of motor proficiency in occupational therapy. *Am J Occup Ther*. 1995;49(1):8-17.
54. Bruininks RH, Bruininks BD. *Bruininks-Oseretsky Test of Motor Proficiency*. 2nd ed. Circle Pines, MN: American Guidance Service Inc; 2005.

PART IX
RESEARCH CONCEPTS USED
WITH ASSESSMENTS

EVIDENCE-BASED ASSESSMENTS USED WITH MENTAL HEALTH

Christine K. Urish, PhD, OTR/L, BCMH

"The conscientious, explicit and judicious use of current best evidence is making decisions about the care of individual patients." Sackett D, Rosenberg W, Gray J, Haynes R, Richardson W. *Evidence based medicine: What it is and what it isn't.* Br Med J. 1996;312:71-72.

Introduction

During the 2000 Eleanor Clarke Slagle Lecture, lecturer Margo B. Holm directed occupational therapy practitioners toward a mandate of becoming evidence-based practitioners.[1] "The fact that patient outcomes are improved with occupational therapy services is no longer sufficient to justify our services, unless we can also explain what we do and how we do it so that others can replicate our interventions and achieve similar outcomes with comparable patients with like needs, wants, and expectations."[1(p576)]

Several official documents exist within the profession of occupational therapy that illuminate the necessity for evidence-based practice. The *Standards for Continuing Competence* developed by the Commission on Continuing Competence and Professional Development state that occupational therapy practitioners are responsible for integration of relevant evidence for the patient populations they serve. The *Standards for Continuing Competence* further indicate that practitioners are responsible for the synthesis and application of evidence from a variety of sources, including collaboration with the patient in making clinical decisions. Lastly, the *Standards for Continuing Competence* direct practitioners to continually update their performance based upon the most current research and evidence available.[2]

The American Occupational Therapy Association (AOTA) *Code of Ethics* affirms the importance of evidence-based practice.[1] In Principle 4E, occupational therapy personnel are directed to achieve and continually maintain standards of competence, including the examination of evidence, so that they may provide services based on current information.[3]

Further, the *Occupational Therapy Practice Framework* directs practitioners to conduct analysis of occupational performance as an evaluative step within the occupational therapy process.[4] During this phase of the occupational therapy process, the patient's assets, problems, or potential problems are identified. Performance skills, performance patterns, context or contexts, activity demands, and patient factors are taken into consideration and the practitioner chooses areas of assessment based on these aspects. Specific patient outcomes are identified. Upon completion of the analysis of occupational performance, an intervention plan is developed. Intervention is implemented and a review of the intervention is conducted to ascertain progress toward targeted outcomes.[4] Therefore, assessment in the occupational therapy process is a mechanism to identify patient functional limitations and facilitate the development of an effective intervention plan, as well as to determine if the intervention that was implemented was effective in the facilitation of improved function and change in occupational performance. During this process, practitioners are directed to use all available evidence from scientific, narrative, pragmatic, and ethical aspects of clinical reasoning to facilitate the selection of assessments and the gathering of evaluation data.[4] Assessments that are utilized during the evaluation process should be valid and reliable, and illuminate the areas of occupational performance in which the patient has limitations. Upon completion of assessment, intervention approaches are chosen based upon best practice and evidence. The intervention plan is to be developed in collaboration with the patient, which is another aspect of the use of evidence-based practice in occupational therapy. In intervention review, the intervention plan is reexamined and patient outcomes are considered to determine whether the plan should be modified and intervention continued, and whether occupational therapy services should be discontinued or the patient referred elsewhere.[4]

WHAT IS EVIDENCE-BASED PRACTICE?

Evidence-based practice in health care service delivery has been identified as an important consideration in psychiatric occupational therapy that should be strengthened.[5] Further, it has been suggested that occupational therapists speak up about their profession and voice the positive outcomes and evidence that exist within the profession.[6] Through presentation of evidence-based information about the profession of occupational therapy, decision makers and patients may come to attach an increased value for the services occupational therapy practitioners provide.[6] Evidence-based practice has been defined within medicine by Sackett et al; however, the definition of evidence-based practice within occupational therapy differs somewhat from Sackett's definition. "An evidence-based occupational therapy practice uses research evidence together with clinical knowledge and reasoning to make decisions about interventions that are effective for specific patient(s)."[7(p131)] The need for evidence-based practice has come from an increased demand for accountability, combined with ongoing restraint in health care spending. These needs have facilitated an increased interest in the use of research evidence within the practice of occupational therapy. The desire for documented outcomes in health care is not a new concept.[8] Payers and policy makers continue to demand objective evidence of treatment efficacy and cost effectiveness of occupational therapy services. Through the utilization of evidence-based practice in occupational therapy, assessment of patient outcomes can provide information regarding the outcomes of a variety of interventions and meet the needs of payers and policy makers.[8] Occupational therapy practitioners have a responsibility to utilize evidence-based perspective. Patients expect this kind of practice; as a profession we have an obligation to ensure we are providing the best practice; furthermore, we need to demonstrate our ability to provide quality services that are of value and provide the best outcomes at minimum cost.[7,8] The goal of evidence-based practice in occupational therapy is to provide improved intervention to the patient that is supported by assessments that are based upon solid evidence.[9] Occupational therapy outcomes in psychiatric occupational therapy need to be documented through research to professionals outside of our discipline.[5] The benefit of research-based, evidence-based practice is that the knowledge obtained from critical review of research can facilitate change that has the potential to expand the body of occupational therapy knowledge.[10] Evidence-based practice in occupational therapy focuses on therapeutic practice that is valid and that considers safety and value. Evidence-based practice is not based solely on opinion, past clinical practice, or precedent.[10]

WHAT IS NOT EVIDENCE-BASED PRACTICE?

One problem in this area is that evidence-based practice has not been well-defined from a universal perspective. As a result, confusion may be present among researchers, practitioners, and payers.[11] Different individuals may feel strongly about one aspect or another from an evidence-based perspective and, as a result, subtle variations of terminology and how terminology is utilized are present within the health care arena.[11] Evidence-based practice in occupational therapy does not mean that the practitioner sets aside his or her own professional knowledge or expertise. Rather, evidence-based practice means that the practitioner focuses on the integration and utilization of research knowledge in conjunction with clinical judgment, expertise, and patient choice.[7] Evidence-based practice does not mean that all patients who come to receive occupational therapy services with similar occupational performance concerns will be provided with the same assessment and intervention.[12] Another myth about evidence-based practice is that it is solely based on research and does not account for the occupational therapy practitioner's knowledge, clinical judgment, or expertise. Evidence-based practice relies on the clinical knowledge and judgment of the practitioner as one piece of the evidence in making clinical decisions.[12] Research and patient contributions are the other essential elements. The goal of evidence-based practice is to provide the best care to the patient through thoughtful consideration and evaluation of all of the evidence available and does not deny the clinical judgment and expertise of the occupational therapy practitioner.[12]

GOAL OF EVIDENCE-BASED ASSESSMENT IN MENTAL HEALTH

The goal of evidence-based practice is to include the best evidence available for the assessment, intervention planning, intervention implementation, and outcomes monitoring for each patient who receives occupational therapy services. The ultimate goal is to provide patients with the most appropriate intervention.[12] When the occupational therapy practitioner uses evidence to choose appropriate areas to assess in the patients he or she is serving, plans interventions based on the outcomes of the assessment, and considers the patient's values, needs, and goals, and the best evidence available, improved function may follow.

IMPROVING INTERVENTION AND OUTCOMES THROUGH ASSESSMENT/INTERVENTION

When assessments are selected that have proven valid and reliable, and are used to facilitate the planning of intervention that has been proven to be effective, ongoing evidence can be generated and added to the body of knowledge within the profession of occupational therapy. This procedure would be described as best practice and occupational therapy practitioners have an obligation to provide therapeutic intervention according to best practice. [7]

Best Practice in Measurement

One of the most essential considerations with regard to evidence-based practice in occupational therapy is the consistent use of outcome measures to evaluate services.[13] Information from outcome measures facilitates decision making as to which programs and services are most effective and adds to the body of knowledge, which builds evidence to support the ongoing provision of occupational therapy interventions. Occupational therapy practitioners are directed to "mine the gold" in considering what researchers in other disciplines have found regarding how individuals interact with their environment to perform tasks. This action can further the profession of occupational therapy through the development of advanced thinking and clinical practices based on the critical review and analysis of available research literature.[13]

Occupational therapy practitioners are directed to become systematic in the choice and utilization of measures that formalize observation and interview data collected within occupational therapy practice. Creating a systematic plan can assist other professionals in viewing the importance and necessity of occupational therapy services. When others cannot understand the how and why of occupational therapy assessment and intervention, our professional practice may be viewed from "folklore" rather than formal professional evidence-based perspective.[13(p42)]

The use of evidence in practice is essential, due to the changes in service delivery, funding mechanisms, and increased pressure to demonstrate service efficacy.[13] Individuals who consume occupational therapy services are more informed regarding their choices through the use of the Internet and various media. This raises the occupational therapy practitioner's need to be knowledgeable of and provide evidence-based assessment and intervention. Use of evidence-based practice provides a means for the occupational therapy practitioner to stay current with regard to what is known about specific conditions and problems. Evidence-based practice offers the practitioner the opportunity to critique and apply relevant research knowledge to clinical practice. Further, the use of evidence-based practice can facilitate critical discussion with the service recipient and the patient's care provider with regard to various interventions. Through this action, the potential risks and benefits of various intervention choices can be discussed and analyzed. Effectiveness of interventions can be considered to determine whether or not changes should be instituted during the course of therapy.[13]

When occupational therapy practitioners utilize measures that were developed by or used within other disciplines, they must be extremely mindful of the need to articulate how occupational therapy views problems or solutions differently than the other disciplines that may utilize these measures.[14] When occupational therapy practitioners use measures that other professionals use, but do not make explicit the significant contribution of occupational therapy from an occupation-focused perspective, others will be unaware of the important contribution that occupational therapists can make. An example would be when considering the context of environment. Social workers may consider environment, but may be more concerned with addressing the social cultural concerns within the environment, whereas from an occupational therapy perspective, the concern may be the physical and temporal features present within the environment that may facilitate or hinder an individual's performance.[14]

It is essential in the context of measurement that we practice from a patient-centered perspective.[14] What this means in terms of assessment is that occupational therapy practitioners need to identify assessments that illuminate the problems experienced by the patient. Occupational therapy practitioners need to direct their resources toward addressing specific concerns regarding the occupational performance raised by the patient and the patient's priorities. The assessments that occupational therapy practitioners choose need to facilitate this process.[14] In considering possible assessments to use, practitioners should first critique the measure in terms of its focus, sensitivity to change, standardization, reliability, validity, strengths, weaknesses, and the overall relevance of the assessment to the problems the therapist wishes to address with the patient.

Assessment from an evidence-based practice perspective provides a means for the occupational therapy practitioner to provide information to the patient about what is known and what is not known about the effectiveness of assessments and interventions.[14] Rapport can be facilitated through this use of evidence-based practice. The therapist is in active dialogue with the patient concerning the outcomes of an assessment and the appropriate interventions to be selected.[14] Utilization of evidence-based practice facilitates a change in the role of the occupational therapist. Occupational therapy practitioners are considered experts in their area of professional knowledge; however, patients need to be considered, as the individual who lives the experience of functional limitation has an increased perspective and should not be discounted from the process.[14] When including the patient in the evidence-based practice process, information needs to be provided in a manner that the patient can easily understand. Extensive use of professional terminology or jargon is not suggested. When using an evidence-based approach, occupational therapy practitioners need to embrace the fact that interventions may evolve from dialogue with the patient. This differs from previous practice, which may not have included the patient in this discussion and in which the therapist selected interventions in advance and in isolation from the patient's input.[14]

Searching and Evaluating the Evidence in Assessment

Developing an effective search and evaluation strategy is an essential component of the utilization of evidence-based practice.[15]

How to Search for Best Evidence

The amount of professional literature available each month to occupational therapy practitioners can make it seem daunting to try to stay current.[14] Colleges or universities may offer assistance to clinicians by providing access to medical and health literature resources including journals, online journals, and computerized databases.[14] To manage the volume of resources available in medical literature, occupational therapy practitioners should consider establishing a surveillance strategy. This means the practitioner chooses a small number of journals whose focus is central to their daily clinical practice and which also review a limited number of more general health-related areas.[16] If there are several therapists in a clinic who have an interest in different areas of clinical practice, but who wish to stay as current as possible with evidence-based literature, they could form a journal club. Using a journal club, occupational therapy practitioners would report on the findings from their review of the literature, and professional discussion could occur regarding the information obtained. Through the use of this mechanism, therapists may be able to better manage the plethora of information they are confronted with in their desire to seek out and consume research information to facilitate evidence-based practice. Collaboration is key to evidence-based practice.[17] Occupational therapy practitioners must collaborate. When a practitioner discovers a resource or new technique or procedure, the practitioner has a duty to share this information with colleagues. Active collaboration and sharing in this manner saves time and no one person may feel as if he or she is reinventing the wheel.[17(p1)] One suggestion for the sharing of knowledge is the development of an EBP tips sheet. When individuals identify new information that could be shared with others, they could record it on a sheet or form and this form is duplicated to share with all staff members.

There are several evidence-based practice databases for occupational therapy practitioners to consider when searching for best evidence regarding potential assessments and interventions they may use with patients. These databases are divided into two basic categories—*unscreened* (unfiltered) and *screened* (filtered)[18] (Table 22-1).

Unscreened databases contain articles from journals that have not been screened according to a predetermined quality standard. Each journal has a peer review process and these reviews provide a primary quality check. MEDLINE and the Cumulative Index of Nursing and Allied Health Literature (CINAHL) are databases of interest to occupational therapists that would fit into this category. Journal articles that are accessed through these sources should be scrutinized by the practitioner to determine the quality of the evidence contained within the article.[18]

Screened databases are prefiltered and articles are selectively chosen for inclusion based on a minimum rating on a scoring system that addresses the scientific rigor of the research. The Cochrane Library is an example of a screened database. Other databases provide a synthesis and/or summarization of evidence and provide recommendations related to clinical practice. OT Seeker and Occupational Therapy Critically Appraised Topics are examples of these types of databases. Clinical guidelines are also available in cyberspace. Clinical guidelines provide the occupational therapy practitioner with recommendations that can be used to assist in clinical decision making. Guidelines are developed by experts within any given field.[18] Systematic reviews and randomized controlled trials are important sources of data utilized in the development of clinical guidelines. The Agency for Health Care Research and Quality has developed clinical guidelines in 22 areas. Evidence-based practice reports in psychiatry exist for attention deficit hyperactivity disorder (ADHD) diagnosis and treatment, pharmacotherapy for alcohol dependence, and depression (both perinatal and post-myocardial infarction).[19] When entering the term "psychiatry" into the National Guidelines Clearinghouse database, 642 related guidelines were identified.[20] Advantages and disadvantages to the use of clinical guidelines exist.[21]

The usefulness of clinical practice guidelines in ongoing clinical practice should be critiqued by occupational therapy practitioners. Clinical practice guidelines may be easier to use with some areas of practice than with others. Guidelines are just that; they may not provide the specific, straightforward solution that the practitioner desires.[21] Most of the guidelines that have been developed are for medicine and nursing for specific conditions. However, when providing intervention for individuals who present with complex and multiple disabilities, the use of clinical practice guidelines may not be as straightforward as the practitioner would like.[21]

EVALUATING THE EVIDENCE

Once studies have been obtained or guidelines secured, occupational therapy practitioners are directed to ask specific questions that can facilitate the review and evaluation of

Table 22-1

Available Websites and Databases for Accessing Evidence-Based Research Literature

Name	URL
American Occupational Therapy Association Evidence Briefs Series (must be an AOTA member to access)	http://www.aota.org/members/area15/index.asp
Occupational Therapy Critically Appraised Topics	http://www.otcats.com/links/cat_banks.html
OT Seeker (Occupational Therapy Systematic Evaluation of Evidence)	http://www.otseeker.com
MEDLINE	http://www.pubmed.com
Database of Abstracts of Reviews of Effects	http://www.york.ac.uk/inst/crd/crddatabases.htm#DARE
Cochrane Collaboration	http://www.cochrane.org/index.htm
Evidence-based Thinking in Healthcare	http://www.jr2.ox.ac.uk/Bandolier/
Clinical Guidelines Clearinghouse	http://www.guideline.gov
Website providing links to evidence-based practice sites on the Internet	http://www.shef.ac.uk/scharr/ir/netting/
Protocols available for review of quantitative and qualitative research	http://www.fhs.mcmaster.ca/rehab/ebp/
Division of Stanford University Libraries that includes 919 journals and 1,196,321 free full text articles	http://highwire.stanford.edu/

information obtained.[15] When researching the literature, if meta-analysis is available, one should attempt to secure research articles of this nature. A meta-analysis can potentially save time, as it summarizes the statistical findings from a large number of individual research studies. Research participants in the studies selected for review need to be critically examined to determine if they are similar to the patient for whom the occupational therapy practitioner will be assessing and providing intervention.[15] Next, the assessment or intervention presented in the article needs to be considered. Would it address the functional concerns of the patient in the area of assessment or the needs and attributes of the patient in the area of intervention? Then the assessment or intervention should be considered for practicality. Is the assessment practical to administer in the practitioner's setting in terms of resources of time, funding, personnel, and equipment? Does it possess good reliability and validity? Lastly, is the outcome obtained from the intervention one that the occupational therapy practitioner intends to work toward with the patients for whom he or she is providing intervention?[14] In considering all these areas, the occupational therapy practitioner must also consider the level of evidence provided by the research.

The American Occupational Therapy Foundation (AOTF) in 2003-2004 hosted an international conference on evidence-based occupational therapy.[22] As a result of this conference, a number of occupational therapists expressed their belief that the strict application and use of levels of evidence in medicine as developed by Sackett were inappropriate for use within occupational therapy. The exclusive reliance on randomized controlled trials was identified as a potential factor that could negate other types of evidence that could be more directly applicable to specific patients. Further, the conference participants objected that, when heavy emphasis is directed toward examination of the study design, other elements, such as the critical evaluation of the validity of the outcome measures utilized within the study, or the value of the outcomes from the patient's perspective, may not be taken into consideration as significantly as desired.[22]

One outcome from this conference was the identification of a need for a classification structure in considering research evidence that was suitable for occupational therapy. The classification system being used by the AOTA within the evidence-based literature review project includes a level of evidence coding format that takes into consideration the design, sample size, internal validity, and external validity of a study to assign a level of evidence.[23] Level of evidence for research design is coded as follows:

- Randomized controlled trial is considered level of evidence I
- Nonrandomized controlled trial with two groups is level of evidence II
- Nonrandomized controlled trial with one group addressing one treatment condition, with a pre-test and post-test, is considered level of evidence III
- A research study with a single subject design is level of evidence IV
- Narratives and case studies are identified as "NA" in the level of evidence for the research design[23]

The sample size of a study also receives a rating. Studies with greater than 20 subjects per condition (experimental and control) receive a level of evidence rating of "A." Studies with less than 20 subjects per condition receive a level of evidence rating of "B." A three-point system has been identified for rating internal validity within a study. Level 1 is assigned to studies with high internal validity that demonstrated no alternative explanation for the outcomes obtained within the study. Level 2 is assigned to studies with moderate internal validity in which the study attempted to control for a lack of randomization. Level 3 is assigned to studies that demonstrated low internal validity, as when two or more serious alternative explanations could be provided for the outcome obtained within the study.[23]

External validity is evaluated as well. Studies that present a high level of external validity, in which subjects represent the populations and interventions were representative of current practice, receive a level of evidence rating of "a." Moderate external validity in a study is assigned a level of evidence rating of "b." Low external validity rating, in which the sample was heterogeneous and one is not able to ascertain whether the outcomes presented within the study were similar for all diagnoses or the intervention provided does not reflect current practice, receives a level of evidence rating of "c."[23]

For example, a study with a level of evidence rating "IA2a" would be a randomized controlled trial with greater than 20 subjects per conditions with a moderate level of internal validity and a high level of external validity.

Although disagreements exist from a variety of different disciplines regarding levels of evidence, there are interventions being utilized widely within clinical practice in psychiatry that have not been supported by research.[24]

Process of Evidence-Based Practice

The ability to obtain research information to facilitate evidence-based practice can be developed through the formation of partnerships with patients, service providers, researchers, payers, and policy makers.[7] The changing nature of mental health services places occupational therapy practitioners at a crossroads, needing to be able to clearly demonstrate the effectiveness of the services being provided. As a result, it is increasingly important for occupational therapists to know how to engage in the process of searching for best evidence to assist them in selecting and implementing the most effective interventions in practice.[25] There are five steps to utilizing evidence-based approach in occupational therapy practice. These steps, in conjunction with patient collaboration and the practitioner's clinical reasoning skills, form the basis for evidence-based occupational therapy practice.[26] These steps include:

1. Formulating clinical questions
2. Searching the literature and sorting the evidence
3. Critically reviewing the evidence
4. Applying applicable findings to practice
5. Evaluating the effect.[26]

FORMULATING CLINICAL QUESTIONS

Questions that arise from everyday clinical practice related to therapy, prevention, etiology and harm, diagnosis, prognosis, and economic analysis can become the basis of a clinical question. The key to effective searching of electronic evidence available on the Internet and through electronic databases is the formulation of a clear question.[26] Questions can relate to assessments, intervention effectiveness, or be descriptive to the gathering of more information about patients with specific occupational performance limitations (eg, Do older adult women in the community with depression experience a difference in activity participation from those who are not diagnosed with depression?).[27] An effective method for the development of a clinical question is the use of *Patient, Problem, or Population; Intervention; Comparison of Intervention; and Outcome* (PICO). Examples of questions are:

P: How could a practitioner describe a group of patients similar to the patient I am interested in securing information about?

I: What intervention am I considering for use?

C: What is the alternative to the intervention I have identified, or what is another intervention for which I would like to make a comparison?

O: What is the outcome I would like to measure, what improvement is desired?[28]

An example of an intervention effectiveness question could be: "What are the most effective interventions for increasing participation in satisfying daily life activities among elderly women with depression who live in the community?"[27(p103)]

SEARCHING THE LITERATURE AND SORTING THE EVIDENCE

Searching the literature was addressed earlier in this chapter. Planning a search strategy through development of a PICO and then keeping a record of the databases searched and the terms utilized is an effective strategy. If occupational therapy practitioners do not have access through their place of employment to medical and health databases, making connections with colleges and universities may yield access to these resources.[26] Some colleges and universities may welcome partnering with practitioners. Students enrolled in educational programs need to learn research strategies and may be available as a resource to access the resources desired and present their findings.

Considering the level of evidence and the type of research findings that relate to the PICO question posed is key. The occupational therapy practitioner needs to be able to effectively rank the research evidence that was available and the ability of the research to answer the PICO question. Secondary evidence through systematic reviews and meta-analysis studies can provide the practitioner with a good deal of information which has been summarized and possibly simplified to provide a trustworthy presentation of previously conducted research in a specific area of interest.[26]

CRITICALLY REVIEWING THE EVIDENCE OBTAINED

To effectively critique evidence obtained, occupational therapy practitioners may need to update their research knowledge.[26] Understanding of various research designs, methodology, and statistics will facilitate effective review and appraisal of available evidence. In appraising the available evidence, the power of a research study, randomization, and clinical significance need to be considered. To determine if an intervention was effective, one must consider if the number of subjects who participated in the study was sufficient to determine statistical significance or the power to detect change.[26] Random assignment is an important consideration when examining the causal relationship between the intervention and the outcome obtained. Statistical significance is most commonly established such that a 95% likelihood exists that the effects obtained were due to the intervention, with a 5% likelihood that the results were due to chance. Clinical significance assists the therapist in examining the results from a different perspective and may seem more practical to the occupational therapy practitioner. Results that do not indicate statistical significance may be deemed clinically significant if some change, but not statistically significant change occurred.[26] Some occupational therapy practitioners have expressed concern with regard to the interpretation of statistics contained within research papers. The Internet is a helpful resource, containing statistical tutorials. Journal articles such as "How to Read a Paper: Statistics for the Non-Statistician I: Different Data Need Different Statistical Tests" and "How to Read a Paper: Statistics for the Non-Statistician II: Significance, Relations and their Pitfalls" by Greenhaigh could be of great assistance.[29,30]

Critical examination of the rigor of the study design, outcome measures chosen to examine the variable of interest, level of evidence, sample size, and internal and external validity need to be considered when reviewing the evidence.[26]

Occupational therapy practitioners can also ask themselves the following questions to facilitate review of literature:

- Were the subjects in the research similar to the patient or patients for whom information is being reviewed?
- Did the intervention presented in the study meet the needs of the therapist and the patient?
- Was the intervention in the study practical to implement in terms of time, money, equipment and required personnel in comparison to other intervention options?
- Was the outcome that was measured an outcome that was identified as important and desired by the patient?[15]

APPLICATION OF RELEVANT FINDINGS TO CLINICAL PRACTICE

It is important that occupational therapy practitioners collaborate to collect and share research evidence and strategies that have proven successful to change practice. Success in this area will assist in ensuring good quality and effective services to patients.[21] Once research findings have been obtained and reviewed, application of these findings depends on patient factors and problems, practitioner clinical reasoning and expertise, and institutional factors.[26] During this step of the process, ongoing and effective communication with the patient is significant. Information needs to relate to the patients' needs and concerns and be presented in a clear manner.[15]

EVALUATING THE EFFECT—REASSESSING THE EVIDENCE-BASED PRACTICE PROCESS

The last step of the process is the evaluation of the entire process. Examination of the procedures undertaken and reflection on the effectiveness or ineffectiveness of the process can facilitate changes and improvements that could be implemented.[26]

It was reported that education-based approaches that incorporated methods to improve the clinician's knowledge and skills, in addition to an organizational approach that facilitated collaboration, teamwork, and effective leadership, were effective for implementing evidence-based practice.[31] In considering professional development and to begin incorporating evidence-based practice into one's clinical repertoire, one should allocate time for reflection on the patients and current practice.[32] Keeping a notebook that clinical questions which arise during assessment and intervention can be one method of facilitating reflection regarding clinical practice.

Collaboration with colleagues on setting clinic priorities and working with one another to share knowledge and research resources is a good suggestion.[32] Practitioners are directed to access quality information and use their skills to critically appraise the information obtained. Some practitioners may need to attend continuing education courses to increase their knowledge of research design and bias in order to increase their ability to determine the quality of the information available.

Practitioners should identify their current practice and compare this practice with a benchmark.[32] In considering where their practice is and where they'd like it to be, practitioners are directed to develop an improvement plan that is reasonable and doable. In consideration of their plan for change, practitioners must identify barriers to making the change and determine how these barriers can be overcome. Development of a plan for ongoing education can include taking continuing education courses, participating in a clinic-based journal club, completing Critically-Appraised Topics (CATs) on the most recently published research literature, and reviewing CATs and disseminating this information to clinic colleagues. Practitioners are encouraged to consistently and continually reassess their progress.[32] Are the assessments chosen yielding valid and reliable results? Are the interventions planned and implemented proving to be effective based on outcomes data?

EVALUATING EVIDENCE USING THE CANADIAN OCCUPATIONAL PERFORMANCE MEASURE

Research for literature assessing the Canadian Occupational Performance Measure (COPM) was conducted online via MEDLINE, CINAHL, and the OTD Base. This research yielded a clinical review of the instrument published in 2004[33] that analyzed research published from January 1991 through July 2003. In addition, a manual search was conducted to secure articles that addressed the COPM that were not included within the database. Articles were considered for this review if the COPM was identified in the article title or abstract, and if the article addressed: (1) the psychometric properties, (2) contribution to research outcomes, or (3) contribution to occupational therapy practice. This review yielded 88 articles, of which 76 could be placed into one of the three categories previously mentioned.[33]

If this review were not available, the occupational therapy practitioner could access similar information regarding the COPM assessment by conducting individual searches using CINAHL or MEDLINE by entering the terms "Canadian Occupational Performance Measure" and other descriptive terms, such as a population of individuals with whom they are working, such as patients with mental health concerns or homeless individuals.[33]

The review included articles on the use of the COPM published in 35 different journals. In considering the psychometric properties of the COPM, 19 articles examined the reliability, validity, and responsiveness of the instrument. The studies reviewed indicated strong test-retest reliability. In general, the studies reviewed indicated the COPM was a valid measure of occupational performance. One study challenged the concurrent validity of the COPM relative to other functional measures. One would anticipate a low correlation with an objective functional measure, as the COPM may not address functional items that would be considered within typical functional measures. The review found the COPM to be sensitive to changes in patient outcomes over time in the areas of perceived performance and satisfaction when examining other functional measures, such as the Health Assessment Questionnaire and the Short Form-36.[33]

In considering occupational therapy research outcomes and the use of the COPM,[33] articles presented in this review identified the use of the COPM as an outcome measure. These studies included six randomized controlled trials, 16 quasi-experimental designs, 10 case studies and two patient surveys. The studies found the COPM to be useful as an outcome measure when examining new therapeutic interventions or specific therapeutic devices. There was most often agreement that the use of the COPM was an effective method for engaging patients in the therapeutic process and setting goals. The review also provided information on the negative aspects or limitations of the COPM. In spite of the limitations, the literature presented in this review indicated that the COPM has been utilized in a successful fashion with a variety of patients, from homeless persons, to outpatients, patients with mental health needs, patients on a neuro rehabilitation unit, and older adults residing in a care facility.[33] Thirty-three articles were reviewed and identified that described the use of the COPM in the provision of patient-centered occupational therapy services from an evidence-based practice perspective.

Overall, this review suggested that the measurement properties of the COPM were repeatedly identified as satisfactory to excellent.[33] The review identified that inter-rater reliability is not testable, as each patient determines specific problems and assigns scores for the patient's own situation. Therefore, consistency of the responses was measured as test-retest reliability. This review presented information from studies that suggested the COPM was not appropriate for patients who lacked insight, who were diagnosed with dementia, or who relied on health care professionals to make decisions.[33]

As a measure, the COPM is effective in identifying patient occupational performance concerns and areas the patient wishes to address within occupational therapy services. Without such measures, how would an occupational therapy practitioner provide patient-centered therapy services? Therefore, the COPM is an assessment that facilitates the identification of performance concerns from the patient's perspective. The performance components that are causing the patient's concerns can then be further evaluated by the occupational therapy practitioner.[33]

The COPM can facilitate the occupational therapy practitioner's use of evidence-based practice, as the measure gains information from the patient's perspective, an essential feature of evidence-based practice. Through use of this measure, occupational therapy practitioners can develop and implement meaningful patient intervention and measure changes that can be attributed to occupational therapy intervention.[33] This review of the COPM highlights the fact that the instrument has become an accepted outcome measure for occupational therapy practitioners.

Review of Outcome Measures

Evidence regarding the effectiveness of therapeutic services is most commonly described according to specific outcome measures.[34] In considering outcome measures, the occupational therapy practitioner is concerned with precision and accuracy.[35]

PRECISION

Precision and the related concepts of reliability and validity are of concern when considering assessments from an evidence-based practice perspective. Reliability and validity are affected by random error. An assessment will be deemed less precise the greater the error.[35] In considering assessment, there are four major sources of error:[36] observer variability, subject variability, instrument variability, and environmental variability. *Observer variability* consists of the variability in measurement that is attributable to the observer and the observer's involvement in the administration process. *Subject variability* is the differences in the subject that may be attributed to fatigue, time of day, mood, or other biological factors. *Instrument variability* is specific to the design of the instrument (eg, rounding scores up). *Environmental variability* includes environmental factors that may change during the course of an assessment, such as noise, temperature, and lighting.[36]

Five guidelines exist for critical evaluation of the precision of an assessment.[35]

1. Are the assessment methods standardized? If so, administration, scoring and interpretation of the measure according to standardized procedures yields increased precision and accuracy of the assessment results and can facilitate the planning of an effective intervention that addresses the patient's functional limitations.[35]

2. Are the individuals administering the assessment trained to perform this function? Appropriate training and qualifications can yield increased precision and accuracy.[35]

3. Has the instrument been well-refined? Some assessments have been developed in a way that has reduced variability. Assessments that have been well-refined yield increased precision and accuracy.[35]

4. Has automation been developed for the assessment? Measures that have been automated reduce the potential for variability and human error. As a result, the measure would be viewed as more precise.[35]

5. Does evidence exist that variability is due to the order of measurements administered? The order of measurements can influence precision by providing a training effect or fatiguing the patient. Considering the order of measurements can increase the precision of the measurements administered.[35]

Occupational therapy practitioners should consider the strategies available to increase the precision of assessments. As a guide, the first two strategies are essential, while the fifth strategy is considered most likely to improve precision, if feasible within the measurement process.[36]

ACCURACY

A measure is identified as accurate if it actually measures what it was intended to measure.[36] Internal and external validity of research are considered relative to accuracy. If the findings of a research study lead to a specific set of inferences, the accuracy of the measure used for the phenomena addressed in the study must be considered. When a measure is accurate, it measures what it is intended to measure, with systematic error being minimal.[35] Having accuracy in measurements can increase the validity of the conclusions drawn from the assessment findings. Comparison of an instrument to a gold standard is the method to assess accuracy of an instrument.

Six guidelines exist for the critical evaluation of accuracy within a measure.[35,36]

1. Was the measurement utilized considered unobtrusive? Patients may bias their own results on a measure if they anticipate pain or other negative factors. Measurements that are designed so that the subject is not aware of the measure eliminate the chance for the subject to bias the assessment results and, therefore, increase the accuracy of the measure.[35]

2. Were the administrators of the outcomes measures independent or masked to the treatment conditions? Individuals who implement the intervention and then assess the subject's progress may bias the results in efforts to make the experimental intervention appear favorable. In reviewing literature regarding intervention effectiveness, outcome measures that have been conducted by individuals who are trained and masked to the treatment conditions can increase the accuracy of the assessment.[35]

3. Have instruments which require calibration been appropriately calibrated? Appropriate calibration increases the accuracy of the assessment results.[35]

4. Does the measure appropriately predict the outcome of concern? If a measure predicts change in the variable of concern, the measure is said to have good predictive validity, and accuracy of the prediction is an important consideration.[35]

5. Does the assessment agree with other approaches available to measure the same variable of concern, and thereby display convergent validity or criterion-related validity? If so, this is another way the attribute measured can be considered from an accuracy perspective.[35]

6. Does the assessment make sense and provide a reasonable approach for measuring the variable of concern? Face validity is the final consideration relative to accuracy.[35]

Precision and accuracy are two important concerns when reviewing outcomes literature. Occupational therapy practitioners can learn not only about assessments utilized, but the outcomes obtained in a particular study through close consideration of the precision and accuracy of the measures used within the study.[35] There are other guidelines that practitioners must consider in critical examination of measurements utilized in outcome studies. First, is the measurement sensitive? Does the measure identify differences when, in fact, differences exist? This is an important consideration when viewing the results of an outcome study. Another consideration in viewing the results of an outcome study is to ascertain if the measurement was responsive to change that may have occurred. A responsive measure would measure change within the variable of interest when, in fact, a change had occurred. Lastly, is the characteristic of interest specific to the measurement chosen? Will the measure detect changes present due to occupational therapy intervention or would psychiatric intervention confound the potential results that could be obtained from the measure?[35]

Occupational therapy practitioners are urged to read outcome studies with caution and to critically analyze the measures chosen in relation to the results.[37] One study reported a randomized controlled trial to examine the effectiveness of a community re-entry program to facilitate effective community functioning in patients diagnosed with schizophrenia and schizoaffective disorder prior to discharge. Intervention groups were occupational therapy or the community re-entry program. In this article, the researchers provided a significant description of the community re-entry program and only a limited description of what was conducted within occupational therapy services. The outcome measure that was selected to determine the effectiveness of the two intervention groups was attendance at the patient's first scheduled outpatient appointment. As a result of this measure the researchers reported a significant difference between individuals who participated in occupational therapy intervention and those who received community re-entry services.[37] Individuals in the community re-entry program who attended the first outpatient appointment came to 85%, whereas individuals who received occupational therapy services and were considered the control group attended the first outpatient appointment at a rate of only 37%. Attendance at the first outpatient appointment, when considered as an outcome measure of the two interventions, was deemed a very limited indicator of community functioning; however, this was not addressed by the researchers. This illuminates the importance of the occupational therapy practitioner critically reading the entire journal article and critically analyzing the outcome measures that were utilized within the research to ascertain if a change as a result of the intervention proposed within the study was valid.[37]

Advantages of Evidence-Based Assessment

Utilizing an evidence-based practice perspective in clinical practice provides the practitioner with information regarding specific interventions and services that have been proven effective.[34] Selecting an assessment that has been proven valid and reliable can enable the occupational therapy practitioner to state that the outcomes obtained from intervention were as a result of the intervention.[33] If services that have been provided are being challenged by a managed care system or other funding agency,[34] use of an evidence-based assessment can provide justification that the results obtained from the assessment were valid and reliable and that treatment works.[33] Through the use of valid and reliable assessments, the occupational therapy practitioner is able to ascertain the functional performance limitations present within the patient and plan intervention according to the patient's values and goals. Including the patient in the implementation of goals and intervention is an important aspect of evidence-based practice. Therefore, assessments should be chosen that illuminate the patient's perceived concerns so that effective intervention can be planned and implemented.

WHY EVIDENCE-BASED PRACTICE MAY NOT BE USED

Occupational therapy practitioners who wish to utilize evidence-based practice may encounter barriers to implementation of this practice within their clinic environment.[38] Some managers may not promote or foster evidence-based practice among their subordinates. There may be misperceptions as to what evidence-based practice is and what it is not, in addition to a lack of understanding of the research that is a portion of evidence-based practice. This lack of understanding related to research can be remedied through participation in continuing professional development, such as coursework and self-study, which is mandated through AOTA's *Standards of Continuing Competence* and the AOTA *Code of Ethics*.[1,2,38]

Some practitioners may be reluctant to utilize evidence-based practice because they are uncertain as to what constitutes "evidence."[38] Another reason why practitioners may not use evidence-based practice is that some research that is conducted is not published or disseminated widely or adequately, and thus practitioners do not have access to the evidence resources that may exist. Some of the research that is published and accessible may be viewed by practitioners as not applicable to their current clinical practice setting, due to the degree of research language utilized within the article. Even when research is written in a clearly applicable manner, some practitioners may resist utilizing the evidence, as the research may be viewed as "too scientific" and a challenge to their professional artistry.[38]

Other factors that have been identified as to why evidence-based practice was not used by occupational therapy practitioners included limited time and resources, insufficient training and support, and personal reasons.[39] Factors identified that enable evidence-based practice included support, resources, personal, time, training, and department development. Despite the barriers, therapists in two studies were generally positive about evidence-based practice, viewing this as a part of their professional responsibility and duty.[39,40] These findings related to the 2000 Eleanor Clarke Slagle Lecture, which directed occupational therapy practitioners to engage in evidence-based practice now and in the future of our profession.[1] Evidence-based practice requires occupational therapy practitioners to shift their thinking. Most practitioners were educated to use specific clinical decision making and thought processes.

Summary

In recent years, clinical decisions relied solely upon clinical expertise, published standards, and opinions of colleagues and experts. Evidence-based practice continues to utilize these sources, in addition to patient input into care, and additionally passes the information through another filter: "On what evidence is this advice based?"[41] One must consider evidence individually, as not all evidence can be considered of the same quality. Evidence from a randomized controlled trial that has been carefully conducted may be considered as more true than evidence based on one practitioner's experience or personal opinion. However, in the giving and receiving of advice, we are encouraged to pause and consider the quality of the underlying evidence more frequently.[41]

References

1. Holm MB. Our mandate for the new millennium: Evidence-based practice. *Am J Occup Ther*. 2000;54(6):575-585.
2. American Occupational Therapy Association. Standards for continuing competence. *Am J Occup Ther*. 2005;59:661-662.
3. American Occupational Therapy Association. Occupational therapy code of ethics. *Am J Occup Ther*. 2005;59:639-642.
4. American Occupational Therapy Association. Occupational therapy practice framework. *Am J Occup Ther*. 2002;56:609-639.
5. Tsang HWH. EBP in psychiatric OT should be strengthened. *Am J Occup Ther*. 2002;56:475.
6. Dickinson R. Occupational therapy: a hidden treasure. *Can J Occup Ther*. 2003;70(3):133-135.
7. Law M, Baum C. Evidence based occupational therapy. *Can J Occup Ther*. 1998;65(3):131-135.
8. Foto M. Outcome studies: the what, why, how and when. *Am J Occup Ther*. 1996;50:87-88.
9. Tickle-Degnen L. Monitoring and documenting evidence during assessment and intervention. *Am J Occup Ther*. 2000;54(4):434-436.
10. Brown TG, Rodger S. Research utilization models: frameworks for implementing evidence based occupational therapy practice. *Occup Ther Int*. 1999;1-23.
11. LaGrossa J. A lesson in evidence based research and practice. *Advance for Occupational Therapy Practitioners*. 2003;17-18,43.
12. Law M. Evidence-based practice: what can it mean for me? OT Practice Online. Available: http://www.aota.org/featured/area2/links/lnk16ar.asp. Accessed July 9, 2001.
13. Law M, Baum C, Dunn W. *Measuring Occupational Performance: Supporting Best Practice in Occupational Therapy*. Thorofare, NJ: SLACK Incorporated; 2000:1-50.
14. Law M, Baum C, Dunn W. *Measuring Occupational Performance: Supporting Best Practice in Occupational Therapy*. 2nd ed. Thorofare, NJ: SLACK Incorporated; 2005:22-47.
15. Tickle-Degnen L. Using evidence in planning treatment for the individual client. *Can J Occup Ther*. 1998;65(3):152-159.
16. Hall-Flavin DK. Resources for accessing evidence-based practice information—Symposium I: translating research into practice. Available: http://www.aaap.org/meetings2001am/proceedings/symposium1.html. Accessed August 15, 2005.
17. Coster W. Facilitating transfer of evidence based practice into practice. *Education Special Interest Section Quarterly*. 2004;14(2):1.
18. Wong R, Barr JO, Farina N, Lusardi M. Evidence-based practice: a resource for physical therapists. *Issues on Aging*. 2000;23:19-26.
19. Agency for Heath Care Research and Quality. Clinical practice guidelines. Available at: http://www.ahrq.gov/clinic/cpgsix.htm. Accessed February 16, 2006.
20. National Guideline Clearinghouse. Welcome. Available at: http://www.guideline.gov. Accessed February 16, 2006.
21. Roberts AEK, Barber G. Applying research evidence to practice. *British Journal of Occupational Therapy*. 2001;65(5):223-227.
22. Coster WJ, Gillette N, Law M, Lieberman D, Scheer J. International conference on evidence based occupational therapy 2004. Available at: http://www.aotf.org/pdf/ahrq_grant.pdf. Accessed February 16, 2006.
23. Liberman D, Scheer J. AOTA's evidence based literature review project: an overview. *Am J Occup Ther*. 2002;56:344-349.
24. Torrey WC, Drake RE, Dixon L, et al. Implementing evidence-based practices for persons with severe mental illnesses. *Psych Services*. 2001;52(1):45-50.
25. Lloyd C, Bassett H, King R. Occupational therapy and evidence-based practice in mental health. *British Journal of Occupational Therapy*. 2004;67(2):83-88.
26. Abreu BC, Chang PF. Getting started in evidence-based practice. AOTA Continuing Education Article. *OT Practice*. 2002;1-8.
27. Tickle-Degnen L. Gathering current research evidence to enhance clinical reasoning. *Am J Occup Ther*. 2000;54:102-105.
28. University Libraries – University of Illinois at Chicago Library of the Health Sciences Peoria. Evidence based medicine: Formulating patience centered questions. April 2005. Available: http://www.uic.edu/depts/lib/lhsp/resources/pico.shtml. Accessed February 16, 2005.
29. Greenhaigh T. How to read a paper: Statistics for the non-statistician I: different data need different statistical tests. *BMJ*. 1997;315:364-366.

30. Greenhaigh T. How to read a paper: statistics for the non-statistician II: significance, relations and their pitfalls. *BMJ*. 1997;315:422-425.
31. Tilley S, Chambers M. The process of implementing evidence-based practice—the curate's egg. *J Psychiatr Ment Health Nurs*. 2004;11:117-119.
32. O'Brien MA. Keeping up-to-date: Continuing education, practice improvement strategies, and evidence-based physiotherapy practice. *Physiother Theory Pract*. 2001;17:187-199.
33. Carswell A, McColl MA, Baptiste S, Law M, Polatajko H, Pollock N. The Canadian occupational performance measure: a research and clinical literature review. *Can J Occup Ther*. 2004;71:210-222.
34. Nemee PB. Evidence-based practice: bandwagon or handbasket? *Rehab Educ*. 2004;18(3):133-135.
35. Helewa A, Walker JM. *Critical Evaluation of Research in Physical Rehabilitation: Towards Evidence-Based Practice*. Philadelphia, PA: W.B. Saunders; 2000:61-70.
36. Hulley SB, Cummings SR. *Designing Clinical Research: An Epidemiological Approach*. Baltimore, MD: Williams & Wilkins; 1988.
37. Mairs H. Evidence-based practice in mental health: A cause for concern for occupational therapists? *British Journal of Occupational Therapy*. 2003;66(4):168-170.
38. Alsop A. Evidence-based practice and continuing professional development. *British Journal of Occupational Therapy*. 1997;60(11):503-508.
39. Curtin M, Jaramazovic E. Occupational therapists' views and perceptions of evidence-based practice. *British Journal of Occupational Therapy*. 2001;64(5):214-222.
40. Dubouloz CJ, Egan M, Vallerand J, vonZweck C. Occupational therapists' perceptions of evidence-based practice. *Am J Occup Ther*. 1999;53:445-453.
41. Geyman JP, Deyo RA, Ramsey SD. *Evidence-Based Clinical Practice: Concepts and Approaches*. Boston, MA: Butterworth-Heinemann; 2000: 23-25.

RESEARCH PRINCIPLES USED IN DEVELOPING ASSESSMENTS IN OCCUPATIONAL THERAPY

Nancy J. Powell, PhD, OTR, FAOTA

"Truth, like infinity, is to be forever approached but never reached." Ayres, AJ. Sensory Integration and Learning Disorders. *Los Angeles, CA: Western Psychological Services; 1972:4.*

Introduction

Occupational therapy assessments are vital to the survival of the profession. If occupational therapy is going to take its unique place among health care providers, therapists must provide valuable evaluation information to the treatment team and be accountable for the outcomes of their intervention. The past two decades have seen an emphasis on the development and use of valid, reliable instruments to assess occupation and related domains of function. Occupational therapists at all levels need to be involved in developing, improving, and evaluating assessment tools.

This chapter has two purposes. The first is to guide potential assessment developers with an overview of the basic information needed. It is hoped that graduate students, practicing therapists, and beginning faculty will find this chapter helpful in learning basic concepts and selected techniques for evaluation tool development. The second is to assist students and therapists in developing a deeper understanding of the research principles underlying the construction of evaluation instruments, so they can examine more critically the tools they choose to use in practice.

Basics of Assessment

DEFINITIONS

It is important to have consistent definitions of assessment, evaluation, and measurement in any research effort. First, *assessment*, according to the *Uniform Terminology for*

Occupational Therapy, Second Edition, is "… the planned process of obtaining, interpreting, and documenting the functional status of the individual."[1] It is a holistic data-gathering process that includes obtaining patient information from records, such as a chart; observing the patient and family; interviewing family members; and administering one or more testing procedures or evaluation tools. By engaging in this process, dysfunction or risk for dysfunction can be identified, and appropriate occupational therapy can be planned.

Evaluation in this chapter refers to gathering data on performance, such as activities of daily living (ADL) or observation, or using a specific tool or tools in one or more areas. Tools used as part of the assessment process will be identified as evaluation instruments in this chapter.

Measurement is "...quantifying or assigning a number to express the degree to which a characteristic is present."[2] In occupational therapy, the phenomena of interest are behaviors or performance of patients and families. Therapists are searching for the accurate amount of some characteristic related to function. A therapist might be evaluating the amount of independence a patient has, the degree to which a patient is oriented, or the number of leisure skills in which a patient participates.

Types of Evaluation in Occupational Therapy

Criterion-referenced tests are those that present predetermined standards or criteria that a patient is expected to achieve. These are the most commonly performed occupational therapy evaluations. Developers of these kinds of evaluation instruments first choose an area or domain that they want to assess, eg, daily living skills. Then skills are selected, such as face washing, hair combing, or shirt buttoning. These may be scored on a nominal scale of satisfactory or not satisfactory.

Norm-referenced evaluation instruments are those in which an individual's performance is compared to the performance of others or normative data. These are the least common in mental health assessment in occupational therapy, probably because they are the most time-consuming and costly to develop. Developers of these kinds of tools decide which performance areas or characteristics they wish to assess. Then they construct test items to assess the characteristics. The norming process consists of administering the instrument to large numbers of the target population for whom the instrument was developed. Procedures in administering and scoring the instrument are standardized. Specifically, testing equipment, instructions to the patient, and contextual elements are all kept the same to ensure that the assessment is always given the same way.

VALIDITY IN EVALUATION DEVELOPMENT

Validity is defined as the extent to which an evaluation measures what it is supposed to measure. In mental health assessment, validity represents the truthfulness of the instrument about a trait or behavior. For example, a therapist might wish to evaluate how oriented mentally impaired patients are to their environments. The tested trait is orientation. The evaluation tool used needs to accurately measure orientation. The Mini-Mental State Examination (MMSE) is one such evaluation.[3]

Types of Validity

Validity can be broken down into several types. The first type is *content validity*. If an evaluation tool has content validity, the content of the test covers aspects of the area being assessed as completely as possible. For example, with reality orientation, the tool must cover orientation to at least person, place, and time, or it would not be comprehensive enough. A test developer is concerned with how many test items are necessary to cover all the major aspects of the behavior or trait being measured, as well as whether the format of the test is suited to gathering information relevant to the trait or behavior.

Construct validity refers to ensuring that a test remains true to the domain it purports to assess. For example, one would not include items about dressing performance on a test of orientation; these would be better suited to a test that assessed occupational performance.

Groth-Marnat explains criterion validity as being "...determined by comparing the test scores with some sort of performance on an outside measure."[4] This author divides criterion validity into two kinds—concurrent and predictive. *Concurrent* occurs when a test is compared to another similar tool that is taken at approximately the same time. For example, the MMSE[3] could be compared to another test of orientation, or scores on two measures of functional performance might be compared.

The second type of validity discussed by Groth-Marnat is *predictive* validity.[4] This kind of validity is established when a test is compared to another similar test taken after a period of time. For example, a patient might be tested on a vocational evaluation, then tested 2 years later on a work-performance evaluation at a job site. Groth-Marnat states that predictive validity is best sought for tests of selection and classification of personnel.[4] Occupational therapists possibly could use this sort of validation of tests used for work placement of patients. Groth-Marnat concludes that concurrent validity might be of most concern to those developing tests that measures a patient's current status on some trait. In occupational therapy, such a trait might be functional performance in self-care.

Aiken[5] states that factors affecting validity include heterogeneity and length of the test. Generally, the shorter and more homogeneous the group taking the test, the less the variability will affect validity.

METHODS TO ESTABLISH CONTENT AND CONSTRUCT VALIDITY

There are a variety of ways that evaluation developers can check the validity of the tools they develop. Content and construct validity can be verified by having a panel of experts examine the test. In relation to content validity, Brown suggests using scales on which judges can rate coverage of the area being tested, the appropriateness of the format of the items, and the emphasis of important points.[6] When using this method, Brown points out that inter-rater reliability can be calculated and then serve as an index of content validity. Aiken also points out that experts can analyze the processes the patients have to go through to respond to the test items.[5] Aiken also urges test developers to use experts to help establish validity as the tool is being developed. This author suggests another specific method to use early on, which is comparing test content to an outline from written works on the subject or to a table of contents of a published work of the domain being tested.

Aiken suggests several methods to use to establish construct validity.[5] Specifically, these are using experts' judgments, analyzing the internal consistency of the test, correlating the test with other related tests and factor analyses of these intercorrelations, and querying the testees and raters about the mental processes they go through in completing the evaluation. Groth-Marnat reports the method for examining the internal consistency of a test is to correlate subtests within the tool to the test's total score.[4] For example, in occupational therapy, a subtest of items related to dressing might be correlated to the full scale of items on a functional performance evaluation.

RELIABILITY IN EVALUATION DEVELOPMENT

After validity, next in importance is the establishment of reliability. Validity cannot ensure reliability; a test can be reliable without being valid.

Definition of Reliability

Reliability is the stability of an evaluation tool over time. It means that barring any intervening factors, a patient will perform in a consistent manner on a test; ie, the test items will produce the same responses. Lack of reliability can result from errors in measurement that are produced by changes in the patient, such as fatigue or pain; or problems in the environment, such as distractions or temperature. The therapist using the evaluation must try to eliminate these sources of unreliability. Lack of reliability can also result from problems in test-item construction, such as the lack of clarity of an item, making interpretation of the item difficult.

Methods of Estimating Reliability

The first method of estimating reliability of any evaluation instrument is test-retest reliability. In this method, a test is given once, then repeated. The two test scores are correlated. Groth-Marnat states that the length of the interval between the two administrations of the test can affect reliability due to a practice effect.[4] In general, Groth-Marnat recommends this kind of reliability assessment for relatively stable traits, such as problem-solving ability, not for traits that are likely to vary due to outside influences, such as work skills.

There are two types of test-retest reliability—alternate and parallel. The *alternate* form has two methods. In the first method, the order of the items is rearranged, eg, making item No. 1 on the initial test item No. 10 on the retest. This may prevent the test taker from remembering the test items. The second method involves using a different form of the same question, eg, by turning the question around.

The second type of test-retest reliability is the *parallel* form. Here, the test writer writes two similar items on the same content, then puts one of the items on the first test and one on the retest. For example, on a test of adaptive behavior, one item could be making change for a 75-cent item from a dollar in quarters. The similar item put on the retest could be making change for a 50-cent item from a dollar in quarters. In contrast to the alternate form, this method eliminates the memory effect. Drawbacks to this method are expense and uncertainty about whether the two tests are parallel.

Another area of testing the reliability of evaluations involves measures of internal consistency. These measurements include split-half reliability, the Kuder-Richardson method, and Cronbach's alpha. Aiken states that these measures of internal consistency do not reflect errors in measurement caused by different conditions and times of measurement, so they are not equivalent to the test-retest methods.[5] The split-half method involves dividing the items in the evaluation into two parts arbitrarily; eg, a test may be divided into Part A, items 1 to 20, and Part B, items 21 to 40. A statistical test of correlation can then be run between the scores on Part A and the scores on Part B. Also, the items on an evaluation could be split by odd- and even-numbered items. This is similar to the parallel form above, except the correlation is between items on a single test, given at one time.

Carey describes the Kuder-Richardson internal consistency reliability index[2] by stating that it is to be used for objective-style tests with items that are scored correct or incorrect. The index compares the sum of the item variances with the total test variance. Factors that affect the score on the index are content homogeneity, group homogeneity, test length, and item difficulty. Kuder-Richardson indices are typically generated by computer-scored tests and range from .00 to 1.00. Carey states that values at about .80 indicate good internal consistency for classroom-type tests.[2]

Cronbach's alpha extends the Kuder-Richardson index in that it can be used for measures other than that of ability.[7] Thorndike explains that this internal consistency measure "...is based on the idea that each item is a parallel form 'minitest,' and the overall reliability is an average of all interitem correlations, corrected to the length of the total test."[7] Carey states that the Kuder-Richardson index and Cronbach's alpha give support for the homogeneity of the test. These two measures can be accessed on computerized statistical programs.[2]

Designing an Evaluation

The concepts of validity and reliability are fundamental to evaluation instrument development. Once these concepts are understood by the would-be evaluation developer, the process of construction can begin. Because this is not a textbook of test construction, the instrument-development process has been condensed to a set of 10 steps that will serve as guidelines for the development of the kinds of evaluations used in mental health assessment. The steps described below are expanded from the work on test construction by Kline.[8] A brief description of each step follows the list.

1. Identify a domain or area to evaluate.
2. Formulate a comprehensive outline of the content or behaviors related to the domain.
3. Select the type of evaluation format best suited to the domain.
4. Write the test items.
5. Perform validity checks.
6. Field-test the instrument.
7. Analyze the instrument.
8. Standardize the evaluation.
9. Write the evaluation manual.
10. Seek a publisher.

IDENTIFY A DOMAIN OR AREA TO EVALUATE

An idea for an evaluation may come from three different sources—a need in one's clinical practice, a needs assessment, or a need written about by experts or other test developers in the mental health occupational therapy literature. Once the area is selected, the literature on assessment of that area or domain should be thoroughly reviewed. Also, a survey of experts or a focused needs assessment for an evaluation instrument can also be done. At this point, funding for evaluation instrument development can be sought. For example, some foundations, such as the American Occupational Therapy Association, might fund the development of a needed evaluation. Other possibilities for funding are publishing houses (see step 10) or government agencies, such as state developmental disabilities councils or departments of mental health.

Formulate a Comprehensive Outline

This step will help ensure content validity. The developer should write a comprehensive outline of areas to be evaluated that are related to the construct of interest. For example, in constructing an assessment of work aptitude, the items related to attendance, punctuality, attitude toward work, ability to relate to people, manual dexterity, and other related areas must be identified.

Select the Type of Evaluation

In this step, the developer needs to decide which kind of evaluation format best fits the kind of behavior or trait that is being examined. Examples of formats are observation checklists, Likert scales, objective tests, or behavioral rating scales. In the above example of a work aptitude evaluation, perhaps an observation checklist would be best. The evaluator would check off items related to performing work duties. On punctuality, the patient might be given a check for an item stating "usually on time."

Write the Test Items

Now the evaluation developer is finally ready to do what some people try to do first—write the test items. Clarity and understandability of the items to patients and evaluators is the key to making the test reliable and valid. The language should be at the reading level of the patients to be tested if reading by them is involved. Professional terminology that is current and accepted in occupational therapy should be used so that an occupational therapist using the instrument can understand what is involved. Two traits or behaviors should not be included in one item. For example, in the work aptitude evaluation discussed above, an item should not state both punctuality and attendance. As these are two different behaviors, interpretation of the item will be difficult. If appropriate, it is also a good idea to include some filler items that everyone can answer correctly, so as not to discourage the test taker (EM Hockman, PhD; personal communication, May 1, 1998).

Perform Validity Checks

Once the evaluation is written, the real work begins. At this point, the developer usually needs to seek help from experts to see if the evaluation instrument completely measures what it is intended to measure. The evaluation should be reviewed by no fewer than three experts.

Field-Test the Instrument

Finally, the valid instrument is ready to try out on real people. Kline stresses that the field-test sample must be similar to the one for which the test is intended.[8] For example, if developing a measure of work aptitude for patients with mental impairment, then field-test the instrument on people with this impairment. Limiting the size of the field-test population to less than 40 is not recommended.[8] This number will enable the developer to use more powerful statistics to analyze the field-test results.

Analyze the Instrument

In this step, the developer will analyze the results of the field test. It is beyond the scope of this chapter to provide in-depth instruction in test analysis, but two methods will be briefly discussed. Kline has described the item-analytic method as the best and simplest way to construct a homogeneous test, ie, one containing items measuring the same characteristic.[8] After field-testing the pool of items, the developer can run a statistical analysis to determine the item difficulty (p) or the item mean for each item, such as an attitude-evaluation item, by asking for a response on a scale of 1 to 5 (EM Hockman, PhD; personal communication, May 1, 1998). P is the proportion who answered the item correctly on a test such as a multiple-choice test. On a test with dichotomous answers, eg, this trait is like me or this trait is not like me, P is the proportion who answered in the scored direction, meaning the proportion who chose the answer representing the trait being measured. For attitude scales, P is the item mean (EM Hockman, PhD; personal communication, May 1, 1998).

Next, a corrected correlation, the Pearson product moment correlation, or r, can be calculated for each item. The Pearson product moment correlation is a correlation between the item response and the sum of the responses to all the other test items minus the item whose correlation is being computed. For example, if on a 10-item test, the developer is trying to correlate item No. 6, this item is correlated with the sum of items 1 through 5, plus 7 through 10 (EM Hockman, PhD; personal communication, May 1, 1998). The correlation should be positive; in Kline's opinion, the correlation should be >0.30.[8] Filler items—the easy items discussed in the Write the Test Items section—are expected to show a very low correlation. Negative item correlations are not acceptable and should be discarded (EM Hockman, PhD; personal communication, May 1, 1998).

If the evaluation is an attitude scale, examine an item receiving a strong negative correlation to determine if the polarity of the response to the item is correct. For example, does the scored response need to be flip-flopped, with the low score on the scale now representing the attitude being evaluated, not the high score on that item? If a scoring problem is apparent, the scoring must be corrected and recomputed (EM Hockman, PhD; personal communication, May 1, 1998).

Also, in Kline's opinion, a p value for an item should be between .20 and .80; however, if the r is high, it is acceptable to keep the item.[8] Kline states that the aim of the test is to discriminate between those with a certain characteristic such as anxiety and those who do not have this trait. An item with a p of .50, therefore, is maximally discriminating.

After checking that all items reach the recommended p and r values, items can be discarded or rewritten. Then it is recommended that a second field test be performed, and the p and r values for rewritten items be rechecked.

The second step in instrument analysis is to compute the Cronbach's alpha. This is the final reliability check. If all items survive, then a reliable and homogeneous evaluation tool has been devised.

Although some measures of validity were initially done in the construction of the evaluation, now, as the final part of this step, the developer may want to perform concurrent validity checks. If another test is available that assesses the same characteristic as the newly developed test, an analysis can be performed to see if scores on the old test and the new test correlate. If the scores correlate, this adds validity to the newly developed instrument.

STANDARDIZE THE EVALUATION

Tallent describes three criteria that evaluations must exhibit to become widely accepted standardized tools: 1) demonstrate adequate validity; 2) have precise instructions that administrators must follow, including strict time limits if applicable; and 3) be normed correctly.[9]

Norming a test involves giving the test to the nondisabled population in, for example, a similar age range. This will enable the scores of persons with suspected disability to be compared to the scores of those without disability. Kline has stated that the two most crucial characteristics of normal samples are large size and representativeness.[8] How large the sample should be depends on the heterogeneity of the sample. Kline's recommendations are from 5000 for a heterogeneous group to 300 if special subgroup norms are formed. In addition, the sample must represent the population as a whole and not be biased by the variable studied. For example, on a test for work aptitude, it must include equal numbers of males and females. Lastly, Kline recommends that the instrument developer decide how best to describe the norms and score the test.[8] For example, would stanines or percentile ranks be best?

Receiver Operating Characteristic Curve Analysis

A final analytical method that can relate validity of the instrument and treatment is the use of the receiver operating characteristic (ROC) curve analysis. Using this statistical tool helps describe what an evaluation tool measures (validity). It also helps establish a score cutoff point that distinguishes those in the tested sample who should receive treatment from those who should not receive treatment. After testing, therapists often ask how the performance on the evaluation (the score) indicates that a patient needs treatment.

A ROC curve analysis will generate a visual curve in the form of a graph that will help a clinician make a decision to treat or not treat a client. For example, if a therapist develops an evaluation of memory skills for persons with suspected dementia in a work task to see how a loss of memory skills affects occupational performance, a ROC curve can determine a cut-off score for those who need work programming treatment to improve their skills from those who do not. Thus, one can determine whether the evaluation correctly identifies true positives (those who actually have memory problems affecting work) from true negatives (those who don't have serious enough memory problems related to work to need treatment).

Let's look at a study using ROC curves to validate use of an evaluation with a specific population. Saremi et al[10] performed a study to validate the CAGE questionnaire with 273 Native Americans. The CAGE is a short test consisting of four questions and detects severe alcohol dependency. When compared to another diagnostic tool for alcoholism, the DSM-III-R, the CAGE was found to be as valid a tool for identifying true positives and true negatives. A cut-off score of 2 or more was established to distinguish between those who were alcohol dependent and those who were not alcohol dependent. This study is an example of how ROC curves can help therapists use evaluation tools that are simpler and less time consuming to administer. (For a technical description of ROC curves, see Metz.[11])

WRITE THE EVALUATION MANUAL

Well-written, complete, and clear user manuals need to accompany all evaluations that are developed. The contents of a manual are described by Kline.[8] Kline's ideas are expanded and applied to occupational therapy evaluation instruments below in the approximate order in which they might best appear.

Introduction and Description

The need for the evaluation, the occupational therapy theory relating to the instrument, and the background of the development of the tool can be described here to orient the user. The domains or areas of human performance should be described in sufficient detail. The aims and purposes of the instrument need to be clearly described. An overview of the contents is designated in this section, as is the length of time needed to administer the instrument.

Population

Describe for whom the test is devised, eg, the parents of children with autism or the adult with schizophrenia, and to whom it should not be given. It is hoped that this latter information will help dissuade misuse of the instrument.

Standardization and Analysis Sections

Give detailed information to the users on the methods used to standardize the test. Include a description of the population used to norm the test. Identify the validity and reliability checks done and report the related statistical results.

Administration Qualifications

Cite the professionals who, by tradition, may be qualified to give the evaluation. Identify if special training is necessary to administer the instrument and where that training is available.

Materials and Environmental Requirements

List and describe any materials needed to give the test, eg, stopwatch, paper, and pencil. Specify where the evaluation is to be given, eg, in a testing room, with a group of patients in a classroom.

Precautions

Point out to the user what precautions need to be taken, if any, during the testing. These precautions can be related to the performance required on test items, test materials used, or physical and mental disabilities the patient may have.

Protocol

Clearly describe the instructions for administering the test. For example, describe what the administrator specifically says and does item by item.

Scoring Instructions

Detail how the evaluation is scored, and include methods and forms that have been developed to help report the outcomes clearly.

SEEK A PUBLISHER

Once you have an idea for developing an evaluation, do a needs assessment to see what has been published. At this time, note which publishers publish the type of instrument you wish to develop. Write to secure the author guidelines, if available, from those publishers you decide are the best. To get the best results, work from the beginning with a representative of the company you choose.

Ethics in Evaluation Development

There are three major ethical considerations in evaluation tool development. The first is the unauthorized use of test items from someone else's evaluation. Whenever a test developer "borrows" items from an instrument developed by another author, credit in the form of a citation must be given to the original author of the item or items, and permission from the publisher must be obtained. In the past, the author has observed that personnel at clinical sites developed and adapted forms of published tests for which no permission had been sought or the original authors cited.

The second ethical issue is the development of evaluation tools that are culturally biased.[4] Developers need to make sure that the language in test items does not disadvantage any group of patients from responding in a truthful and complete way. When devising scoring procedures, developers need to take into consideration various responses related to culture. In the evaluation manual, developers need to point out any limitations, including the lack of generalizability of the instrument to ethnic and other groups.[12]

The third issue is developing an evaluation that is on another professional's turf. For example, an occupational therapist might attempt to develop an intelligence evaluation, which traditionally is in the area of psychology. Occupational therapy has had an especially difficult time in this area due to perceived or actual lack of definition of the profession and its boundaries. Scholars are ever expanding the theory of occupational therapy, and we need to keep pace with new, updated assessment and concomitant evaluation instrument development. We need to remain vigilant about the development of instruments in areas that are traditionally occupational therapy areas by others who are less qualified. Function suddenly appeared to be every professional's area in the '90s, possibly resulting in more multidisciplinary evaluation tools.

Summary

Future assessment studies in occupational therapy would do well to investigate treatment utility. Hayes et al have defined this as "...the degree to which assessment is shown to contribute to beneficial treatment outcome."[13] As Silva has stated, evaluators need to move from looking at whether assessment versus no assessment is desirable to improve treatment outcomes, to which specific assessment is most useful.[14] This calls for refinement and updating of existing evaluation tools and the assessment process in occupational therapy. More patient-centered, functional evaluation instruments are needed to provide better usefulness and guidance for therapists to design effective treatment procedures.

As occupational therapists, we need to move away from the medical model of developing evaluation tools, and move toward community-based types of evaluation that enable or empower patients and their families. Evaluation can enable patients to obtain proper treatment, demonstrate when improvement has occurred, and capitalize on abilities. Evaluations must lead to clear treatment goals and objectives from which clearly discernable outcomes can be derived. In this age of cost containment, the benefits and outcomes of treatment are of utmost importance. Therefore, evaluation developers and users alike need to work with their professional organizations on outcomes research to ensure quality development and the appropriate use of evaluations.

Acknowledgment

The author wishes to thank Elaine M. Hockman, PhD, Adjunct Assistant Professor, School of Natural Resources and Environment, University of Michigan, Ann Arbor, MI, for her assistance with sections of this chapter.

References

1. American Occupational Therapy Association, Uniform Terminology Task Force and the Commission on Practice. Uniform Terminology for Occupational Therapy, second edition. In: Hopkins HL, Smith H, eds. *Willard and Spackman's Occupational Therapy.* 8th ed. Philadelphia, PA: JB Lippincott Co; 1993.
2. Carey L. *Measuring and Evaluating School Learning.* 2nd ed. Boston, MA: Allyn and Bacon Inc; 1994:76.
3. Folstein MF, Folstein S, McHugh PR. Mini-mental state: a practical method of grading the cognitive state of patients for the clinician. *J Psychiatr Res.* 1975;12:189.
4. Groth-Marnat G. *Handbook of Psychological Assessment.* New York, NY: Van Norstrand Rheinhold Co Inc; 1984:15.
5. Aiken LR. *Psychological Testing and Assessment.* 8th ed. Boston, MA: Allyn and Bacon Inc; 1994.
6. Brown FG. *Principles of Educational and Psychological Testing.* 3rd ed. New York, NY: Holt, Reinhart and Winston; 1983.
7. Thorndike RM. Reliability. In: Bolton B. *Handbook of Measurement and Evaluation in Rehabilitation.* 2nd ed. Baltimore, MD: Paul Brookes Publishing Co; 1987:31.
8. Kline P. How tests are constructed. In: Beech JR, Harding L. *Testing People: A Practical Guide to Psychometrics.* Windsor, England: The Neer-Nelson Publishing Co Ltd; 1990.
9. Tallent N. *The Practice of Psychological Assessment.* Englewood Cliffs, NJ: Prentice Hall; 1992.
10. Saremi A, Hanson RL, Williams DE, et al. Validity of the CAGE Questionnaire in an American Indian population. *Journal of Studies in Alcohol.* 2001;62:294-300.
11. Metz CE. Basic principles of ROC analysis. *Seminars of Nuclear Medicine.* 1978;8:283-298.
12. Canter MB, Bennett BE, Jones SE, Nagy TF. *Ethics for Psychologists: A Commentary on the APA Ethics Code.* Washington, DC: American Psychological Association; 1994.
13. Hayes SC, Nelson RO, Jarrett RB. The treatment utility of assessment: a functional approach to evaluating assessment quality. *American Psychologist.* 1987;42:963-974.
14. Silva F. *Psychometric Foundations and Behavioral Assessment.* Thousand Oaks, CA: Sage Publications; 1993.

APPENDICES

APPENDIX A

Journaling Resources

Adams K. *Journal to the Self: Twenty-Two Paths to Personal Growth.* New York, NY: Warner Books; 1990.

Kathleen Adams is cited by other authors as contributing much to the application of the journal process both in personal and professional/therapist venues. This book is written from the perspective of a therapist regarding the transformative powers of a journal. The writing and format are easy to read. Several suggestions and tools are given related to the art of journal writing. *Special Note:* Much of this book refers to and builds upon the works of Progoff.

Adams K. *Mightier Than the Sword: The Journal as a Path to Men's Self-Discovery.* New York, NY: Warner Books; 1994.

Kathleen Adams discusses how journal writing may be used by men to work through issues caused by role models who may have taught emotional restriction. The author cites the book as "practical, immediately useful ways to use a journal for personal growth, problem solving, stress management, creative expression, and a whole host of other applications."

Adams K. *The Way of the Journal: A Journal Therapy Workbook for Healing.* 2nd ed. Baltimore, MD: Sidran Institute Press; 1998.

A series of exercises are presented and designed to help the reader come to self-understanding, deal with personal conflicts, and work towards personal growth. The book may be helpful to use in conjunction with Adam's *Journal to the Self.*

Baldwin C. *One to One: A New and Updated Edition of the Classic Self-Understanding Through Journal Writing.* New York, NY: M. Evans and Company; 1991.

This book is a revision of a previous book written by Christina Baldwin. It provides a general overview of journal writing, as well as exercises and discussions of how to promote self-awareness and personal growth through the use of the journal.

Baldwin C. *Life's Companion: Journal Writing as a Spiritual Quest.* New York, NY: Bantam; 1991.

Christina Baldwin discusses the inner process and spiritual journey of journal writing as it contributes to the development of the self in life's journey. Baldwin uses a split format for the book, writing the actual text on the right hand side of the book, and offering quotes, journal excerpts, and exercises on the left hand side of the book. The book itself is written as a journey through life, and a journey through writing.

Bender S. *A Year in the Life: Journaling for Self-Discovery.* Cincinnati, OH: Walking Stick Press; 2000.

This book provides a basic overview of journaling in the first three chapters, followed by a series of chapters that include multiple exercises designed to take the journal writer through a year of structured writing. Each exercise includes additional suggestions for variations on the central theme.

Bolton G, Howlett S, Lago C, Wright JK, eds. *Writing Cures: An Introductory Handbook of Writing in Counseling and Therapy.* New York, NY: Brunner-Routledge; 2004.
A compilation of authors presents the therapeutic benefits of writing in a variety of venues including poetry, journal writing, expressive techniques, and reflective writing. The theoretical background and research findings are presented, along with writing applications within theoretical frameworks. This book is well suited to health care practitioners who wish to utilize writing in the healing process.

Bouton EE. *Journaling from the Heart: A Writing Workshop in Three Parts.* San Luis, CA: Whole Heart Publications; 2000.
This book is set up as a three-part writing workshop designed to take the journal writer through a series of exercises for personal use and reflection. The exercises range from light to fairly heavy and deep, and are focused quite heavily on introspection.

Capacchione L. *The Creative Journal: The Art of Finding Yourself.* Hollywood, CA: New Castle Publications; 1989.
This book presents ideas for personal creativity designed to teach the journal writer about the self through drawing and writing.

Heart RD, Strickland A. *Harvesting Your Journals: Writing Tools to Enhance Your Growth and Creativity.* Santa Fe, NM: Blessingway Books; 1999.
The authors provide various exercises and ideas for personal learning through the use of the journal. The focus is often on re-reading and learning from past journal writing.

Jacobs B. *Writing for Emotional Balance.* Oakland, CA: New Harbinger Publications; 2004.
This book provides guided journal exercises, many of which come out of techniques similar to cognitive behavioral therapy, in order to facilitate self-understanding and self-control over emotions. The book provides a background of each concept presented, followed by exercises designed to help emotional regulation.

Mallon T. *A Book of One's Own: People and Their Diaries.* St. Paul, MN: Hungry Mind Press; 1995.
Mallon presents an interesting book on the importance of diaries. This book is often cited by others, and offers information from published diaries.

Neubauer JN. *The Complete Idiot's Guide to Journaling.* Indianapolis, IN: Alpha; 2001.
Neubauer's book is a general elementary overview of principles for journaling. The book does not go into great detail or depth and therefore is best suited for the beginning journalist who has little to no experience with journal/diary writing. For those most serious with journaling, I would recommend some of the other books over this selection.

Phifer N. *Memoirs of the Soul: Writing Your Spiritual Autobiography.* Cincinnati, OH: Walking Stick Press, 2002.
This book takes a powerful look at writing one's memoirs. The content differs some from reflections on journals and diaries in that the writing of memoirs may involve sharing with others and/or production of a lasting product, and therefore the development of memoirs involve more drafts and editing than may otherwise be used within a personal journal or diary.

Progoff I. *At a Journal Workshop: Writing to Access the Power of the Unconscious and Evoke Creative Ability*. New York, NY: Penguin Putnam Books; 1992.

Ira Progoff is often considered one of the key contemporary writers on the journal process. He combines psychological roots with an intensive prescriptive process for journal writing. Ira spends a fair amount of time discussing how each phase/section of the journal relates to life and the development of the self. This book is a compilation of his previous classic works on journal writing.

Rainer T. *The New Diary: How to Use a Journal for Self-Guidance and Expanded Creativity*. Los Angeles, CA: Jeremy P. Tarcher Inc; 1978.

While Rainer's book is dated, much of the information presented holds true for present day journaling and diary techniques. Rainer uses the term diary interchangeably with journal and provides extensive insights into the history, techniques, and practical suggestions for diary writing. At times she indicates favor of maintaining a diary in chronological order and cites concerns about Progoff's numerous sections, as she contends the use of numerous sections can be difficult to use when re-reading and reflecting on the diary contents within the continuity of the individual's life.

Ramsland K. *Writing to Find Your True Self: Bliss*. Cincinnati OH: Walking Stick Press; 2000.

This book takes a look at the role of writing and self-reflection in finding one's direction in life. The concept of flow is discussed, as is the pursuit of bliss, which is identified as coming to know what is meant to be for one's life. Ramsland offers a number of exercises for individual and group reflection.

Woodward P. *Journal Jumpstarts: Quick Topics and Tips for Journal Writing*. Fort Collins, CO: Cottonwood Press; 1996.

This book is fairly small and simple and compiles a series of questions the journal writer may use as "jumpstarts" to journal writing.

Zukav G. *The Mind of the Soul: Responsible Choice*. New York, NY: Free Press; 2003.

Zukav's book is a New York Times best-seller. The book has information and exercises focused on personal choices, personal control, and means to facilitate responsible choice. The book may be used alone, or in conjunction with the *Self-Empowerment Journal*.

Zukav G, Francis, L. *Self-Empowerment Journal: A Companion Guide to the Mind of the Soul: Responsible Choice*. New York, NY: Free Press; 2003.

This journal workbook provides a series of exercises designed to go along with Zukav's book. The exercises are easy to read and provide clear directions for use.

APPENDIX B

Comprehensive Occupational Therapy Evaluation Scale (COTE Scale)

I. General Behavior	Date	Date	Date
Therapist's signature			
A. Appearance			
B. Non-Productive Behavior			
C. Activity Level * (A or B)			
D. Expression			
E. Responsibility			
F. Punctuality/Attendance			
G. Reality Orientation			
H. Conceptualization			
Subtotal			
II. Interpersonal Behavior			
A. Independence			
B. Cooperation			
C. Self Assertion* (A or B)			
D. Sociability			
E. Attention-Getting Behavior			
F. Negative Response from Others			
Subtotal			
III. Task Behaviors			
A. Engagement			
B. Concentration			
C. Coordination			
D. Follow Directions			
E. Activity Neatness/Attention to Detail* (A or B)			
F. Problem Solving			
G. Complexity and Organization of Task			
I. Initial Learning			
J. Interest in Activity			

continued

III. Task Behaviors	Date	Date	Date
K. Interest in Accomplishment			
L. Decision Making			
M. Frustration Tolerance			
Subtotal			
TOTAL			

Scale: 0 = Normal; 1= Minimal; 2 = Mild; 3 = Moderate; 4 = Severe
* Rate either Activity Neatness or Attention to Detail, not both

Comments:

Therapist Signature _____

Date _____

APPENDIX C

Definitions of Terms for the COTE Scale

I. General Behaviors

A. Appearance

The following six factors are involved: 1) clean skin, 2) clean hair, 3) hair combed, 4) clean clothes, 5) clothes neat, and 6) clothing suitable for the occasion.

0-No problems in any area

1-Problem in 1 area

2-Problem in 2 areas

3-Problem in 3 or 4 areas

4-Problem in 5 or 6 areas

B. Non-Productive Behavior

(Rocking, playing with hands, repetitive statements, appears to be talking to self, preoccupied with own thoughts, etc.)

0-No non-productive behavior during session

1-Non-productive behavior occasionally during session

2-Non-productive behavior for half of the session

3-Non-productive behavior for three-fourths of the session

4-Non-productive behavior the entire session

C. Activity Level (A or B)

(A)

0-No hyperactivity

1-Occasional hyperactivity

2-Hyperactivity attracts the attention of other clients but participates

3-Hyperactivity level such that can only participate with great difficulty

4-So hyperactive that client cannot participate

(B)

1-No hypoactivity

2-Occasional hypoactivity

3-Hypoactivity level such that can participate but with great difficulty

4-So hypoactive that the client cannot participate

D. Expression

0-Expression consistent with situation and setting

1-Communicates with expression, occasionally inappropriate
2-Shows inappropriate expression several times during session
3-Show of expression but inconsistent with situation
4-Extremes of expression—bizarre, uncontrolled, or no expression

E. Responsibility
0-Takes responsibility for own actions
1-Denies responsibility for 1 or 2 actions
2-Denies responsibility for several actions
3-Denies responsibility for most actions
4-Denial of all responsibility (messes up project and blames others)

F. Attendance/Punctuality
0-Consistently ready for therapy
1-Needs encouragement 20% of the time
2-Needs encouragement 50% of the time
3-Refuses up to 50% of the time
4-Refuses more than 50 % of the time

G. Reality Orientation
0-Complete awareness of person, place, time, and situation
1-General awareness but inconsistency in 1 area
2-Awareness of only 2 areas
3-Awareness in 1 area
4-Lack of awareness of person, place, time, and situation

H. Conceptualization
0-Demonstrates abstract thinking
1-Responds abstractly 1+ times
2-Relevant concrete responses
3-Responds concretely 1+ times
4-Responses unrelated to situation

II. Interpersonal Behaviors

A. Independence
0-Independent functioning
1-Only 1 or 2 dependent actions
2-50% independent and 50% dependent actions
3-Only 1 or 2 independent actions
4-No independent actions

B. Cooperation

    0-Cooperates with program

    1-Follows most directions, opposes less than 50%

    2-Follows 50%, opposes 50%

    3-Opposes 75% of the session

    4-Opposes all directions/suggestions

C. Self-Assertion

    (A)

    0-Assertive when appropriate

    1-Passive less than 50% of the session

    2-Passive 50% of the session

    3-Passive more than 50% of the session

    4-Passive the entire session

    (B)

    0-Assertive when appropriate

    1-Dominant less than 50% of the session

    2-Dominant 50% of the session

    3-Dominant more than 50% of the session

    4-Dominantes aggressively

D. Sociability

    0-Socializes with staff and other clients

    1-Socializes with staff and occasionally with other clients or vice versa

    2-Socializes only with staff or only with clients

    3-Socializes only if approached

    4-Does not join others in activities, unable to carry on casual conversation even if approached

E. Attention-Getting Behavior

    0-No unreasonable attention-getting behavior

    1-Less than 50% of the time spent in attention-getting behavior

    2-50% of the time spent in attention-getting behavior

    3-75% of the time spent in attention-getting behavior

    4-Verbally or non-verbally demands constant attention

F. Negative Response from Others

    0-Evokes no negative responses

    1-Evokes 1 negative response

2-Evokes 2 negative responses

3-Evokes 3 or more negative responses during the session

4-Evokes numerous negative responses from others, and therapist must take some action

III. Task Behaviors

A. Engagement

0-Needs no encouragement to begin task

1-Encourage once to begin activity

2-Encourage 2 or 3 times to engage in activity

3-Engages in activity only after much encouragement

4-Does not engage in activity

B. Concentration

0-No difficulty concentrating during session

1-Off task less than 25% of the time

2-Off task 50% of the time

3-Off task 75% of the time

4-Loss of concentration on task in less than 1 minute

C. Coordination

0-No problems with coordination

1-Occasionally has trouble with fine detail, manipulating tools and materials

2-Occasionally has trouble manipulating tools and materials but has frequent trouble with fine detail

3-Some difficulty in gross movement—unable to manipulate some tools and materials

4-Has great difficulty in movement (gross motor), virtually unable to manipulate tools and materials.

D. Follow Directions

0-Carries out directions without problems

1-Carries out simple directions, has trouble with 2-step directions

2-Carries out 1 direction, has trouble with 2

3-Can carry out only very simple 1-step directions (demonstrated, written, or verbal)

4-Unable to carry out any directions

E. Activity Neatness/Attention to Detail

(A)

0-Activity neatly done

1-Occasionally ignores fine detail

2-Often ignores fine detail and materials are scattered

3-Ignores fine detail and work habits disturbing to those around

4-Unaware of fine detail; so sloppy that therapist has to intervene

(B)

0-Pays attention to detail appropriately

1-Occasionally too concise

2-More attention to several details than is required

3-So concise that project will take twice as long as expected

4-So concerned that project will never get finished

F. Problem-Solving

0-Solves problems without assistance

1-Solves problems after assistance is given once

2-Can solve only after repeated instructions

3-Recognizes a problem but cannot solve it

4-Unable to recognize or solve a problem

G. Complexity and Organization of Task

0-Organizes and performs tasks given

1-Occasionally has trouble with organization of complex activities that should be able to do

2-Can organize simple but not complex activities

3-Can do only very simple activities with organization imposed by therapist

4-Unable to organize or carry out an activity when all tools, materials, and directions are available

H. Initial Learning

0-Learns a new activity quickly and without difficulty

1-Occasionally has difficulty learning a complex activity

2-Has frequent difficulty learning a complex activity

3-Unable to learn complex activities, occasionally has difficulty learning simple activities

4-Unable to learn a new activity

I. Interest in Activities

0-Interested in a variety of activities

1-Occasionally not interested in a new activity

2-Shows occasional interest in a part of an activity

3-Engages in activities but shows no interest

4-Does not participate

J. Interest in Accomplishment

0-Interested in finishing activities

1-Occasional lack of interest or pleasure in finishing a long-term activity

2-Interest or pleasure in accomplishment of a short-term activity, lack of interest in a long-term activity

3-Only occasional interest in finishing an activity

4-No interest or pleasure in finishing an activity

K. Decision Making

0-Makes own decisions

1-Makes own decisions but occasionally seeks therapist's approval

2-Makes own decisions but often seeks therapist's approval

3-Makes decisions when given only 2 alternatives

4-Cannot make or refuses to make any decision

L. Frustration Tolerance

0-Handles all tasks without becoming overly frustrated

1-Occasionally becomes frustrated with 1 or more complex tasks; can handle simple tasks

2-Often becomes frustrated with more complex tasks, but is able to handle simple tasks

3-Often becomes frustrated with any task but attempts to continue

4-Becomes so frustrated with simple tasks that refuses or is unable to function

APPENDIX D

COLLABORATIVE
ADAPTIVE
PLANNING
ASSESSMENT

The Collaborative Adaptive Planning Assessment (CAPA) is designed to organize a collaborative process between client and therapist to develop plans for the future following major life changes

**Developed by the CAPA Project Group
School of Occupational Therapy
Texas Woman's University**

Personal Information	ID#:		Name:
Initial Assessment Date:	**Planning Reassessment Date:**		**Reassessment Date:**

Address:

Age:	Gender:	Marital Status:	Ethnicity:

Living Arrangement: Choose one:	Choose one:	Choose one:
❑ Apartment	❑ Own	❑ Rural
❑ Home	❑ Rent	❑ Urban

Members of Household:	**Key Family Members:**
* Relationships and approximate ages	* Relationships & locations
Other Major Sources of Support:	**Disability and Date of Onset:**
Adaptive Equipment:	**Other Health Problems:**
Source of Income:	**Support for Health Care Expenses:**
	* Inpatient services, outpatient services, equipment

Perceived Adequacy of Income:		
❑ Comfortable	❑ Adequate for meeting needs	❑ Inadequate for meeting needs

Self-reported coping style:

* What have you done in the past when you ran into difficulties in life?

Occupational Areas		Client Rating Summary (Information from the Occupation Cards of the client)							
		Occupation Time Spent		Persons Participation		Environment Negotiability		Value Importance	
Indicate occupations to be examined:		1 = Initial Assessment (month 1)				2 = Reassessment (month 2)			
		1	2	1	2	1	2	1	2
Work	Full-time paid employment	___	___	___	___	___	___	___	___
	Part-time paid employment	___	___	___	___	___	___	___	___
	Volunteer work	___	___	___	___	___	___	___	___
	School/university	___	___	___	___	___	___	___	___
Leisure	Identify activity:								
	1. _____	___	___	___	___	___	___	___	___
	2. _____	___	___	___	___	___	___	___	___
	3. _____	___	___	___	___	___	___	___	___
	4. _____	___	___	___	___	___	___	___	___
	5. _____	___	___	___	___	___	___	___	___
Household Management	General shopping	___	___	___	___	___	___	___	___
	Grocery shopping	___	___	___	___	___	___	___	___
	Health care	___	___	___	___	___	___	___	___
	Meal preparation	___	___	___	___	___	___	___	___
	Housecleaning	___	___	___	___	___	___	___	___
	Outside maintenance	___	___	___	___	___	___	___	___
	Laundry	___	___	___	___	___	___	___	___
	Financial management	___	___	___	___	___	___	___	___
	Using telephone	___	___	___	___	___	___	___	___
	Using computer	___	___	___	___	___	___	___	___
	Care giving	___	___	___	___	___	___	___	___
Self care	Eating	___	___	___	___	___	___	___	___
	Dressing	___	___	___	___	___	___	___	___
	Bathing	___	___	___	___	___	___	___	___
	Grooming	___	___	___	___	___	___	___	___
	Toileting	___	___	___	___	___	___	___	___
	Taking medications	___	___	___	___	___	___	___	___
Rest	Sleep at night	___	___	___	___	___	___	___	___
	Daytime rest	___	___	___	___	___	___	___	___

Rating Index:
Occupation   1 = Very unsatisfied with time spent   10 = Very satisfied with time spent

Persons	1 = Very unsatisfied with own participation	10 = Very satisfied with own participation
Environment	1 = Environment unfamiliar or difficult to negotiate	10 = Environment familiar or easy to negotiate
Value	1 = Not important to continue	10 = Important to continue or substitute

Occupational Areas		**Client Rating Summary** (Information from the Occupation Cards of the client)							
		Occupation Time Spent		**Persons** Participation		**Environment** Negotiability		**Value** Importance	
Indicate occupations to be examined:		3 = Reassessment (month 3)				4 = Reassessment (month 6)			
		3	4	3	4	3	4	3	4
Work	Full-time paid employment	—	—	—	—	—	—	—	—
	Part-time paid employment	—	—	—	—	—	—	—	—
	Volunteer work	—	—	—	—	—	—	—	—
	School/university	—	—	—	—	—	—	—	—
Leisure	Identify activity:								
	1. _____	—	—	—	—	—	—	—	—
	2. _____	—	—	—	—	—	—	—	—
	3. _____	—	—	—	—	—	—	—	—
	4. _____	—	—	—	—	—	—	—	—
	5. _____	—	—	—	—	—	—	—	—
Household Management	General shopping	—	—	—	—	—	—	—	—
	Grocery shopping	—	—	—	—	—	—	—	—
	Health care	—	—	—	—	—	—	—	—
	Meal preparation	—	—	—	—	—	—	—	—
	Housecleaning	—	—	—	—	—	—	—	—
	Outside maintenance	—	—	—	—	—	—	—	—
	Laundry	—	—	—	—	—	—	—	—
	Financial management	—	—	—	—	—	—	—	—
	Using telephone	—	—	—	—	—	—	—	—
	Using computer	—	—	—	—	—	—	—	—
	Care giving	—	—	—	—	—	—	—	—
Self care	Eating	—	—	—	—	—	—	—	—
	Dressing	—	—	—	—	—	—	—	—
	Bathing	—	—	—	—	—	—	—	—
	Grooming	—	—	—	—	—	—	—	—
	Toileting	—	—	—	—	—	—	—	—
	Taking medications	—	—	—	—	—	—	—	—
Rest	Sleep at night	—	—	—	—	—	—	—	—
	Daytime rest	—	—	—	—	—	—	—	—

Rating Index: Rate each on a scale of 1 to 10

Occupation	1 = Very unsatisfied with time spent	10 = Very satisfied with time spent

Persons	1 = Very unsatisfied with own participation	10 = Very satisfied with own participation
Environment	1 = Environment unfamiliar or difficult to negotiate	10 = Environment familiar or easy to negotiate
Value	1 = Not important to continue	10 = Important to continue or substitute

Planning Report	• Major occupations expected to change following onset of disability • Integrated pictures of client's adaptation • Collaborative process • Major goals and needed forms of support * narrative summary of occupation cards
Initial Assessment (Month 1):	**Reassessment (Month 2):**

Estimation of future ability to follow through with implementation of plans:

	Expected to need extensive support			Able to manage implementation without help	
Initial Assessment (month1):	1	2	3	4	5
Reassessment (month2):	1	2	3	4	5

Planning Report	• Major occupations expected to change following onset of disability • Integrated pictures of client's adaptation • Collaborative process • Major goals and needed forms of support * narrative summary of occupation cards
Initial Assessment (Month 3):	**Reassessment (Month 6):**

Estimation of future ability to follow through with implementation of plans:

	Expected to need extensive support			Able to manage implementation without help	
Reassessment (month 3):	1	2	3	4	5
Reassessment (month 6):	1	2	3	4	5

APPENDIX E

Community Adaptive Planning Report Format

Major Occupations Performed Regularly Before Onset of Disability

Activities, persons, environments, and value for each

Occupational Ratings for Each Major Occupation (Optional)

Rating by client on a scale from 1 (low) to 10 (high), satisfaction with time spent, satisfaction with degree of participation, negotiability of environment, importance of continuing occupation

Integrated Picture of Client's Community Adaptation

Overall Round of Occupations

Balance among work, leisure, activities of daily living, and rest satisfactory to client and others; ability to manage overall round of occupations

Social Network

Persons client interacts with regularly, inside and outside of household; key support resources

Personal Territory

Where does client go to perform major occupations? How does client get to these locations?

Value

What occupations would client be most willing to give up? What occupations does client most want to hold on to? What opportunities does client want to pursue in the future?

Major Occupations Expected to Change After Onset of Disability

Expected losses, expected gains, future-planning goals for each major occupation

Internal or External Sources of Structure

Level of Involvement in Collaborative Planning Process

Emotional commitment or psychic energy devoted by client to planning process; completeness of client's account of previous occupations; relative contributions of client and therapist to the planning process

Ability to Make Sense of Current Therapy

Ability to use therapy experience to anticipate future capabilities; ability to see connections between current therapy and future goals

Estimation of Future Ability to Follow Through With Implementation of Plans

> Rating by therapist on a scale from 1 (expected to need extensive support) to 5 (able to manage implementation without help)

Summary of Major Goals and Needed Forms of Support

APPENDIX F

Task Skills Scale

Client _____ Date _____ Staff_____

Task Behavior	Rating	Comments
1. Willingness to engage in doing tasks. Avoids engaging in tasks, talks more than engages in productive activity, needs prompting or encouragement to engage in task, seems fearful when engaging in tasks		
2. Physical capacity: includes posture, strength, and gross and fine motor coordination. Is unable to assume and/or maintain a posture that is conducive to successful completion of the task, tires very easily and/or asks for or takes an inordinate number of rest periods, clumsy carrying out tasks and/or performs tasks very slowly because of need to concentrate on coordinated movements.		
3. Ability to maintain concentration on task. Short attention span, spends most of the time engaged in nontask-oriented behavior (eg, walking around), frequently changes tasks, leaves tasks uncompleted.		
4. Ability to organize task in a logical manner. Appears not to think about task prior to beginning, does not have all the items needed for task completion close at hand, does not consider what should be done first, second, and so forth.		
5. Ability to follow directions. Unable to comprehend directions, unable to follow directions without assistance, repeatedly asks for directions when these have been given and/or when available, does not return to directions to check whether the task is being done correctly.		

6. Rate of performance. Unable to work at a steady pace, is excessively slow in performing a task so that little is accomplished in comparison to others, or is excessively fast so that quality is sacrificed, spends considerable time on tasks but is not productive.		
7. Attention to detail. Excessive attention to detail, is not certain what aspects of a task are more or less important, conversely there may be excessive disregard of details, hurries through tasks with little attention to details.		
8. Tolerates frustration. Becomes upset when confronted with a problem, has difficulty in accepting delays, becomes agitated when he or she makes a mistake, has difficulty in accepting negative feedback, does not like to repeat steps or to do something again.		

1=Significantly below essential performance standards = Significantly fails to achieve standards defined for the group (eg, does not work on the task, may show deviant or abusive behaviors toward the task).
2=Below essential performance standards = Fails to meet standards defined for the group (eg, needs assistance to productively engage in the task).
3=Meets essential performance standards = Meets, but does not exceed, standards defined for the group (eg, engages in the task as required or appropriate for the activity).
4=Above essential performance standards = Exceeds standards defined for the group (eg, readily and independently engages in task and exceeds level of performance required for task).
5=Significantly above essential performance standards = Significantly exceeds standards defined for the group (eg, can teach and supervise others in task completion, assistant to the group leader).

Additional Comments:

Adapted with permission from Mosey AC. *Psychosocial Components of Occupational Therapy.* New York: Raven Press; 1986: 322. Copyright 1986 by Raven Press.

APPENDIX G

Interpersonal Skills Scale

Client _____ Date _____ Staff_____

Interpersonal Behavior	Rating	Comments
1. Ability to initiate, respond to, and sustain verbal interactions Has difficulty in spontaneously initiating a conversation with another person, does not spontaneously respond to others, cannot carry on a conversation, is not able to participate in normal give-and-take of conversation.		
2. Keeps all statements appropriate to context. Cannot follow thread of discussion, makes statements that are inappropriate or irrelevant to subject matter, is unable to keep statements appropriate despite redirection.		
3. Communicates accurately and expresses self clearly. Does not communicate in a way that is sensible to the listener, communicates false statements, expresses ideas in a circuitous or tangential manner.		
4. Interacts comfortably with staff. Is overly shy, friendly or in need of constant attention from staff, is not able to request or receive assistance from staff, is not able to follow direction, rules, or procedures from staff.		
5. Interacts comfortably with peers. Is overly shy, aggressive, or inappropriate with peers, acts as though he or she has not considered the needs or feelings of others, is not able to work collaboratively with peers, is not able to accept help from peers.		
6. Uses appropriate nonverbal behavior and tone of voice (Invades the space of others, tone of voice and/or nonverbal gestures are inconsistent or inappropriate to verbal content or context of the situation.		

7. Cooperates as a member of a group. Avoids interacting in groups, acts independently in situations where cooperation is required, treats cooperative situations as if they were competitive, has difficulty being the winner or the loser in a competitive group situation.		
8. Controls impulsive, offensive, and/or annoying behavior. Hastily acts out toward self or others in a negative or harmful manner, intentionally irritates, torments, teases, or causes anguish to others, is verbally degrading or abusive to others.		

1=Significantly below essential performance standards = Significantly fails to achieve standards defined for the group (eg, does not interact with others, may show deviant or abusive behaviors toward others).

2=Below essential performance standards = Fails to meet standards defined for the group (eg, needs assistance for productive interaction with others).

3=Meets essential performance standards = Meets, but does not exceed, standards defined for the group (eg, engages in interaction as required or appropriate for the activity; is not disruptive to the group process).

4=Above essential performance standards = Exceeds standards defined for the group (eg, readily engages others in interactions, is helpful to others).

5=Significantly above essential performance standards = Significantly exceeds standards defined for the group (eg, assumes appropriate group leadership role, assistant to the group leader).

Additional Comments:

Adapted with permission from Mosey AC. *Psychosocial Components of Occupational Therapy.* New York: Raven Press; 1986: 324. Copyright 1986 by Raven Press; Rogers ES, Sciarappa K, Anthony WA. Development and evaluation of situational assessment instruments and procedures for persons with psychiatric disabilities. *Vocational Evaluation and Work Adjustment Bulletin.* 1991(Summer):61-67.

APPENDIX H

School Scale

Client _____ Date _____ Staff_____

School Behavior	Rating	Comments
1. Class attendance. Frequently does not go to class, does not attend all classes, is late for and/or leaves early from class.		
2. Group behavior. Does not pay attention, disturbs other students, does not do tasks, does not participate in discussions.		
3. Relationship with teachers. Does not want to do what the teacher asks, ignores or is insolent to teacher, does not ask for guidelines or assistance when needed, cannot adapt to the style of some teachers, or is overly dependent on teacher.		
4. Relationship with classmates. States that he or she has no friends in class, is excessively shy with classmates, is a loner, or provokes classmates, acts as if superior to others, is not liked by classmates.		
5. Academic Performance. Grades are below what one would expect given the individual's apparent abilities, grades are markedly uneven across subjects and/or grading periods, does not seem to put forth much effort, blames poor academic performance on others.		
6. Participation in academic evaluations. Does not study adequately for tests, hurries through examinations without giving appropriate attention to each item, or becomes excessively anxious prior to or during test, is overly preoccupied with grades.		

1=Significantly below essential performance standards = Significantly fails to achieve standards defined for school (eg, does not work on the task, may show deviant or abusive behaviors toward the task).

2=Below essential performance standards = Fails to meet standards defined for school (eg, needs assistance to productively engage in the task).

3=Meets essential performance standards = Meets, but does not exceed, standards defined for school (eg, engages in the task as required or appropriate for the assignment).

4=Above essential performance standards = Exceeds standards defined for school (eg, readily and independently engages in the task and exceeds level of performance required for the task).
5=Significantly above essential performance standards = Significantly exceeds standards defined for school (eg, can teach and supervise others in task completion, assistant to the teacher).

Additional Comments:

Adapted with permission from Mosey AC. *Psychosocial Components of Occupational Therapy.* New York: Raven Press; 1986: 322. Copyright 1986 by Raven Press.

APPENDIX I

Work Scale

Client _____ Date _____ Staff_____

Work Behavior	Rating	Comments
1. Attendance. Attendance at work is irregular, frequently late to work, leaves work early, has difficulty tolerating a full session of work.		
2. General attitude. Does not feel the role of worker is an important social role, does not see self as a worker, is happier when not working.		
3. Performance. Manifests fear or anxiety as a response to the demand to be productive, does not organize tasks relative to priority, does not work at increased speeds when required, does not easily return to work after interruptions, does not plan work periods so that required amount of work is accomplished, avoids responsibility, does not complete assigned tasks in an acceptable manner, completes assigned tasks late.		
4. Take direction from work supervisor. Acts in a hostile or aggressive manner when assigned work, does not follow directions given, unable to accept constructive criticism, or is overly dependent on supervisor.		
5. Relationship to co-workers. Is overly dependent, does not give assistance when requested, is unable to carry on a casual conversation with co-workers, responds to co-workers in a belligerent manner, makes derogatory remarks to co-workers, avoids co-workers during breaks and lunch hour, acts in a way that makes co-workers uncomfortable.		
6. Response to norms of the work setting. Does not dress appropriately, selects inappropriate topics of conversation, pace of work is markedly different from workers, acts as if the work setting is designed to suit needs that are more appropriately satisfied in other settings, does not conform to the rules of the setting, cannot differentiate between formal and informal structure.		

1=Significantly below essential performance standards = Significantly fails to achieve standards defined for work (eg, does not work on the task, may show deviant or abusive behaviors toward the task).

2=Below essential performance standards = Fails to meet standards defined for work (eg, needs assistance for to productively engage in the task).

3=Meets essential performance standards = Meets, but does not exceed, standards defined for work (eg, engages in the task as required or appropriate for the activity).

4=Above essential performance standards = Exceeds standards defined for work (eg, readily and independently engages in task and exceeds level of performance required for the task).

5=Significantly above essential performance standards = Significantly exceeds standards defined for the group (eg, can teach and supervise others in task completion, assistant to the group leader).

Additional Comments:

APPENDIX J

Group Membership

Client _____ Date _____ Staff_____

Group Membership Behavior	Rating	Comments
1. Group attendance. Frequently does not go to group, does not attend all group sessions, is late for and/or leaves early from group sessions.		
2. Group behavior. Does not pay attention, disturbs other group members, does not do tasks, does not participate in discussions.		
3. Relationship with group leaders. Does not want to do what the group leader asks, ignores or is insolent to group leader, does not ask for guidelines or assistance when needed, cannot adapt to the style of some group leaders, or, is overly dependent on group leader.		
4. Relationship with group members. States that he or she has no friends in group, is excessively shy, avoids others during breaks, is unable to carry on a casual conversation, does not give assistance when requested, responds to others in a belligerent manner, makes derogatory remarks, acts as if superior to others, is not liked by group members.		
5. Performance. Manifests fear or anxiety as a response to the demand to be productive, does not organize tasks relative to priority, does not work at increased speeds when required, does not easily return to work after interruptions, does not plan work periods so that required amount of work is accomplished, avoids responsibility, does not complete assigned tasks in an acceptable manner, completes assigned tasks late.		
6. Response to norms of the setting. Does not dress appropriately, selects inappropriate topics of conversation, pace of task completion is markedly different from peers, does not conform to the rules of the setting.		

1=Significantly below essential performance standards = Significantly fails to achieve standards defined for the group (eg, does not work on the task, may show deviant or abusive behaviors toward the task).

2=Below essential performance standards = Fails to meet standards defined for the group (eg, needs assistance for to productively engage in the task).

3=Meets essential performance standards = Meets, but does not exceed, standards defined for the group (eg, engages in the task as required or appropriate for the activity).

4=Above essential performance standards = Exceeds standards defined for the group (eg, readily and independently engages in the task and exceeds level of performance required for the task).

5=Significantly above essential performance standards = Significantly exceeds standards defined for the group (eg, can teach and supervise others in task completion, assistant to the group leader).

Additional Comments:

APPENDIX K

Family Member – Parent Role

Client _____ Date _____ Staff_____

Family Member Behavior – Parent Role	Rating	Comments
1. Child's physical needs. Does not provide adequate food, clothing, and shelter; does not secure periodic physical, dental, and eye examinations; does not maintain a safe home; does not secure adequate child-care assistance (baby sitter, child care centers, etc.).		
2. Child's emotional needs. Is not able to demonstrate affection, is apparently unaware of the child's emotional needs, avoids interaction with child, expresses strong negative feelings toward the child.		
3. Play/recreational activities with child. Does not provide appropriate toys, is unconcerned about the child's recreational activities, does not see play/recreation as part of a parental role.		
4. Communication. Does not communicate in a clear manner, gives conflicting messages to the child, denies child opportunity to discuss matters of concern, communication is not geared to the child's lever of understanding and interests, unnecessarily limits expression of own thoughts and feelings.		
5. Discipline. Does not set forth specific behavioral expectations, is not consistent in disciplining the child relative to expectations, does not maintain adequate balance between giving the child freedom and imposing limits, is not able to maintain self-control when child does not meet behavioral expectations, abuses child.		

6. Education. Does not demonstrate concern for the child's education, knows little or nothing about the child's academic performance or behavior in school, does not assist in or provide guidelines for the child's completion of homework assignments, has not contact with the school, does not encourage the child to attend school on a regular basis.		
7. Responsibilities. Does not give the child appropriate self-care and household responsibilities, allows the child to be excessively dependent, give the child responsibilities beyond his or her capacity, does not adequately reward the child for taking appropriate responsibilities.		
8. Encourage appropriate independence. Does not encourage child's independence, rewards dependent behavior, makes demands on the child for need satisfaction which are inappropriate to a parent-child relationship, demands independence of the child before he/she is ready for such an independence		

1=Significantly below essential performance standards = Significantly fails to achieve standards defined for work (eg, does not work on the task, may show deviant or abusive behaviors toward the task).

2=Below essential performance standards = Fails to meet standards defined for work (eg, needs assistance for to productively engage in the task).

3=Meets essential performance standards = Meets, but does not exceed, standards defined for work (eg, engages in the task as required or appropriate for the activity).

4=Above essential performance standards = Exceeds standards defined for work (eg, readily and independently engages in task and exceeds level of performance required for the task).

5=Significantly above essential performance standards = Significantly exceeds standards defined for the group (eg, can teach and supervise others in task completion, assistant to the group leader).

Additional Comments:

Adapted with permission from Mosey AC. *Psychosocial Components of Occupational Therapy.* New York: Raven Press; 1986: 322. Copyright 1986 by Raven Press.

APPENDIX L

Family Member – General Family Interaction

Client _____ Date _____ Staff_____

Family Member Behavior	Rating	Comments
1. Quantity of roles. Does not have a satisfying number of roles appropriate to one's age, gender, and family situation.		
2. Quality of family roles. Does not feel the family member roles are important social roles, does not see self as a family member or in family roles, experiences conflict in family member roles, is not invited to be a family member by other members of the family.		
3. Communication with family members. Is unable to communicate ideas and feelings in an appropriate manner; is not able to give or receive emotional support.		
4. Relationship to partner. Is not able to take on acceptable degree of responsibility for the relationship; is overly dependent and/or demanding; treats partner in a demeaning fashion; is physically, sexually, or psychologically abusive; is unable to engage in mutual satisfaction of sexual needs.		
5. Relationship to family members. Is not able to take on acceptable degree of responsibility for the relationship; is overly dependent and/or demanding; is physically, sexually, or psychologically abusive; is not able to engage in activities of daily living that are appropriate to the relationship.		

1=Significantly below essential performance standards = Significantly fails to achieve standards defined for work (eg, does not work on the task, may show deviant or abusive behaviors toward the task).
2=Below essential performance standards = Fails to meet standards defined for work (eg, needs assistance for to productively engage in the task).
3=Meets essential performance standards = Meets, but does not exceed, standards defined for work (eg, engages in the task as required or appropriate for the activity).
4=Above essential performance standards = Exceeds standards defined for work (eg, readily and independently engages in task and exceeds level of performance required for the task).

5=Significantly above essential performance standards = Significantly exceeds standards defined for the group (eg, can teach and supervise others in task completion, assistant to the group leader).

Additional Comments:

Adapted with permission from Mosey AC. *Psychosocial Components of Occupational Therapy.* New York: Raven Press; 1986: 322. Copyright 1986 by Raven Press.

APPENDIX M

Friendships

Client _____ Date _____ Staff_____

Friendship Behavior	Rating	Comments
1. Initiates friendships. States that he or she has no friends, does not know how to go about establishing friend relationships, states that there is no one that he or she can talk to.		
2. Maintains friendships. Spends little if any time with other people outside of the context of school/work/groups, has friendships for only a short period of time.		

1=Significantly below essential performance standards = Significantly fails to achieve standards defined for the group (eg, does not interact with others, may show deviant or abusive behaviors toward others).

2=Below essential performance standards = Fails to meet standards defined for the group (eg, needs assistance for productive interaction with others).

3=Meets essential performance standards = Meets, but does not exceed, standards defined for the group (eg, engages in interaction as required or appropriate for the activity; is not disruptive to the group process).

4=Above essential performance standards = Exceeds standards defined for the group (eg,.readily engages others in interactions, is helpful to others).

5=Significantly above essential performance standards = Significantly exceeds standards defined for the group (eg, assumes appropriate group leadership role, assistant to the group leader).

Additional Comments:

Adapted with permission from Mosey AC. *Psychosocial Components of Occupational Therapy.* New York: Raven Press; 1986: 322. Copyright 1986 by Raven Press.

APPENDIX N

Community Member

Client _____ Date _____ Staff_____

Community Member Behavior	Rating	Comments
1. Leisure/Recreation. Minimal engagement in leisure/recreational activities, little variety in leisure/recreational activities, complains of boredom, states that leisure activities are not satisfying, leisure/recreational activities are not within the bounds considered acceptable by one's cultural group, activities are potentially self-destructive.		
2. Community activities. Minimal engagement in community activities, states that he/she does not feel accepted by the community, community activities are not within the bounds considered acceptable by one's cultural group.		

1=Significantly below essential performance standards = Significantly fails to achieve standards defined for the group (eg, does not interact with others, may show deviant or abusive behaviors toward others).

2=Below essential performance standards = Fails to meet standards defined for the group (eg, needs assistance for productive interaction with others).

3=Meets essential performance standards = Meets, but does not exceed, standards defined for the group (eg, engages in interaction as required or appropriate for the activity; is not disruptive to the group process).

4=Above essential performance standards = Exceeds standards defined for the group (eg,.readily engages others in interactions, is helpful to others).

5=Significantly above essential performance standards = Significantly exceeds standards defined for the group (eg, assumes appropriate group leadership role, assistant to the group leader).

Additional Comments:

APPENDIX O

Health Maintenance

Client _____ Date _____ Staff_____

Health Maintenance Behavior	Rating	Comments
1. Ability to understand what health is and what is required to maintain health. Is not able to define healthy living or the components of healthy living. Describes a lifestyle that is unhealthy in the areas of diet, exercise. Lacks information pertinent to individual needs about illnesses and diseases.		
2. Ability to understand how to maintain medication management. Is unable to state medications currently prescribed, as well as the dosing requirements, effects, side effects, and precautions. Does not know how to locate information about medications or is unable to locate the information.		
3. Ability to understand how to maintain a healthy well-balanced diet. Is unable to describe the 4 basic food groups or the food that constitutes a healthy diet. Describes a diet that is unhealthy or has more than recommended amounts of fat, sugar, carbohydrates, and calories. Is unable to state how diet can contribute to illness and disease.		
4. Ability to understand how to maintain an appropriate exercise program. Is unable to state exercise or fitness routine that would contribute to an appropriate exercise program. Does not engage in recommended amount or type of fitness or exercise activity.		

1=Significantly below essential performance standards = Significantly fails to achieve standards defined for the group (eg, does not interact with others, may show deviant or abusive behaviors toward others).

2=Below essential performance standards = Fails to meet standards defined for the group (eg, needs assistance for productive interaction with others).

3=Meets essential performance standards = Meets, but does not exceed, standards defined for the group (eg, engages in interaction as required or appropriate for the activity; is not disruptive to the group process).

4=Above essential performance standards = Exceeds standards defined for the group (eg,.readily engages others in interactions, is helpful to others).
5=Significantly above essential performance standards = Significantly exceeds standards defined for the group (eg, assumes appropriate group leadership role, assistant to the group leader).

Additional Comments:

Adapted with permission from Mosey AC. *Psychosocial Components of Occupational Therapy.* New York: Raven Press; 1986: 322. Copyright 1986 by Raven Press.

APPENDIX P

Home Maintenance

Client _____ Date _____ Staff_____

Home Maintenance Behavior	Rating	Comments
1. Meal planning, preparation, and cleanup. Ability to plan, prepare, and serve well-balanced, nutritional meals and cleanup food and equipment after meals. Is not able to define components of meal planning, serving, and cleanup. Describes a lifestyle that does not incorporate adequate meal planning, serving and cleanup. Lacks information pertinent to individual needs about meal planning, serving, and cleanup.		
2. Shopping. Ability to understand how to prepare a shopping list, select and purchase items, select method of payment, and complete money transaction. Is unable to state steps for and/or demonstrate actions for preparing a shopping list, selecting and purchasing items, selecting method of payment, and completing money transaction.		
3. Home establishment and management. Ability to develop and maintain personal and household possessions and environment (eg, home, yard, garden, appliances, vehicles), including maintaining and repairing personal possessions (clothing and household items) and knowing how to seek help or whom to contact. Is unable to describe steps or demonstrate actions regarding developing and maintaining personal and household possessions and environment (eg, home, yard, garden, appliances, vehicles), including maintaining and repairing personal possessions (clothing and household items) and knowing how to seek help or whom to contact.		

4. Safety. Ability to know and perform preventive procedures to maintain a safe environment as well as recognizing sudden, unexpected hazardous situations and initiating emergency action to reduce the threat to health and safety. Is able to describe steps or demonstrate actions regarding knowing and performing preventive procedures to maintain a safe environment as well as recognizing sudden, unexpected hazardous situations and initiating emergency action to reduce the threat to health and safety.		

1=Significantly below essential performance standards = Significantly fails to achieve standards defined for the group (eg, does not interact with others, may show deviant or abusive behaviors toward others).

2=Below essential performance standards = Fails to meet standards defined for the group (eg, needs assistance for productive interaction with others).

3=Meets essential performance standards = Meets, but does not exceed, standards defined for the group (eg, engages in interaction as required or appropriate for the activity; is not disruptive to the group process).

4=Above essential performance standards = Exceeds standards defined for the group (eg,.readily engages others in interactions, is helpful to others).

5=Significantly above essential performance standards = Significantly exceeds standards defined for the group (eg, assumes appropriate group leadership role, assistant to the group leader).

Additional Comments:

Adapted from American Occupational Therapy Assocation. Occupational Therapy Practice Framework. *Am J Occup Ther.* 2002;56(6):620.

APPENDIX Q

Role Checklist Summary Sheet

DATE: June 2005

NAME: Doris Ross   AGE: 78

Sex: ☐ Male   ☑ Female   Retired: ☑ Yes   ☐ No

Martial Status: ☐ Single ☐ Married ☐ Separated ☐ Divorced ☑ Widowed

Overview   **Perceived Incumbency**   **Value Designation**

Role	Past	Present	Future	Not At All	Somewhat	Very
Student	✓			✓		
Worker	✓			✓		
Volunteer	✓		✓			
Caregiver	✓		✓			
Home maintainer	✓	✓	✓		✓	
Friend	✓		✓			✓
Family member	✓	✓	✓			✓
Religious partici-pant	✓		✓			✓
Hobbyist/ Amateur	✓		✓			✓
Participant in organizations	✓			✓		
Other _____						

APPENDIX R

Studies That Used the Role Checklist as a Part of the Methodology

Baker F, Curbow B, Wingard JR. Role retention and quality of life of bone marrow transplant survivors. *Social Science and Medicine*. 1991;32:697-704.

This study presents the results of a survey of survivors of bone marrow transplants to determine if role retention is significantly related to quality of life. The Role Checklist was used as one of the measures, although it was adapted. Participants were asked if they performed the role before their transplant, performed it currently, and then rated each role on a 7-point scale before and after the transplant. Quality of life measurements were also administered. Role losses were in roles of student and worker and the least amount of changes were in family member, friend, and home maintainer. The main hypothesis, that role retention is related to higher quality of life, was supported. The results also indicated that there are sex differences in the patterns of role retention.

Barris R, Dickie V, Baron K. A comparison of psychiatric patients and normal subjects based on the model of human occupation. *Journal of Occupational Therapy Research*. 1988;8:3-23.

The past and future roles were used as one of several variables in a regression analysis to examine the empirical validity of the Model of Human Occupation in psychosocial occupational therapy. Subjects included normal adults and adolescents, young adults with chronic conditions, patients with eating disorders, and adolescents with psychiatric disorders. The present roles could not be used in comparison since hospitalized individuals would have different roles in the present as a result of their environment and not because of an actual difference between groups. Together with the other variables, past roles accounted for some of the variance in productive role performance for young adult patients with chronic conditions and for variance in social role performance for adolescents hospitalized for psychiatric disorders.

Barris R, Kielhofner G, Martin RMB, Gelinas I, Klement M, Schultz B. Occupational function and dysfunction in three groups of adolescents. *Occupational Therapy Journal of Research*. 1986;6:301-317.

This exploratory study presented the characteristics of occupational function and dysfunction in adolescents with psychophysiological illnesses compared to those with psychiatric illness and to normal high school students. The role checklist was used as part of the study of the habituation system. There were no differences among the groups until a discriminant function analysis was completed and variables were treated as an aggregate. That model accurately discriminated between all normal subjects from the patient groups using several variables. From the Role Checklist, the variables included the number of non-valued roles and number of past roles.

Brånholm IB, Fugl-Myer AR. Occupational role preferences and life satisfaction. *Occupational Therapy Journal of Research.* 1992;12:159-171.

A modified Role Checklist was used in this study to compare the roles of men and women at various ages (25-, 35-, 45-, and 55-year-olds) and was compared with an assessment of life satisfaction. The results suggested that family, leisure, and vocational roles are closely linked to overall levels of happiness. The study supports the assumptions that a person's ability to sustain meaningful and realistic occupational roles is closely related to her or his general satisfaction with life. The researchers then discuss and suggest that identification of role preferences is one of the important aspects upon which to build occupational therapy intervention.

Branholm IB, Fugl-Meyer AR. On non-work activity preferences: relationships with occupational roles. *Disability and Rehabilitation.* 1994;16:205-216.

This study used factor analysis to examine the inter-relationships between activity preferences and the possible effects of those preferences on self-reported occupational role internalization. The study did not actually use the Role Checklist, but the role titles were apparently originally delineated from the Checklist. Results indicated that preferences were more gender-dependent than age-dependent. The authors suggest that activity preferences affect occupational roles which lead to domain-specific life satisfaction and ultimately overall happiness.

Crowe TK, VanLeit B, Berghmans KK, Mann P. Role perceptions of mothers with young children: The impact of a child's disability. *Am J Occup Ther.* 1997;51:651-661.

This study used the Role Checklist as a tool to examine the roles of mothers with children with disability compared the mothers with children without disability. The mothers with normally developing children had significantly more roles than the mothers with children with disabilities although both groups had a significant number of roles from the past to present (after the birth of the child). Mothers give up discretionary roles in order to meet their caregiving roles and there was no difference in the value of roles between the groups.

Dickerson A, Oakley F. Comparing the roles of community-living persons and patient populations. *Am J Occup Ther.* 1995;49:221-228.

This study used the Role Checklist to compare the occupational roles of community-living persons without disabilities with a population of clients with psychosocial or physical disabilities. Community-living individuals were matched with patient groups in terms of gender, age, race, and education. Analyses indicated that roles were not significantly different in the past (with the exception of worker), but were significantly different in the present and future. The value of roles for the two groups were also different. The paper examines the differences as well as the differences between role incumbency for individuals with physical disabilities and individuals with psychosocial disabilities.

Duellman MK, Barris R, Kielhofner G. Organized activity and the adaptive status of nursing home residents. *Am J Occup Ther*. 1986; 40: 618-622.

In this study of 44 residents in three nursing homes, the relationship between the amount of organized activities and the residents' perception of their roles in the present and future was examined. The Role Checklist was used as one of instruments. There was a positive relationship between the amount of organized activity in the institution and the role that elderly people perceived themselves as occupying in both the present and the future supporting the hypothesis that when activity is available, individuals will form and maintain images of themselves as actively engaged in the environment.

Ebb EW, Coster W, Duncombe L. Comparison of normal and psychosocially dysfunctional male adolescents. *Occupational Therapy in Mental Health*. 1989;9:53-74.

This study used the Role Checklist as well as four other assessments to examine whether variables from these assessments could discriminate between normal and psychosocially dysfunctional groups of male adolescents. The variables were defined as critical from the Model of Human Occupation and included personal causation, values, interests, roles, habits, communication skills, and process skills. The results showed that the number of current roles, future roles, and strong interests were the most valuable variables to differentiate between the two groups of adolescents.

Egan M, Warren SA, Hessel PA, Gilewich G. Activities of daily living after hip fracture: pre- and post-discharge. *Occupational Therapy Journal of Research*. 1992;12:342-356.

In this study, the researchers were examining whether the independence of individuals with hip fractures had the same independence at discharge as 3 weeks after discharge. The Role Checklist, Part 1, was one of several assessments used. The relationship between role loss, depression, mental status, health status, age, gender, and social support were examined in terms of increased post-discharge dependence. Only gender was significantly related to greater dependence in ADL post-discharge.

Elliott MS, Barris R. Occupational role performance and life satisfaction in elderly persons. *Occupational Therapy Journal of Research*. 1987;7:215-224.

In this study, the Role Checklist was used as a tool to examine if life satisfaction with elderly persons is positively correlated with the number of occupational roles performed and whether meaningful role involvement is more strongly correlated with life satisfaction than the number of roles performed. A life satisfaction tool was also used. Results show that in both hypotheses, life satisfaction was positively correlated with the number of occupational roles performed. Although the level of involvement in meaningful life roles and life satisfaction, it was not stronger than the number of roles performed and life satisfaction. What the results did suggest is that occupation can maintain and restore health.

Frosch S, Gruber A, Jones C, Myers S, Noel E, Westerlund A, Zavisin T. The long term effects of traumatic brain injury on the roles of caregivers. *Brain Injury.* 1997;11:891-906.

This was a study to examine the effects of traumatic brain injury on the roles of caregivers over the long term. A questionnaire was developed and included the Role Checklist. Respondents were 155 caregivers of survivors of traumatic brain injury. Results showed a significant change in roles of caregivers between before the injury and currently. Additionally, there were greater changes with caregivers who provided care in the home versus those who did not. A trend existed between the number of role changes and the behavioral effects of the survivors of brain injury as well as a relationship between participation in support systems.

Hallett JD, Zasler ND, Maurer P, Cash S. Role change after traumatic brain injury in adults. *Am J Occup Ther.* 1994;48:241-246.

This study used the Role Checklist to examine role changes after traumatic head injury. Twenty-eight adults with traumatic head injury were interviewed and completed the Checklist. Analysis showed that the more severe the disability, the more evident the change in life roles. All subjects reported role changes in their lives after at least 8 months post hospitalization and the majority of role changes were lost roles. The role of worker showed the most loss, the home maintainer showed the most gains, and the home maintainer and friend showed the most continuous role patterns.

Kusznir A, Scott E, Cooke RG, Young LT. Functional consequences of Bipolar Affective Disorder: An occupational therapy perspective. *Can J Occup Ther.* 1996;63:313-322.

A study to examine the functional consequences of clients with bipolar disorder was completed in Canada. The investigators used the Role Checklist as a basis to develop a questionnaire renamed the Occupational Performance Questionnaire. The roles were the same as the Role Checklist, but this questionnaire was designed to describe and rate adaptive functioning derived from ratings of involvement, satisfaction, functioning, and importance. The study showed that even when the client with bipolar disorder may have a remission of symptoms, they still may have impaired occupational functioning.

Lederer JM, Kielhofner G, Watts JH. Values, personal causation and skills of delinquents and nondelinquents. *Occupational Therapy in Mental Health.* 1985;5:59-77.

In this study, four assessments were used to compare adolescent delinquents with age-matched non-delinquents on variables of occupational behavior. The second part of the Role Checklist was used to compare how the two groups valued roles. Although there were no differences in standards of performance or values, internal/external locus of control or personal causation, or perceptual motor skills of the two groups, it was found that the delinquent adolescent valued different roles and devalued roles found to be valuable by the non-delinquent adolescents. The results suggest delinquents may seek meaning in solitary or deviant roles.

Oakley F, Kielhofner G, Barris R. An occupational therapy approach to assessing psychiatric patients' adaptive functioning. *Am J Occup Ther.* 1985;39:147-154.

In this study, the Role Checklist was used as one of six assessments to look at the utility of the Model of Human Occupation with persons with mental disorders. The subjects were 30 persons with a diagnosis of mental disorder and between the ages of 18 and 59 years. For the Role Checklist specifically, all subjects had at least one disrupted role and few of the subjects performed roles on a continuous basis.

Prusti S, Branholm IB. Occupational roles and life satisfaction in psychiatric outpatients and vocational disabilities. *Work.* 2000; 14: 145-149.

The objective of this study was to investigate the internalization of occupational roles and levels of life satisfaction for clients with psychiatric disorders with vocational disability. The twenty subjects were administered the Role Checklist, which was modified to a four point scale with the roles mixed with the role value (ie, I do not have a role, I have the role, but it is not at all valuable, I have the role, but it is somewhat valuable, etc.). A life satisfaction scale was developed and compared to the Checklist. The subjects had low levels of satisfaction with life as a whole and various domains. Results suggest that the low number of meaningful occupational roles with this group support the association between occupational roles and life satisfaction.

Rust KM, Barris R, Hooper FH. Use of the model of human occupation to predict women's exercise behavior. *Occupational Therapy Journal of Research.* 1987;7:23-35.

In this study, the Role Checklist was one tool of several used to answer the question of whether the Model of Human Occupation could be used to predict engagement in exercise by adult women. 140 questionnaires were collected and used in regression analyses. Results offered some support for the validity of the model as a framework for examining occupational behavior, but there was much variability unexplained. Thus, further research would need to be done.

Tompson H, Werner J. The impact of role conflict/facilitation on core and discretionary behaviors: Testing a ediated model. *Journal of Management.* 1997;23:583-601.

In this study, the Role Checklist was not used as an assessment, but the list of roles for the Checklist was used to measure inter-role conflict and facilitation in a matrix format. Each role was compared to the others in terms of if the role facilitated achievement of success in the comparison role or if participation of the role conflicted with the comparison role. Other assessments were used in this study to illustrate a model of organizational citizenship behaviors with students in business administration programs. The results indicated that even individuals with high role conflict will carry out their expected job requirements, however, when it comes to discretionary behaviors, role conflict/facilitation was significantly related to citizenship dimensions.

Vause-Earland T. Perceptions of the role assessment tools in the physical disability setting. *Am J Occup Ther.* 1991;45:26-31.

This national survey of occupational therapists examined practitioners' knowledge of four published role assessment tools, the frequency of the use of the tools, and their perception of the importance of role function of clients. The Role Checklist was one of the identified assessment tools. 88% of the respondents believed that identifying a patient's role function was an important function. Ten percent of the respondents indicated they had access to the Role Checklist and only 3% used it. Twenty-two percent used a role assessment tool developed by their department while 81% indicated they used an informal interview approach to obtain the information.

Watson MA, Lager CL. The impact of role valuation on performance on life satisfaction in old age. *Physical and Occupational Therapy in Geriatrics*. 1991;10(1):27-62.

This study used the Role Checklist as a tool to compare the relationship between frequency of performance of valued roles and life satisfaction in older adults. The Checklist was revised to rank the value on a five-point scale instead of three and were asked to rate how often they performed each role on a 6-point scale. A global life satisfaction scale was used. The results of 75 older adults between 50 and 90 years of age only the role of home maintainer had a positive and significant correlation between the role and life satisfaction. However, there was positive and significant correlation with all but one role between value scores and frequency of performance, indicating that valued roles were being undertaken.

APPENDIX S

Studies Supporting the Validity and Reliability of the Role Checklist

Colon H, Haertlein C. Spanish translation of the Role Checklist. *Am J Occup Ther.* 2002;56:586-589.

This case report describes the validity and reliability study of converting the Role Checklist into the Spanish language to create a content valid and reliable Spanish Version of the Role Checklist. The English and Spanish versions were evaluated using 14 bilingual college students over a 2-week interval. The intra-language correlation was .907 for Part 1 and .798 for Part II.

Gillard M, Segal M. Social roles and subjective well-being in a population of nondisabled older adults. *OTJR: Occupation, Participation, and Health.* 2002;22:96S.

This is a one-page summary of a study that used the Role Checklist to determine if two occupational therapy measures were related to a well-known life satisfaction scale with 52 non-disabled older adults. Results showed that when social roles were weighted by their value as measured by the Checklist, they were moderately correlated with life satisfaction.

Hachey R, Boyer G, Mercier C. Perceived and valued roles of adults with severe mental heath problems. *Can J Occup Ther.* 2001;68:112-120.

This article analyzes the results of two studies that used the Role Checklist. The studies were related to the French translation of the Role Checklist and a study related to the perception of roles and quality of life. All the subjects were adults with schizophrenia. The Role Checklist was analyzed here, interpreting the results for this population for perception of roles and role patterns. Results indicated that this population has many role losses and the worker role is the one in which most change is desired. Most role losses were in productive roles, and the roles of friend and family member were the most consistent and valued roles.

Hachey R, Jumoorty J, Mercier C. Methodology for validating the translation of test measurements applied to occupational therapy. *Occupational Therapy International.* 1995;2:190-203.

This study described methods to validate the translation of the Role Checklist into French, as well as the results of such as study. The same analyses were used as the original work, with sixteen bilingual participants. Overall results were good, but part two of the Checklist (value of roles) needs to be used cautiously.

Oakley F, Kielhofner G, Barris R, Reichler R. The role checklist: Development and empirical assessment of reliability. *Occupational Therapy Journal of Research*. 1986;6:157-170.

This was the first study that describes the development and the empirical use of the Role Checklist. Data from the Role Checklist indicate an individual's role incumbency, valuation of roles, role balance, and role continuity. It was the preliminary study of the test/retest reliability, which demonstrated satisfactory stability with a group of normal adults.

APPENDIX T

Descriptions of the Use of the Role Checklist as a Therapeutic Tool or Outcome Measure

Bavaro SM. Occupational therapy and obsessive-compulsive disorder. *Am J Occup Ther.* 1991;45:456-458.

This is a case study of a client with obsessive-compulsive disorder using the Model of Human Occupation for an intervention plan. The Role Checklist, as well as other assessments, were used and discussed.

Oakley F. Clinical application of the model of human occupation in dementia of the Alzheimer's type. *Occupational Therapy in Mental Health.* 1987;7:37-50.

This article describes a case study of a client with dementia of the Alzheimer's type using the Model of Human Occupation as the framework for intervention. The Role Checklist was used as one of the assessments. Evaluation results and intervention is described.

Pizzi M. The model of human occupation and adults with HIV infection and AIDS. *Am J Occup Ther.* 1989;44:257-264.

This article argues that HIV or AIDS affects all components of an individual's life and given their needs, the client must be comprehensively evaluated. Using the Model of Human Occupation, a case study of assessment and treatment is illustrated. The Role Checklist is one of the primary assessments used in the case.

Ponsford J, Olver J, Nelms R, Curran C, Ponsford M. Outcome measurement in an inpatient and outpatient traumatic brain injury rehabilitation programme. *Neurosychological Rehabilitation.* 1999;9:517-534.

This is a description of a 5-year outcome study of individuals with traumatic brain injury. The Role Checklist was used as one of several outcome measures to compare methods to evaluate progress in attaining the goals of the program by individuals. They found that emotional adjustment has a significant influence on self-reporting of problems and changes and recommended that objective measures be used in addition to self report measures.

Sepiol JM, Froehlich J. Use of the role checklist with the patient with multiple personality disorder. *Am J Occup Ther.* 1990;44:1008-1012.

This article describes the use of the Role Checklist with clients with the diagnosis of multiple personality disorder. The authors describe some background of evaluation of the disorder and the lack of adequate evaluations tools. A case study is used to describe how on client with multiple personality disorder choice to have several Role

Checklists completed, one for each personality. Other clients refused to do more than one evaluation. The authors conclude that the client will tell the therapist what they need and the Role Checklist can be a useful treatment planning tool.

Stoffel VC. The Americans with disabilities act of 1990 as applied to an adult with alcohol dependence. *Am J Occup Ther.* 1992;46:640-644.

This article is a case study of a client with alcohol dependence. A Role Checklist was used as the primary assessment tool within the Model of Human Occupation. The evaluation, treatment plan, and follow-up are described within the framework of Model of Human Occupation and the Role Checklist specifically.

APPENDIX U

Excerpts of OT FACT Psychosocial Categories and Definitions

I. ROLE INTEGRATION	Functions appropriately in all life roles and balances roles in unified life activity. Doesn't demonstrate overemphasis or skill in some roles to the deficit of others.
A. ROLE PERFORMANCE	Functions adequately in each applicable life role, encompassing all aspects of each role.
1. Personal Maintainer	Takes care of self (self-care and health management).
2. Student	Performs all functions required of a student.
3. Worker/Volunteer	Contributes time and skills to complete tasks toward vocational/volunteer goals.
4. Caregiver	Provides necessary nurturance and support to those requiring care.
5. Employer	Responsibly recruits and maintains employees to secure short- and long-term needs for self and employees.
6. Citizen/Neighbor	Participates in societal activities and interacts respectfully as next-door and world neighbor.
7. Player/Recreator	Initiates, develops, and participates in individual and social leisure activities to self satisfaction.
8. Friend/Companion	Develops, maintains, and participates in non-family social relationships.
9. Significant Other	Participates effectively in an intimate relationship with another.
10. Family Member	Participates constructively in family. Interacts with parents, siblings, in-laws, etc. as appropriate.
11. Consumer	Makes knowledgeable purchases to meet needs and interests.
B. INTEGRATES SELF/ EXTERNAL ROLES	Coordinates physical, social, and cultural expectations with internal role expectations.
C. BALANCES ROLES	Balances number and time allocation among life roles to prevent role overload, role conflict, or role deprivation.
1. Role Overload	Limits number of roles to maintain quality of life and effective role functioning.

2. Role Conflict	Roles coexist without interference among them.
3. Role Deprivation	Effectively assumes an adequate number of roles.
D. INTEGRATES ROLES OVER TIME	Experiences no disruption among past, present, and future roles.

II. ACTIVITIES OF PERFORMANCE
  A. PERSONAL CARE ACTIVITIES

1. Cleanliness, Hyg. & Appear.	Bathes, performs toilet and oral hygiene activities, and dresses as needed.
a. Bathing	Obtains and uses supplies; doffs clothing; achieves bathing position; maintains bathing position; soaps, rinses, dries all body parts; leaves bathing position.
b. Toilet Hygiene	Obtains and uses supplies; achieves toileting or elimination position; maintains position; cleans; leaves toileting or elimination position.
c. Hand Washing	Obtains and uses supplies; regulates water; soaps, scrubs, and rinses, shuts water off; dries hands.
d. Oral Hygiene	Obtains and uses supplies; cleans mouth and teeth; rinses pertinent to natural teeth or dentures.
e. Grooming	Obtains and uses supplies; shaves; applies and removes cosmetics; combs and brushes hair.
1) Cares for hair	Obtains needed tools and supplies; combs/brushes, styles hair.
2) Fingernails	Obtains needed tools and supplies; cares for fingernails.
3) Toenails	Obtains needed tools and supplies; cares for toenails.
4) Shaves	Obtains supplies; shaves face, legs, axilla as needed.
5) Cosmetics	Applies and removes cosmetics (obtains materials, applies appropriate amount in an acceptable fashion).
6) Deodorant	Obtains and applies deodorant.
f. Dressing	Selects appropriate clothing; obtains clothing from storage area; sequentially dons and doffs all items including appliances (eg, glasses, prostheses, orthoses), underwear, shoes, outerwear, and accessories; adjusts clothing; and fastens and unfastens.

g. Nose Blowing	Grasps tissue or handkerchief; blows and wipes nose.
2. Medical and Health Mgmt. Act.	Performs exercise programs, uses medication, manages unhealthy behavior, and communicates in emergencies as needed.
a. Health Maint. and Improvement	Manages healthy routines to maintain or improve status; avoids unhealthy practices.
1) Exercise Program/ Routine	Performs prescribed physical and psychosocial health promotion routines, eg, functional exercise program, pressure-relief activities, splint-wearing schedules.
2) Manages unhealthy behaviors	Regulates unhealthy practices including smoking, alcohol and drug use, food consumption, and sexual activities ignoring self-health and welfare.
aa. Smoking	Regulates smoking.
bb. Alcohol and drug use	Regulates alcohol and drug use.
cc. Food consumption	Regulates quantities of food consumption.
dd. Sexual practices	Avoids sexual activities that ignore self-health and welfare, including those that lead to infectious disease and unwanted pregnancy.
b. Medication Routine	Obtains medication, accesses container, takes appropriate quantities using correct schedule, and exhibits knowledge of side effects and precautions.
1) Schedule	Uses correct schedule.
2) Obtains medication	Obtains medication from storage location.
3) Containers	Opens and closes containers.
4) Selects/measures	Selects/measures appropriate amount of medication.
5) Administers/takes	Administers/takes medication in available form (manipulates pills, swallows, places under tongue, IM, etc.).
6) Stores medication	Stores medication properly.
7) Manages side effects	Takes action as necessary when dosage problems arise.
c. Emergency Communication	Performs steps required to obtain appropriate help at all times of the day or night.

3. Nutrition Activities	Prepares and cleans up meals; eats as needed.
4. Sleep and Rest Activities	Plans and takes sleeping and rest breaks, relaxes; sleeps in appropriate locations and positions; has established cycle and sufficient amount of sleep and rest for normal daily routine.
5. Mobility Activities	Moves indoors, outdoors with private transportation, and outdoors with public transportation as needed.
6. Communication Activities	Speaks, writes, reads, uses the telephone, and expresses self sexually as needed.
a. Speaking	Intelligibly expresses basic needs orally, gesturally, or symbolically without documentation, including identifying need and obtaining equipment when needed.
b. Writing	Legibly writes, prints, or types appropriate person, place, and time information and short message.
c. Reading	Comprehends public signs and messages and follows simple step-by-step written directions, including identifying need to read and obtaining equipment when needed.
d. Telephone	Manages steps in sending and receiving phone calls; accesses the phone; uses proper social etiquette; selects telephone use when appropriate.
e. Sexual Expression	Recognizes, communicates, and performs sexual behaviors appropriate for individual and environment.
7. Assistive Device Repair & Maint.	Cares for assistive technology devices such as wheelchair or communication aid to avoid damage; replaces and fixes broken devices; cleans devices as needed; or obtains appropriate assistance for these functions.

B. OCCUPATIONAL ROLE-RELATED ACTS

1. Home Management Activities	Acquires home, plans meals, cares for clothing, cleans the home, repairs and maintains the facility and contents, keeps the home safe, and manages the yard as needed.
a. Home Acquisition	Finds an apartment/home that is suited to geographic, economic, mobility, and personal preferences; uses newspaper

	ads or agencies as needed; and appropri- ately interacts with potential landlords and banks.
b. Menu Planning	Plans nutritional meals within budget; coordinates grocery needs with food required; plans meals over an extended period of time (ie, more than just one meal at a time).
c. Care of Clothing/ Launderables	Launders, stores, and mends clothing and other launderables. Arranges for dry-cleaning.
d. Cleaning	Picks up; dusts; removes garbage; main- tains sinks, tub, shower, and toilet; vacuums; sweeps; scrubs/mops; and makes bed.
e. Household Repair & Maint.	Repairs and maintains items in the living environment as needed, eg replac es lightbulbs and fuses; fixes broken appliances, furniture, and other house- hold items; paints/weatherizes and/or obtains appropriate assistance for these functions.
f. Household Safety	Recognizes and prevents hazards such as fire, slipping, extreme air temperatures, and extreme utensil temperatures. Also secures doors and windows.
1) Safe building/ facility	Recognizes and prevents damage to home (eg, fires, fire hazards, water damage, intruders, etc.).
2) Safe contents	Recognizes and prevents loss of material goods (secures/locks doors and windows, turns off equipment).
3) Safe for people	Recognizes danger and prevents harm to self or others (from hot appliances, pans, food, extreme air temperatures, intruders, etc.).
g. Yard Work	Picks up, mows, trims, shovels, and gardens.
2. Consumer Activities	Purchases items and manages money as needed.
a. Purchasing Acts	Shops for food, clothing, and supplies; handles money transactions; finds, obtains, and transports needed items in store; negotiates store geography; uses catalogs as needed.
b. Money Mgmt. Acts	Budgets, uses bank, and buys within means; allocates money for all necessary

	areas of expense; uses credit prudently; and conserves money before next income arrives.
1) Banking	Uses bank; balances accounts (eg, checking, savings, loans).
2) Budgeting	Budgets (buys within means, conserves money, allocates money for all necessary areas of expense).
3. Educational Activities	Participates in a school/campus environment and school-sponsored activities; attends educational activities regularly and on time; studies; performs homework; physically negotiates campus.
4. Employmt. & Voluntr. Acts.	Functions in appropriate work-related activities: determines interests, selects and locates job opportunities, develops appropriate skills, performs tasks of job.
5. Caregiving Activities	Functions in appropriate nurturance activities: provides both necessary physical care and emotional support.
a. Physical Nurturance	Feeds, bathes, and provides other necessary physical care for a child, sibling, adult (if appropriate), and/or pet.
b. Emotional Nurturance	Provides love, security; meets realistic psychological needs of a child, sibling, adult and/or pet.
6. Community Activities	Participates and functions as citizen and in local organizations as needed.
7. Avocational Activities/Play	Participates and functions in solitary and social leisure activities/play as needed.
a. Solitary Leisure Acts	Productively uses free time alone; may include hobbies, reading, TV, etc. Person considers it consistent with abilities; leisure is not likely to conflict with the environment or to create maladaptation within individual.
1) Explores activities	Explores objects, space, places, new experiences as appropriate.
2) Chooses	Chooses satisfying activities.
3) Gets materials	Obtains needed materials and resources for activities.
4) Performs	Performs play or leisure activities, both sedentary and nonsedentary, alone.
5) Puts away	Returns materials to appropriate storage.
b. Social Leisure Activities	Productively engages in leisure/play with other people. Person considers it consistent with abilities; leisure is not likely to conflict with the environment or to create maladaptation within individual.

8. Employer Activities	Recruits, selects, and retains employees as needed.

III. INTEGRATED SKILLS OF PERFORMANCE

A. MOTOR INTEGRATION SKILLS	Moves body parts effectively in activities.
B. SENSORY-MTR. INTEGRATION SKILLS	Incorporates sensory information effectively into coordinated mental and motor processes.
C. COGNITIVE INTEGRATION SKILLS	Comprehends, synthesizes, evaluates environmental information and incorporates results into behavior.
D. SOCIAL INTEGRATION SKILLS	Skills that enable successful interaction in peer relationships, work, and family, including one-to-one relationships as well as group interaction; involves ability to give and take in social situations.
1. Peer Interactions	Negotiates, compromises, competes, and cooperates with peers (eg, other children, co-workers, neighbors).
a. Initiates interaction	Starts a peer interaction or joins an exist ing one.
b. Manages own behavior	Independently manages own behavior and displays no inappropriate aggressive behaviors during peer interactions.
c. Follows rules	Follows documented or undocumented rules of activities involving peers.
d. Provides positive feedback	Provides positive feedback and reinforcement to other peers, eg, smiles, helps out, compliments.
e. Provides negative feedback	Provides negative feedback or consequences to other peers, eg, ignores inappropriate activity, politely asserts self, offers alternate opinions.
f. Obtains and integrates cues	Obtains and responds to relevant situational cues in the social environment.
g. Offers information/ assistance	Provides information and assistance to peers.
h. Obtains information/ assistance	Solicits and accepts assistance from peers when needed.
i. Adjusts to negative situations	Exhibits alternative strategies to cope with negative peer social situations.
j. Terminates interaction	Terminates or withdraws from a peer interaction.

2. Authority/Subord. Interactions	Negotiates, compromises, competes, and cooperates with individuals in authority and with individuals under one's authority.
3. Family Interactions	Negotiates, compromises, competes, and cooperates with family members; maintains satisfactory relationships with family members; recognizes own role in contributing to family dynamics; achieves individualization from family if appropriate.
4. Pet and Animal Interactions	Approaches and interacts with pets and animals.
E. PSYCHOLOGICAL INTEGRATION SKILLS	Includes ability to respond to environmental demands in a personally and socially satisfying manner.
1. Coping/Stress Management	Can modulate responses to environmental demands such that problem-solving skills remain evident; has identified and uses mechanisms for reducing stress; is able to function under a range of environmental conditions.
2. Time Use/Planning	Develops plans to accomplish tasks; meets obligations on time; is generally on time for appointments.
a. Plans	Develops plans to accomplish tasks.
b. Timely	Is generally on time for appointments.
c. Meets obligations	Meets obligations on time. Delivers by due date.
3. Initiation and Termination of Acts	Starts and stops activities when necessary. (Inability in this area is not to be confused with components such as perseveration or motivation. Cause is not defined.)
4. Maintains Physical Integrity	Acts in ways that will not cause physical harm to own body
IV. COMPONENTS OF PERFORMANCE A. NEUROMUSCULAR COMPONENTS	Effective musculoskeletal and neuromuscular functioning.
B. SENSORY AWARENESS COMPONENTS	Fundamental sensory processes such as tactile, proprioceptive, ocular control, vision, vestibular, auditory, olfactory, and gustatory.

C. SOCIAL COMPONENTS	Includes oral and gestural communication, nonverbal communication; includes component skills for group and dyadic roles.
1. Group Interaction	Takes on a variety of roles as necessary for maintenance of a group; cooperates with others; shares in responsibility for decision making and task completion; uses appropriate verbal and nonverbal communication.
a. Environment Interactions	Respects property and objects including things belonging to self, neighbors, community, or general environment (eg, does not unwarrantedly destroy or break things in the environment.)
b. Personal Behaviors	Manages personal behaviors in social situations in an acceptable manner (eg, avoids behaviors that are socially or culturally offensive such as picking one's nose, expelling gas, touching genitals, talking too loudly).
2. Dyadic Interaction	Interacts in one-to-one relationships with peers, authority, etc.; uses appropriate verbal and nonverbal communication; modulates behavior to reflect changing dynamics in relationships.
D. PSYCHOLOGICAL COMPONENTS	Ability to establish a positive self-concept and take action.
1. Personal Responsibility	Accountable for one's actions and contributing accomplishments.
2. Self-Image	Realistic appraisal of self; accepts own personal qualities and limitations.
3. Value Identification	Identifies values that are important, admirable, or worthy of emulating.
4. Interest Identification	Identifies interests related to leisure and work; identifies stronger and weaker interests. Interests are appropriate to life situation.
5. Goal Setting	Has short- and long-term goals that reflect values, interests, and environmental expectations; goals are within the realm of possibility.
V. ENVIRONMENT A. SOCIAL/CULTURAL ENVIRONMENT	Appropriate and sufficient resources and organizational structures required for personal care and occupational role-related environments are available.

1. Resources	Appropriate social support, financial and medical resources for adequate performance in personal care and occupational role-related activities are available.
a. Social Support System	Appropriate family, friends, community, service providers, and advocates are available, share values and support goals; reliable people are available to help out when things go wrong or for emergencies.
b. Financial Resources	Has adequate funds (wages, supplemental income, insurance) to engage in valued activities including emergency resources (eg, parent, friend, insurance) and basic necessities of life, medical, educational, and recreational needs.
c. Medical Resources	Has access to needed medical care. Adequate emergency, primary care, specialty, rehabilitative, and long-term care, including therapy, is available within reasonable distance.
d. Educational Resources	Adequate formal and informal regular educational, special educational, and training programs are available to meet the particular needs of this individual.
2. Organizational System	Organizational structures required to support individual in personal care and occupational role-related activities are available.
B. PHYSICAL ENVIRONMENT	Appropriate and sufficient accessibility, accomodation, and access to tools and technologies to meet individual needs of user.

APPENDIX U

OT FACT Profile for an Individual With Early Alzheimer's Behaviors

BACKGROUND

This 82-year-old woman named Grandmother was living in a supported retirement efficiency apartment in a facility called Pleasant Manor. Her family resided across several nearby states and included a daughter living in the same town. They became concerned about the failure of her involvement in many of the social activities she had performed regularly for decades. Initially, this included performance changes such as ceasing to make regular phone calls to family, failing to write weekly letters, a disinterest in family members' visits, forgetfulness of appointments and scheduled social events, empty descriptions of recent social activities, and some confabulation to fill in the gaps in her recollection of recent social activities. Later, the memory difficulties shifted to major personality changes such as a shift from being fastidious in self-care, highly inhibited, and controlling of social behavior, to one who did not bathe and publicly exhibited expressions of intimate social interaction. These functional changes became major sources of frustration for her children, who increasingly related being aggravated in interpersonal interactions with their mother, being unprepared for helping a family member with these behaviors, and a total feeling of helplessness in keeping Mom like Mom. This resulted in the suggestion of an overall occupational performance assessment to quantify Grandmother's current performance and to highlight possible interventions to improve both Grandmother's and her concerned children's quality of life.

INTERESTS AND OCCUPATIONS

Grandmother has a master's degree in music education and once was a proficient keyboard player (piano and organ). She has been an avid reader, listener of music, knitter, cook, and companion. Recently, knitting and cooking became too complex, and using a radio or the television was also too complicated. She attended events in the senior center when possible and continued to actively participate in group activities. She remained fully ambulatory and physically able to perform all daily activities appropriate for an individual in her eighth decade. However, independent attendance to social activities or initiating solitary activities became extremely limited to totally absent. She was widowed a number of years ago, but since then was easily able to renew old friendships and develop new casual friendships, including one intimate relationship. She continued to actively participate effectively in one-to-one social interactions. Her participation in the social activities continued to be appropriate with the exception of recent uninhibited behaviors, where she exhibited social hugging and kissing in environments where more conservative social behaviors are expected. She ate meals in a common dining room with other residents in her facility, eating at assigned seats, served by individualized menus. Mealtimes provide a scheduled structure for her day as well as the other residents in her facility.

THE OT FACT QUANTIFIED PROFILE

Data were collected for OT FACT by some of her children. The discussion that transpired during the data collection process highlighted a mix of frustration of Grandmother's inability to perform activities juxtaposed to her abilities to physically perform virtually all categories of tasks in OT FACT. Her general profile reveals a severe disability across all areas of all domains of function. Careful examination of the activities of performance reveals that Grandmother exhibited significant functional performance deficits across most activities in personal care and occupational role-related activities. These performance deficits are further explained by examining the skills and components of performance. In the skills level, it is apparent that Grandmother's assets include most areas of her neuromotor and musculoskeletal performance with her most significant deficits in the psychosocial and cognitive areas. Further scrutiny of OT FACT details in the psychosocial area indicates her high degree of skill in some social areas, yet a very low skill in others. This comparison of different social skills also highlights the psychometric characteristics of OT FACT where scoring is contextual. While Grandmother's social skills are considered a strength in most social situations, it is within a more conservative social environment where her more intimate behaviors are considered inappropriate in that context. Examination of the components of performance level again illustrates the contrasting abilities between various areas of underlying pathology.

RECOMMENDATIONS

This administration of OT FACT resulted in specific discoveries leading to a set of recommendations. These recommendations included:

1. Design an intervention to help coach Grandmother and her new intimate friend on which behaviors are appropriate in which social environments.

2. Discuss these findings with the facility staff to increase the support from the facility to achieve these recommended goals.

3. Administer OT FACT using three co-variates to obtain a focused baseline of performance, isolating and quantifying the contribution of a) memory, b) social skills deficits and c) family support to her overall functional performance deficits. The rationale for performing these co-variate assessments is as follows:

   • Obtain a baseline for comparing the rate and extent of Alzheimer-related problems

   • Specifically quantify social skills to monitor any progress in the social intervention area

   • Identify the contribution of the family support to Grandmother's functional performance to demonstrate that Alzheimer's symptoms are not a result or the "fault" of family support of Grandmother

4. Specific social intervention strategies could include increasing the discussions with Grandmother from family, facility staff, and friends about the appropriateness of her uninhibited social behaviors in public situations. Additionally, increase the external stimuli for Grandmother pertaining to her past social behaviors (such as memorabilia of her family, activities with her deceased husband, church activities of conservative religious background, and previous lifestyle and personality characteristics). Grandmother seems to be forgetting who she was. External and more frequent information may assist the linkage of past behaviors to present.

APPENDIX W

Occupational Wellness Assessment (OWA) Interview Questions

Directions: For each question below, check all the items that apply. List additional responses as "Other." To score, first circle the total number of activities checked (1-4) for each question. If more than 4 responses were checked, circle 4+. To get the total number of responses within each of the categories, Occupations, Values, and Control, add the circled numbers. For a total assessment score, add these three numbers.

OCCUPATIONS   NOTES

1. What activities do you do with other people that you
    find satisfying?
    _____ being with friends away from home
    _____ being with friends at home
    _____ driving where I need or want to go
    _____ attending church services
    _____ working or job
    _____ volunteering
    _____ visiting with family and relatives
    _____ engaging in leisure activities (movies, ball games,
            concerts, social meetings, gardening)
    _____ other_____

0   1   2   3   4+

2. Which activities/tasks that are important to you, do you
    find you have the energy to do?
    _____ visiting with friends at home
    _____ driving where need or want to go
    _____ attending church services
    _____ working or job
    _____ volunteering
    _____ visiting with family and relatives
    _____ engaging in leisure activities (movies, ball games,
            concerts, social meetings, gardening)
    _____ doing housework
    _____ doing home maintenance
    _____ other_____

0   1   2   3   4+

3.   What kinds of activities (solitary or group) did you do for pleasure prior to your illness/disability? (List activities)

                        Solitary (1 or 2 persons)   Group
_____ Home_____
_____ Neighborhood_____
_____ Community_____
_____ Other_____

0   1   2   3   4+

4.   In what kinds of activities (solitary or group) are you interested currently?

                        Solitary (1 or 2 persons)   Group
_____ Home_____
_____ Neighborhood_____
_____ Community_____
_____ Other_____

0   1   2   3   4+

5.   What kinds of activities (solitary or group) do you plan do to in the future?

                        Solitary (1 or 2 persons)   Group
_____ Home_____
_____ Neighborhood_____
_____ Community_____
_____ Other_____

0   1   2   3   4+

6.   If you cannot do some of the activities you used to do, what new activities would you like to try?
_____ Work/Productivity
_____ Self-care/ADL
_____ Play/Leisure
_____ Other_____

0   1   2   3   4+

7.   In what ways do you perceive you life will be more different now than it was before your illness/disability?

Change in: More___   Less___
home making_____
home maintenance_____
socializing with friends outside home_____
visiting with friends at home_____
being able to drive self_____
being able to do own self-care_____
going to work or job_____
doing volunteer service_____
visiting with family and relatives away from home_____
going to leisure activities outside home (movies, ball games,

social meetings)_____

attending church_____

other_____

8. If you cannot do some of the activities you used to do, which do you consider most important to do?

_____ work/productivity

_____ self-care/ADL

_____ play/leisure

_____ other_____

0	1	2	3	4+

9. Assuming you are living at home, what kinds of work (paid or unpaid) do you believe you are able to do right now?

_____ paid work that I did in the past

_____ other kinds of work that would be paid

_____ house work

_____ home maintenance

_____ volunteering to help neighbors

_____ volunteering to help family members

_____ volunteering in the community with social agencies

_____ other_____

0	1	2	3	4+

10. In what activities did you participate on a typical week day in the past (Mon-Fri)?

_____ socialized with friends away from home

_____ visited with friends at home

_____ drove self

_____ went to church services

_____ went to work or job

_____ went to volunteer services

_____ visited with family and relatives

_____ went to leisure activities outside home (movies, ball games, social meetings)

_____ self-care

_____ home making

_____ home maintenance

_____ other_____

0	1	2	3	4+

11. In what activities did you participate on a typical weekend in the past (Sat, Sun)?

_____ socialized with friends away from home

_____ visited with friends at home

_____ drove self

_____ went to church services

_____ went to work or job

_____ went to volunteer services
_____ visited with family and relatives
_____ went to leisure activities outside home (movies, ball games, social meetings)
_____ self-care
_____ home making
_____ home maintenance
_____ other_____

| 0 | 1 | 2 | 3 | 4+ |

12.   In what activities do you plan to participate on a typical weekday (Mon-Fri) in the future?
_____ socialize with friends away from home
_____ visit with friends at home
_____ drive self
_____ go to church services
_____ go to work or job
_____ go to volunteer services
_____ visit with family and relatives
_____ go to leisure activities outside home (movies, ball games, social meetings)
_____ self-care
_____ home making
_____ home maintenance
_____ other_____

| 0 | 1 | 2 | 3 | 4+ |

Total Score for Occupations _____

VALUES

1.   What is your proudest accomplishment? Add anything else?
_____ making money
_____ making friends
_____ skills in sports
_____ ability to do "something"
_____ having a specific talent (artist, musician, etc.)
_____ other_____

| 0 | 1 | 2 | 3 | 4+ |

2.   In the roles you have fulfilled in your life, what about them is the most meaningful?
_____ pride
_____ respect
_____ economic returns
_____ friends

_____ match for my abilities
_____ the working situation
_____ other_____

0	1	2	3	4+

3. If there are activities you can no longer do, which do you miss the most?
_____ socializing with friends away from home
_____ visiting with friends at home
_____ being able to drive self
_____ being able to do own self care
_____ going to church services
_____ going to work or job
_____ doing volunteer service
_____ visits with family and relatives
_____ going to leisure activities (movies, ball games, concerts, social meetings)
_____ other_____

*0	1	2	3	4+

4. In the past when you went out, with whom did you go?
_____ family members
_____ friends
_____ social groups
_____ co-workers
_____ neighbors
_____ hired companion
_____ health care worker
_____ other_____

0	1	2	3	4+

5. Do you have responsibility for any animal, garden flowers, grandchildren to babysit, or person other than yourself whom you value?
_____ pets
_____ grandchildren
_____ family member (adult)
_____ neighbors
_____ relatives
_____ fellow veterans
_____ garden flowers
_____ other_____

0	1	2	3	4+

6. What roles that you perform contribute the most to your community or the world?
_____ contribute through developing own self
_____ contribute through producing creative work (literally, artistic, musical, etc)
_____ contribute through children/family

_____ contribute in the neighborhood
_____ contribute through workplace
_____ contribute through social causes
_____ contribute through enjoying life
_____ other_____

*0	1	2	3	4+

7.   If you perceive that the quality of your life has changed within the past year, what about it has changed? If it has not changed, give 0 points and go on to the next question; otherwise answer the question.
_____ socializing with friends away from home
_____ visiting with friends at home
_____ being able to drive self
_____ being able to own self care
_____ going to work or job
_____ doing volunteer service
_____ visiting with family and relatives
_____ going to leisure activities outside the home (movies,   ball games, concerts, social meetings)
_____ self-care
_____ home making
_____ home maintenance
_____ other_____

*0	1	2	3	4+

8.   Are you satisfied with how things are going in your present situation? (Check if satisfied.)
_____ socializing with friends away from home
_____ visiting with friends at home
_____ being able to do self care
_____ doing volunteer service
_____ visiting with family and relatives
_____ doing leisure activities in the home
_____ home making
_____ home maintenance
_____ other_____

0	1	2	3	4+

9.   What goals do you have for yourself?
_____ self-care
_____ work (paid or unpaid)
_____ leisure
_____ other_____

0	1	2	3	4+

10. In a crisis situation, whom could you call upon to help you?

_____ spouse
_____ family member
_____ relatives
_____ friends
_____ neighbor
_____ community resources
_____ professional services
_____ other_____

| 0 | 1 | 2 | 3 | 4+ |

11. What services do you feel that the person (in 10) would be willing to provide for you?

_____ personal care
_____ problem-solving
_____ housework
_____ home maintenance
_____ transportation
_____ professional knowledge
_____ counseling
_____ spiritual guidance
_____ other_____

| 0 | 1 | 2 | 3 | 4+ |

12. What kinds of spiritual beliefs (beliefs about life) or practices help you in times of need?

_____ prayer   _____ belief in a higher power
_____ attending church   _____ changes in nature
_____ meditating   _____ being connected to others
_____ reading the Bible
_____ sharing the problems with a close friend
_____ other_____

| 0 | 1 | 2 | 3 | 4+ |

Total Score for Values_____

CONTROL

1. Who are the people to whom you are the closest?

    _____ spouse   _____ in-law
    _____ parent   _____ aunt/uncle
    _____ sibling   _____ nephew/niece
    _____ friend   _____ health care professional
    _____ cousin   _____ social service worker
    _____ child   _____ neighbor
    _____ other_____

    0   1   2   3   4+

2. How do you try to overcome your problems?

    _____ use cognitive approaches
    _____ use emotional approaches
    _____ use advice from family
    _____ use advice from friends
    _____ use advice from professionals
    _____ use prayer/meditation
    _____ use faith that problems will solve themselves
    _____ other_____

    0   1   2   3   4+

3. Name activities or tasks that are good for your health that you do.

    _____ walking
    _____ exercising
    _____ eating right
    _____ visiting with others
    _____ gardening
    _____ being good to myself
    _____ attending church
    _____ working
    _____ other_____

    0   1   2   3   4+

4. What activities or tasks which are bad for your health do you do?

    _____ eating foods that are not right
    _____ smoking
    _____ overeating
    _____ drinking excessively
    _____ sitting around too much
    _____ other_____

    *0   1   2   3   4+

5.   In your neighborhood, what physical and social aspects help you get along in your everyday life?
_____ needed resources (food, medical care, leisure activities)
_____ transportation when needed
_____ safe environment
_____ help in emergencies when needed
_____ an aesthetically pleasing environment (parks, plants, etc.)
_____ ease of movement (getting up and down stairs, hills in rainy weather, snow, etc.)
_____ friends
_____ other_____

| 0 | 1 | 2 | 3 | 4+ |

6.   What did you contribute in your neighborhood that helps you get along in everyday life?
_____ help when needed in emergencies
_____ transportation when needed
_____ friendship
_____ other_____

| 0 | 1 | 2 | 3 | 4+ |

7.   What people and pets depend on you for support and assistance?

_____ spouse	_____ in-law
_____ parent	_____ aunt/uncle
_____ sibling	_____ nephew/niece
_____ friend	_____ health care professional
_____ cousin	_____ social service worker
_____ neighbor	_____ pets
_____ other_____	

| 0 | 1 | 2 | 3 | 4+ |

8.   Which of the activities that you do on a typical day do you make the decision to do?
_____ socializing with friends away from home
_____ visiting with friends at home
_____ driving self
_____ going to church services
_____ going to work or job
_____ doing volunteer service
_____ visiting with family and relatives
_____ going to leisure activities outside the home (movies, ball games, concerts, social meetings)
_____ self-care
_____ home making

_____ home maintenance
_____ other_____

0	1	2	3	4+

9.   With whom do you like to spend leisure time?
     Spend leisure time by yourself? 2 points
_____ spouse
_____ family
_____ friends
_____ social groups
_____ public entertainments (concert, ball games, etc.)
_____ other_____

0	1	2	3	4+

10.   In what activities that you presently do, do you feel you have a choice?
_____ socializing with friends away from home
_____ visiting with friends at home
_____ being able to drive self
_____ being able to do own self care
_____ going to work or job
_____ doing volunteer work
_____ visiting with family and relatives
_____ going to leisure activities outside the home (movies, ball games, concerts,
       social meetings)
_____ home making
_____ home maintenance
_____ other_____

0	1	2	3	4+

11.   What obstacles get in the way of your being able to do activities right away?
_____ do not have the physical resources
_____ do not have the cognitive resources
_____ do not have the financial resources
_____ do not feel motivated
_____ feel powerless
_____ other_____

0	1	2	3	4+

12.   If you could choose how to spend your day, what would you do?
_____ socialize with friends away from home
_____ visit with friends at home
_____ drive self
_____ going to church services

_____ going to work or job
_____ doing volunteer service
_____ visits with family and/or relatives
_____ going to leisure activities outside the home (movies, ball games, concerts, social meetings)
_____ self-care
_____ home making
_____ home maintenance
_____other

0	1	2	3	4+

Total Score for Control_____

Total Score for All Categories____

INDICES

Assessment Index

Author Index

Subject Index

WAIT

...There's More!

SLACK Incorporated's Health Care Books and Journals offers a wide selection of products in the field of Occupational Therapy. We are dedicated to providing important works that educate, inform and improve the knowledge of our customers. Don't miss out on our other informative titles that will enhance your collection.

Please visit
www.slackbooks.com
to order any of these titles!
24 Hours a Day...7 Days a Week!

Attention Industry Partners!
Whether you are interested in buying multiple copies of a book, chapter reprints, or looking for something new and different — we are able to accommodate your needs.

Multiple Copies
At attractive discounts starting for purchases as low as 25 copies for a single title, SLACK Incorporated will be able to meet all of your needs.

Chapter Reprints
SLACK Incorporated is able to offer the chapters you want in a format that will lead to success. Bound with an attractive cover, use the chapters that are a fit specifically for your company. Available for quantities of 100 or more.

Customize
SLACK Incorporated is able to create a specialized custom version of any of our products specifically for your company.

Please contact the Marketing Communications Director of the Health Care Books and Journals for further details on multiple copy purchases, chapter reprints or custom printing at 1-800-257-8290 or 1-856-848-1000.

*Please note all conditions are subject to change.

CODE: 328

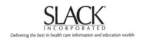
SLACK
INCORPORATED
Delivering the best in health care information and education worldv

SLACK Incorporated • Health Care Books and Journals
6900 Grove Road • Thorofare, NJ 08086
1-800-257-8290 or 1-856-848-1000
Fax: 1-856-848-6091 • E-mail: orders@slackinc.com • Visit: www.slackbooks.com